This is a true second edition, with six new chapters! The applications for working with toddlers and tweens are specific, detailed, and wonderful. The discussion of how neuroscience aligns with CPRT is insightful. An exploration of CPRT research, along with the evidence-based designation, adds informative value. Other additions for using CPRT with adoptive families, teachers, and discussion of cultural issues round out the core chapters for the 10-session model! It is a treat to read and experience!

—Linda E. Homeyer, PhD, LPC-S, RPT-S,
distinguished professor emerita at Texas State University
and director emerita at the Association for Play Therapy

In their new edition, Landreth and Bratton build on their groundbreaking original CPRT treatment approach to provide an updated and expanded model that is practical, evidence-based, and applied to parents of toddlers through preadolescents as well as adoptive families and other systemic partners. Additionally, the authors have integrated interpersonal neurobiology and recent treatment research to provide rationale that makes a difference for child-parent relationships.

—Dee C. Ray, PhD, LPC-S, NCC, RPT-S,
distinguished teaching professor and director of the
Center for Play Therapy, University of North Texas

CPRT has been empirically demonstrated to improve child-parent relationships and child behaviors. This protocol for therapists provides the essentials needed to implement the program successfully. The notebook for parents expands on the principles, allowing parents to apply them to home situations. These resources enable users to experience the full value of CPRT.

—Louise Guerney, PhD, RPT-S,
professor emerita at Penn State University,
co-developer of Filial Therapy, and faculty
member of the National Institute of
Relationship Enhancement (NIRE)

CHILD-PARENT RELATIONSHIP THERAPY (CPRT)

Child-Parent Relationship Therapy (CPRT), grounded in the attitudes and principles of Child-Centered Play Therapy (CCPT), is based on the belief that a parent acting as an agent for change in place of a play therapist has potential for significant and lasting therapeutic gains. This newly expanded and revised edition of *Child-Parent Relationship Therapy (CPRT)* describes training objectives, essential skills and concepts taught in each session, as well as the format for supervising parents' play sessions. Transcripts of actual sessions demonstrate process and content in the 10 CPRT training sessions. Research demonstrating the effectiveness of CPRT on child and parent outcomes is presented in support of CPRT's designation as an evidence-based treatment model.

This second edition is updated to include six new chapters exploring the topics of cultural considerations for working with ethnically and racially diverse families, neuroscience support for CPRT, and adaptions for specific populations including parents of toddlers, parents of preadolescents, adoptive families, and the teacher/student relationship. The authors' expertise and experience results in a book that is essential reading for both students and professionals. By using this text and the accompanying treatment manual, filial therapists will have a complete package for training parents in the CPRT model.

Garry L. Landreth, EdD, LPC, RPT-S, is regents professor emeritus, department of counseling and higher education, and founder and director emeritus, Center for Play Therapy at the University of North Texas.

Sue C. Bratton, PhD, LPC-S, RPT-S, is professor emerita, department of counseling and higher education, and director emerita, Center for Play Therapy at the University of North Texas.

Child-Parent Relationship Therapy (CPRT)

An Evidence-Based 10-Session Filial Therapy Model

2nd Edition

Garry L. Landreth
and Sue C. Bratton

Routledge
Taylor & Francis Group
NEW YORK AND LONDON

Second edition published 2020
by Routledge
52 Vanderbilt Avenue, New York, NY 10017

and by Routledge
2 Park Square, Milton Park, Abingdon, Oxon, OX14 4RN

Routledge is an imprint of the Taylor & Francis Group, an informa business

First edition published by Routledge 2006

Library of Congress Cataloging-in-Publication Data
A catalog record for this book has been requested

ISBN: 978-1-138-68902-2 (hbk)
ISBN: 978-1-138-68903-9 (pbk)
ISBN: 978-1-315-53794-8 (ebk)

Typeset in ITC Garamond Std Light
by Apex CoVantage, LLC

Printed and bound by CPI Group (UK) Ltd, Croydon, CR0 4YY

CONTENTS

PREFACE

This book is about changing the mental health structure of families, communities, and ultimately society, by changing the nature of relationships in families through a process of helping parents become therapeutic agents in their children's lives. From ongoing research, we now know that in a matter of a few weeks, parents are quite capable of learning and incorporating into their relationships with their children and spouses therapeutic skills once thought to require years of graduate education and training.

What we have written in this book about Child-Parent Relationship Therapy (CPRT): An Evidence-Based 10-Session Filial Therapy Model is an extension of our experiences with children in play therapy as they expressed themselves through the process of play in the safety of a caring relationship that released their inner dynamic potential that had been previously unknown to significant adults in their lives. We have long held a deep and abiding belief in the ability of parents to establish the same kind of therapeutic relationship with their own children by learning and incorporating the basic attitudes and skills of Child-Centered Play Therapy in special play relationships, referred to as filial therapy.

We believe the mental health of future adult populations lies squarely on the shoulders of mental health procedures that empower parents to become therapeutic agents with their own children. We must not wait until children become adults to attempt to impact their mental health, for by then a lifetime of less than the best has been lived out. That is not a very progressive or satisfying way for a society to go about the experience of living life. Mental health professionals must actively engage in the process of giving their skills away to families—that is the future.

We are indebted to the many parents who have shared their lives with us in our CPRT groups. From those parents, we have learned how to be more facilitative in our roles as filial therapists and how to use ourselves more fully in developing relationships with parents in our CPRT training groups. From parents, we have learned what works and what does not work very well in the training process. In general, parents have helped to perfect the 10-session filial therapy model into a dynamic, therapeutic, and educational process that changes lives.

The intent of this text is to provide the essential structure, skills, materials, and resources needed to learn how to effectively conduct CPRT training. To that end, some of the unique features of this book are:

- Specific instructions for implementing the group process and teaching components of the 10-session CPRT model.
- Detailed instructions for structuring the 10 sessions of CPRT training.
- Insights of filial therapists in training about difficult dimensions to pay attention to in facilitating a CPRT group.
- Transcripts of the interactions in 10 CPRT sessions for one group of parents afford an opportunity to experience the filial therapy training process.
- One mother's personal struggles are highlighted in each of the filial therapy training transcripts, revealing her development of insight and the dynamic changes in her attitude and behavior.
- Transcripts of parent-child play sessions provide insight into how parents apply the skills learned.

- Answers to questions parents ask about CPRT training.
- Suggested solutions to problems that arise in CPRT training.
- Application of the 10-session CPRT model in various settings is explained.
- Four-year and 13-year follow-up interviews provide an unusual opportunity to evaluate the continuing and long-range effects of the 10-session CPRT model.
- A review of research on the 10-session CPRT model, which is helpful in justifying CPRT to individuals and insurance panels who make decisions regarding children's mental health care.

Since the publication of the first edition of the CPRT text, important happenings include the national recognition of CPRT as an evidence-based practice by the National Registry of Evidence-based Programs and Practices (NREPP) and by the California Evidence-Based Clearinghouse (CEBC) for Child Welfare. Specific to helping adoptive families, the Donaldson Adoption Institute released a report in 2014 in which CPRT was evaluated as the parent-child intervention that demonstrated the most robust research support for this population of parents and children. We have continued to experience the exciting life-changing impact of CPRT on families in ways that have increased the depth of our understanding and expanded our perception of CPRT's potential. The result has been the addition of six new chapters to this second edition authored by experienced CPRT therapists with expertise in their topic areas:

- Neuroscience and CPRT
- Adapting CPRT for Parents of Toddlers
- Adapting CPRT for Parents of Preadolescents
- Adapting CPRT for Adoptive Families
- Adapting CPRT for Teachers
- Culturally Responsive CPRT

READERS' NOTE

To conduct CPRT, therapists will need to purchase this book's companion, *Child-Parent Relationship Therapy (CPRT) Treatment Manual: An Evidence-Based 10-Session Filial Therapy Model, 2nd Edition* (2019) published by Routledge. The treatment manual contains treatment outlines, a therapist study guide, parent handouts, CPRT resources, and supplemental training materials needed for conducting the 10-session training model. The *CPRT Treatment Manual, 2nd Edition* is also accompanied by a Companion Website allowing the therapist to print the therapist notebook, parent notebook, and all additional material needed.

ACKNOWLEDGMENTS

The rewarding shared opportunity with our spouses, Monica and David, to be parents is the most significant experience in which we have invested our lives. Our children, Kimberly, Karla and Craig (G.L.L.) and Lauren (S.C.B.), have made the journey through parenting a wonderful experience as we have struggled to live out the principles of Child-Parent Relationship Therapy on a daily basis with them. They have reaffirmed our faith in the process. This book is dedicated to Monica and David, our children, and our grandchildren. Without their inspiration, love, and encouragement, this book would not have been possible.

We would also like to acknowledge the contributions of our graduate students whose enthusiasm about CPRT and its positive impact on families has been a significant factor in writing this book. We are especially grateful to our many doctoral students who have contributed to the research on the effectiveness of this model. A special thanks to our contributing authors, Mary Morrison Bennett, Kara Carnes-Holt, Peggy Ceballos, Wendy Pretz

Helker, Yung-Wei Lin, Kristin Meany-Walen, Raissa Miller, Yumiko Ogawa, Kristie Opiola, Angela Sheely-Moore, and Alyssa Swan, whose experience and expertise in their topic areas provide a significant addition to the second edition. We are also indebted to Lauren Dimon, Alyssa Swan, and Rinda Thomas-Stein for assistance in preparing and editing the manuscript. Finally, we wish to acknowledge and thank Theresa Kellam and Sandy Blackard for their inspiration, contributions, and feedback throughout the process of writing the first edition of this book.

CONTRIBUTING AUTHORS

Mary Morrison Bennett, PhD, LPC-S, RPT-S, is a Fellow, Institute for Play Therapy at Texas State University and in private practice in Austin, Tx.

Kara Carnes-Holt, PhD, LPC, RPT-S, is associate professor, school of counseling, leadership advocacy, and design, and founder and director, Rocky Mountain Center of Play Therapy Studies at the University of Wyoming.

Peggy L. Ceballos, PhD, NCC, is associate professor and school counseling coordinator, department of counseling and higher education, University of North Texas

Wendy Pretz Helker, PhD, LPC-S, RPT-S, is Certified School Counselor and adjunct faculty, department of counseling and higher education, University of North Texas.

Yung-Wei Dennis Lin, PhD, is assistant professor, department of counselor education at New Jersey City University.

Kristin Meany-Walen, PhD, LMHC, RPT-S, is Mental Health Coordinator, Waterloo Community School District, Iowa and adjunct faculty at University of Northern Iowa.

Raissa M. Miller, PhD, LPC, is assistant professor, department of counselor education, and coordinator of the addiction counseling program, at Boise State University.

Yumiko Ogawa, PhD, LPC, ACS, RPT-S, is associate professor, department of counseling education, and director, Center for Studies of Play Therapy at the New Jersey City University.

Kristie K. Opiola, PhD, LPC, RPT, is assistant professor, department of counseling and higher education at the University of North Carolina at Charlotte.

Angela I. Sheely-Moore, PhD, is associate professor, department of counseling and educational leadership, at Montclair State University.

Alyssa M. Swan, PhD, LPC, RPT, is Associate Clinical Director at Childrens Home of Poughkeepsie in Poughkeepsie, NY.

CHAPTER 1

HISTORY, DEVELOPMENT, AND OBJECTIVES OF CHILD-PARENT RELATIONSHIP THERAPY (CPRT): A 10-SESSION FILIAL THERAPY MODEL

In *Play Therapy: The Art of the Relationship*, Landreth (2012) stated that if the mental health of future adult populations is to be significantly impacted in positive ways, greater effort must be made to substantially improve the mental health of all children. His position was that the skills of those in the mental health professions must be given away through training to parents, who are in the best position to profoundly impact the lives of future adults. Therapists helping parents to become therapeutic agents in their children's lives is the most efficient way to significantly improve the mental health of adult populations of the future. CPRT is grounded in child-centered/person-centered theory and consistent with the principles of child development and attachment theory.

Child-Centered Play Therapy

CPRT/filial therapy applies the constructs and skills of Child-Centered Play Therapy (CCPT) to parent and child relationships in a manner similar to the relationship between a play therapist and a child. As in CCPT, the parent is taught to facilitate a permissive and growth-producing atmosphere in which the child can reach her full potential. Child-Centered Play Therapy is based upon the theoretical constructs of nondirective therapy developed by Carl Rogers (1942) and further developed and expanded by Rogers (1951) as client-centered therapy. CCPT is grounded in a belief in the innate human capacity of the child to strive toward growth and maturity and an attitude of deep and abiding belief in the child's ability to be constructively self-directing. Rogers (1986) summarized the essence of the approach:

> The person-centered approach, then, is primarily a way of being that finds its expression in attitudes and behaviors that create a growth-producing climate. It is a basic philosophy rather than simply a technique or a method. When this philosophy is lived, it helps the person expand the development of his or her own capacities. When it is lived, it also stimulates constructive change in others. It empowers the individual, and when this personal power is sensed, experience shows that it tends to be used for personal and social transformation. (p. 199)

It is this *formative tendency* that all persons—indeed, all of nature—possess that forms the foundation for the child-centered approach to working with children (Rogers, 1951).

These constructs were applied to working with children through play therapy by Virginia Axline (1969), a student and colleague of Rogers. She successfully applied nondirective (client-centered) therapy principles (i.e., belief in the individual's capacity for self-direction) to children in nondirective play therapy. Her approach was later referred to as client-centered play therapy and then as Child-Centered Play Therapy. Axline (1950) summarized her concept of play therapy:

> A play experience is therapeutic because it provides a secure relationship between the child and the adult, so

> that the child has the freedom and room to state himself in his own terms, exactly as he is at that moment in his own way and in his own time. (p. 68)

The child-centered approach to play therapy, like client-centered therapy with adults, is based upon a process of **being with children** as opposed to a procedure of application. It is not so much a process of reparation as it is a process of becoming. Thus, **the focus is on the child, not the problem.** The child-centered play therapist makes no effort to control or change the child, based on the theory that the child's behavior is at all times internally motivated toward self-realization, positive growth, improvement, independence, maturity, and enhancement of self. The child's behavior in this process is goal directed in an effort to satisfy personal needs, as experienced in the unique phenomenal field that for that child constitutes reality. A fundamental rule of thumb in Child-Centered Play Therapy is that the child's perception of reality is what must be understood if the child and behaviors exhibited by the child are to be understood (Landreth, 2012). (*This concept that the child's phenomenal field constitutes reality for the child is central to Child-Parent Relationship Therapy and is the basis for the structure of much of the training.* ***Rule of Thumb: Look through the child's eyes.*** *The parent is to avoid judging or evaluating even the simplest of the child's behaviors, e.g., painting or stacking blocks, and works hard to try to understand the internal frame of reference of the child.*)

In Child-Centered Play Therapy, it is the relationship that is the agent of change. Child-Centered Play Therapy is an experience for children in which the therapeutic process emerges from a shared living relationship developed based on the therapist's consistently conveyed acceptance of children and confidence in their ability to be of help to themselves, thus freeing children to risk using their own strengths. Virginia Axline (1969) concisely clarified the fundamental principles that provide guidelines for establishing and maintaining a therapeutic relationship and making contact with the inner person of the child in the play therapy experience. Landreth (2012, p. 80) revised and extended Axline's eight basic principles as follows:

- The therapist is genuinely interested in the child and develops a warm, caring relationship.

- The therapist experiences unqualified acceptance of the child and does not wish that the child were different in some way.
- The therapist creates a feeling of safety and permissiveness in the relationship so the child feels free to explore and express self completely.
- The therapist is always sensitive to the child's feelings and gently reflects those feelings in such a manner that the child develops self-understanding.
- The therapist believes deeply in the child's capacity to act responsibly, unwaveringly respects the child's ability to solve personal problems, and allows the child to do so.
- The therapist trusts the child's inner direction, allows the child to lead in all areas of the relationship, and resists any urge to direct the child's play or conversation.
- The therapist appreciates the gradual nature of the therapeutic process and does not attempt to hurry things along.
- The therapist establishes only those therapeutic limits that help the child accept personal and appropriate relationship responsibility.

These principles all point to the development and maintenance of a strong therapeutic relationship. Moustakas (1959) further emphasized the therapeutic value of children experiencing this kind of relationship: "Through the process of self-expression and exploration within a significant relationship, through realization of the value within, the child comes to be a positive, self-determining, and self-actualizing individual" (p. 5).

Filial Therapy: A Radical Approach

The development of filial therapy was an evolutionary process for Bernard Guerney (1964), a child-centered play therapist who ascribed to the theoretical principles of client-centered therapy as conceptualized by Carl Rogers and the play therapy principles of Virginia Axline. Early in his professional career, in the 1950s and early 1960s, Guerney (personal communication, October 22, 1992) viewed parents as potential effectual allies in the treatment of their children and began to contemplate the need to involve parents more directly in the therapeutic process. Guerney's first step in the process of involving parents in the therapeutic process of helping their children was to include parents in the playroom as observers, followed by discussions with parents to explain what they had witnessed in the play sessions. His next step in the evolutionary process was to give parents more of a role in the therapeutic process.

These successful experiences led him to conceptualize a training program in which parents would be trained in basic Child-Centered Play Therapy skills to become the therapeutic agent in their children's lives, based on the view that play is the primary way children express themselves and work through issues. Guerney's premise for his innovative approach was that children's problems are often the product of parental lack of parenting knowledge and skill. Furthermore, he proposed that children's problematic behaviors that were influenced by parental attitudes could be more effectively ameliorated under similar conditions. This was a revolutionary idea, because a prevailing attitude in the mental health field in the 1950s and early 1960s was that children's problems are usually a product of the pathology of the parents. This shift from viewing the parents as pathological to being the primary therapeutic agent of change in their child's life was a radical departure for the time.

In 1964, Bernard Guerney published the first article, "Filial Therapy: Description and Rationale," explaining the principles and results of filial therapy. In that article, he described the importance of parents as key to the filial therapy approach:

> The parent-child relationship is nearly always the most significant one in a child's life. Therefore, if a child were provided the experiences of expression, insight, and adult acceptance in the presence of such powerful people as parents, every bit of success the parent achieves in carrying out the therapeutic role should be many more times more powerful than that of a therapist doing the same thing . . . a relatively small amount of affection, attention, interest, and so on, from the parent can be expected to be more therapeutic than a larger amount from a therapist. (p. 309)

Because the parent potentially has more emotional significance to the child than does the therapist, the objective of this approach is to help the parent become the primary change agent in the child's life by using the naturally existing bond between parent and child; thus, the term *filial therapy* was coined by the Guerneys. (Louise Guerney participated with her husband in the early research and development of filial therapy at Rutgers University and has continued as one of the leading proponents of this innovative approach to helping children and families.) Stover and Guerney (1967) proposed further advantages of using filial therapy over play therapy. Utilizing parents as the agent of change would empower parents, reducing feelings of guilt and helplessness parents may experience when dependent upon a professional to help their child. Additionally, as parents learn more effective ways of interacting with their child, there is greater potential for long-lasting change as parents continue to utilize these acquired skills and attitudes throughout their child's life.

The next step in development of this revolutionary approach was the establishment of a sound research program to verify the effectiveness of this program of parent training. The Guerneys' early research results on filial therapy were highly encouraging and provided a strong foundation for the research that followed (Chapter 26 provides an overview of their groundbreaking research).

In the initial stages of development, the Guerneys (personal communication, March 8, 1995) conceptualized filial therapy as a structured treatment program for children with emotional problems and accepted only couples for filial therapy training. Using a small group format, parents were trained in basic Child-Centered Play Therapy principles and skills. Husbands and wives were not placed in the same groups, though, because there were concerns about marital issues dominating the training sessions. Experience and success with their model quickly resulted in a shift in attitude, and they found that when couples were allowed in the same group, they could deal with some marital issues appropriately.

Another important learning was that filial therapy groups composed of parents whose children all had similar personality dynamics, such as acting-out behaviors, were not very effective because the parents had similar dynamics of their own, and they reinforced each other's negative behaviors because they had difficulty viewing each other's children from a different perspective as parents who have children with other kinds of problems might do. This same concern does not apply to groups composed of parents whose children have a similar issue that has nothing to do with dynamics: children with learning disabilities, children with chronic diabetes, etc. These children share a common problem, but they are different in terms of their personality and dynamics. Heterogeneous groups are preferred.

Originally, the Guerneys met with filial groups for 2 hours once a week for about a year. Their experience and success led them to streamline training procedures so that groups now meet 2 hours once a week for about 5 to 6 months. Research on these shorter groups has produced comparable results to those of the longer groups. Ginsberg (1997) and VanFleet (1994), both protégés of the Guerneys, have successfully adapted the Guerneys' model for use with individual parents.

Development of the Child-Parent Relationship Therapy (CPRT) 10-Session Filial Therapy Model

I (first author) have, throughout my professional career as a high school counselor, university professor, and consultant, been involved in working with parents through counseling and training experiences. For many of my early years as an assistant professor teaching play therapy and carrying play therapy cases, I was involved in teaching parents "Lessons from Play Therapy for Parents" but without any emphasis on having playtimes. I had an intensifying belief that if what I did in the playroom was helpful to children, then parents could develop those same kinds of attitudes and learn to utilize those same kinds of skills with their children. Play therapists should be giving their skills away to parents and teachers. We should not hide our skills behind the door of the playroom. When I read the Guerneys' work in filial therapy, I immediately resonated to this dynamic structure of training and supervising parents that incorporated the facets of teaching, supervision, play therapy, and group process, dimensions that are exciting to me and have occupied my professional focus. Here was a model that allowed me to meld my fascination with group process, my passion for play therapy, and my love of teaching. Filial therapy was a natural fit.

Long-term therapy has always been a problematic concern for me, as I believe we do not fully comprehend the potential of the human organism for growth and change. My doctoral dissertation focused on the effects of collapsing the time between group counseling sessions in time-limited settings. Therefore, I was naturally attracted to the possibility of reducing the number of filial therapy training sessions from what was at that time typically a year of training. I had already learned from my counseling experiences—with parents in the Albuquerque, New Mexico, public schools and parents who brought their children for counseling and play therapy sessions at the University of New Mexico counseling clinic where I was a graduate assistant and intern—that it was very difficult for parents to stay committed for long periods of time. I had similar experiences with parents in the Pupil Appraisal Center (later named the Child and Family Resource Clinic), which employed a multidisciplinary approach to children with learning problems and that I helped found in 1967 at the University of North Texas. In public schools, the typical semester of 15 to 17 weeks is a natural break, and many parents have difficulty carrying through with a commitment beyond that time frame. Therefore, my first filial therapy groups were structured around a 15-week model.

Although these experiences were rewarding, maintaining consistent attendance at training sessions in the last four or five sessions was very difficult; I began to experiment with 12 sessions, but still had problems with dropouts. A 3-month commitment seemed to parents to be much too long, so I decided to try 10 sessions and had immediate attendance success. During these early experiences with filial therapy, I was encouraged to find Arthur Kraft's (1973) book, which provided a case description of his use of 10 sessions of filial therapy training.

The immediate problem confronting me in developing my 10-session model was how to efficiently cover all the material and training experiences I thought necessary in only 10 2-hour sessions. The training content, method, and style of presentation, as well as the sequence of training in the 10-session model, was greatly influenced by my years of experience teaching master's- and doctoral-level courses in Child-Centered Play Therapy and by my experiences in play therapy in the Pupil Appraisal Center at the University of North Texas, where I joined the faculty as an assistant professor in 1966.

The process element, that is, the involvement of parents in the learning process, facilitation of interaction within the group, utilization of a therapeutic modality, and general emphasis on group process, in the 10-session model was an outgrowth of my experiences in teaching master's- and doctoral-level courses in group counseling. In the early years of developing the 10-session model, I trained a multitude of filial therapy groups primarily in off-campus settings in my role as a consulting supervisor in private counseling agencies in the late 1970s. Refinement of the 10-session model was a function of my experiences in these settings. Because the term *filial therapy* was not familiar to parents, in the late 1980s I began to market my approach to parents as Child-Parent-Relationship (C-P-R) Training. Later, after successful experiences with filial therapy in these private counseling agencies, I began to teach graduate courses in filial therapy in my department on the University of North Texas campus. Further refinement of the 10-session structure led to formally naming the model Child-Parent Relationship Therapy (CPRT) to distinguish it from other filial therapy models. The resulting structure of the 10-session CPRT training model is described in detail in later chapters.

The second task was to verify the effectiveness of the 10-session CPRT model through rigorous research. Beginning with Bratton and Landreth's (1995) investigation of the effects of CPRT with single parents reporting child behavior problems, the CPRT filial therapy model has been researched in 32 outcome studies representing a wide range of child and parent populations. Of these, 22 studies are controlled outcome studies published in peer-reviewed journals. Many of the studies used the rigorous dimension of blinded rater analysis of video-recordings of parent and child play sessions to evaluate parents' demonstrated ability to apply the empathic skills of Child-Centered Play Therapy. Chapter 26 provides the reader with summary findings for published controlled outcome studies conducted on this model.

Definition of CPRT/Filial Therapy

Since the use of filial therapy is rapidly becoming an accepted practice in the mental health field, it seems important to provide a definition that identifies and standardizes the practice of filial therapy. In the CPRT model, *filial therapy is defined as*

> *a unique approach used by professionals trained in play therapy to train parents to be therapeutic agents with their own children through a format of didactic instruction, demonstration play sessions, required at-home laboratory play sessions, and supervision in a supportive atmosphere. Parents are taught basic child-centered play therapy principles and skills including reflective listening, recognizing and responding to children's feelings, therapeutic limit setting, building children's self-esteem, and structuring required weekly play sessions with their children using a special kit of selected toys. Parents learn how to create a nonjudgmental, understanding, and accepting environment that enhances the parent-child relationship, thus facilitating personal growth and change for child and parent.*

Objectives of CPRT

The focus of CPRT is on the importance of the relationship between the parent and child and on the inner person of the child, what the child is capable of becoming. This relationship is viewed as the vehicle for the process of change. Therefore, the objective is to help the parent relate to the child in ways that will release the child's inner directional, constructive, forward-moving, creative, self-healing power. As in Child-Centered Play Therapy, **CPRT is not focused on solving specific problems** or a "quick fix," but rather is structured to enhance the relationship—in this case between the parent and child, with the parent serving as the therapeutic agent of change.

The overall aim of CPRT is to enhance and strengthen the parent-child relationship through improved family interactions and problem-solving strategies and through increased feelings of familial affection, warmth, and trust. CPRT offers significant benefits for both children and parents. Therapeutic goals for children are similar to those for children in play therapy, including a reduction of symptoms, development of coping strategies, and an increase in positive feelings of self-worth and confidence. Broad therapeutic goals for parents include a greater understanding and acceptance of the child's emotional world, the development of more realistic and tolerant perceptions and attitudes toward both self and child, the development of more effective parenting skills based on developmentally appropriate strategies, and last, but not least, to help parents recapture the joy in parenting.

Specific play session objectives include helping parents (a) understand and accept their child, (b) develop sensitivity to their child's feelings, (c) learn how to encourage their child's self-direction, self-responsibility, and self-reliance, (d) gain insight into self in relation to the child, (e) change their perception of their child, and (f) learn Child-Centered Play Therapy principles and skills. Through didactic instruction, demonstration play sessions with children, viewing of video-recordings, role-playing, and supervision of parents' play sessions, parents' sensitivity to their children is enhanced, and parents learn how to create a nonjudgmental, understanding, and accepting environment in which children feel safe enough to explore other parts of themselves as persons and other ways of relating to their parents.

References

Axline, V. (1950). Entering the child's world via play experiences. *Progressive Education*, *27*, 68–75.

Axline, V. (1969). *Play therapy: The inner dynamics of childhood*. Cambridge, MA: Houghton Mifflin.

Bratton, S., & Landreth, G. (1995). Filial thereapy with single parents: Effects on parental acceptance, empathy, and stress. *International Journal of Play Therapy*, *4*(1), 61–80.

Ginsberg, B. G. (1997). *Relationship enhancement family therapy*. New York, NY: John Wiley & Sons.

Guerney, B. (1964). Filial therapy: Description and rationale. *Journal of Consulting Psychology*, *28*(4), 303–310.

Kraft, A. (1973). *Are you listening to your child? How to bridge the communication gap through creative play sessions*. New York, NY: Walker.

Landreth, G. (2012). *Play therapy: The art of the relationship* (3rd ed). New York, NY: Routledge.

Moustakas, C. (1959). *Psychotherapy with children: The living relationship*. New York, NY: Harper & Row.

Rogers, C. (1942). *Counseling and psychotherapy*. Boston: Houghton Mifflin.

Rogers, C. (1951). *Client-centered therapy*. Boston: Houghton Mifflin.

Rogers, C. (1986). Client-centered therapy. In I. Kutash & A. Wolf (Eds.), *Psychotherapist's casebook* (pp. 197–208). San Francisco: Jossey-Bass.

Stover, L., & Guerney, B., Jr. (1967). The efficacy of training procedures for mothers in filial therapy. *Psychotherapy: Theory, Research, and Practice, 4*, 110–115.

VanFleet, R. (1994). *Filial therapy: Strengthening parent-child relationships through play*. Sarasota, FL: Professional Resource Press.

CHAPTER 2

NEUROSCIENCE AND CPRT

Raissa M. Miller

Child-Parent Relationship Therapy (CPRT) is a well-established approach to working with families (Cornett & Bratton, 2013; Landreth & Bratton, 2019). The many chapters in this text and accompanying manual provide ample evidence of the efficacy of CPRT with a wide range of populations and presenting issues. Although CPRT was developed long before neuroscience terminology and conceptualizations began to enter into counseling, the approach is consistent with a number of findings from developmental, affective, and relational neuroscience fields. Examining links between neuroscience and CPRT can add further depth of understanding and credibility to the approach. Furthermore, relevant neuroscience principles can give counselors another language from which to connect and communicate with clients. Mental health professionals have reported a number of positive outcomes from learning neuroscience and integrating neuroscientific information into their work with clients, including increased empathy, renewed focus on the therapeutic relationship, and increased confidence as a counselor (Badenoch, 2008; Cozolino, 2010; Miller & Barrio Minton, 2016).

The field of neuroscience is still in its relative infancy, and counselors must use caution interpreting and relating such findings to counseling. Individuals are unique, and brain structures and functions are infinitely complex (Perry, 2009). It is for this reason that this chapter will primarily focus on broad meta-concepts within neurobiology that are well established and broadly supported, including the nature of brain development and neuroanatomy of emotion and memory. I will also briefly discuss neuroscience principles of learning as they relate to the structure and implementation of CPRT.

Nature of Brain Development

Hierarchical Progression

The brain develops sequentially, beginning with lower, more primitive regions (e.g., brain stem and diencephalon) and progressing to higher, more advanced regions (e.g., limbic and cortical areas) (Gaskill & Perry, 2014; Siegel, 2012). Lower brain structures primarily develop in utero and are responsible for regulating core body functions, such as heart rate, sleep/wake cycles, temperature, respiration, and so forth (Siegel, 2012). These structures also play an important role in survival responses and physiological regulation. The loosely defined limbic region develops next, forming primarily from birth to age 5. Siegel (2012) noted that this part of the brain permits "the integration of a wide range of basic mental processes, such as the appraisal of meaning, the processing of social signals, and the activation of emotion" (p. 18). Integration of memory and the attachment system, largely mediated in the hippocampus and amygdala, are believed to originate from this central brain region. The thalamus and hypothalamus are also in the limbic region, serving as information links between the body proper and the brain (Sprenger, 2008).

The cerebral cortex is the last developing region of the brain (Perry, 2009). The brain structures in this "higher" part of the brain begin developing in early childhood but do not fully form and integrate with other regions until early adulthood (Siegel, 2012). The cortex is believed to be responsible for more complex executive functioning (e.g., working memory, attention and focus, planning, and response flexibility), abstract reasoning, problem solving, and inhibition of subcortical impulses.

The hierarchical nature of brain development has a number of implications for child and family therapy. Perhaps most importantly, interventions should match and appropriately scaffold children's cognitive, affective, and behavioral capacities (Perry, 2009). Perry (2009) developed a neurosequential developmental model of therapeutics, in which he suggests a sequence of therapeutic interventions based on children's developmental capabilities and domains of functionality. Perry noted that play therapy approaches are most useful in supporting the development of the limbic system, fostering secure attachments and emotional regulation. The limbic system is the dominant brain region throughout much of early childhood. Therapeutic interventions that primarily rely on verbal dialogue (e.g., cognitive, behavioral, and psychodynamic approaches) are often less effective with young children because they rely heavily on a part of the brain that is not fully developed or integrated, the cortex.

Child-Parent Relationship Therapy includes a number of principles and practices that demonstrate neurodevelopmental sensitivity. Perhaps most significantly, the approach helps parents learn principles of play therapy and engage children in relational connection rather than verbal discussions. This emphasis on relationship is well matched to the part of the brain that is dominant in early to mid-childhood, the limbic system. Neurodevelopmental sensitivity is also reflected in at least two Rules of Thumb: Big choices for big kids, little choices for little kids and If you can't say it in 10 words or less, don't say it. These Rules of Thumb honor the still developing nature of the cortex by not overwhelming children with too many words (i.e., language-based communication) and not expecting children to process too many pieces of information at once.

Neuroplasticity

The brain changes in response to experience throughout the lifespan (Kleim & Jones, 2008; Perry, 2009; Siegel, 2012). Cozolino and Sprokay (2006) defined neural plasticity as "the ability of neurons to change their structure and relationships to one another in an experience-dependent manner according to environmental demands" (p. 12). Put most simply, neuroplasticity is the way the brain learns (Sprenger, 2008). Neurons and neural pathways that are regularly activated will strengthen and become more automatic and efficient, whereas neurons and neural pathways that are less used will eventually weaken and die (i.e., apoptosis, pruning). Siegel (2012) referred to this process as "use it or lose it." Although individuals are born with certain genetic predispositions and potentialities, experiences influence which genes are turned off or on (i.e., epigenetics). Experiences early in life disproportionally impact specific regions and resulting functions of the developing brain. Negative early experiences can significantly impact the integrative fibers of the brain, deeply impacting stress response systems and self-regulation capacities (Andersen et al., 2008).

The concept of neuroplasticity has significant implications for work with parents. Relationships with caregivers are some of the first experiences humans encounter and are thus central to brain development. The types of experiences parents facilitate, and the frequency of those experiences, will directly impact their children's genetic expression and developing neural structures. Most parents want their children to develop characteristics of self-reliance, compassion, resilience, flexibility, emotion regulation, and so forth. However, many parents do not know the optimal ways to promote neural learning in these areas.

CPRT both enhances and utilizes the brain's natural capacity for neuroplasticity. As noted above, healthy relationships, a key focus in CPRT, support the brain's capacity to learn. Porges (2009) noted that when individuals have a neuroception of safety, their social engagement system is turned on, fostering calm bodily (e.g., slow heart rate, reduced inflammation, and low levels of stress response hormones, such as cortisol) and behavioral (e.g., improved listening, expressions of empathy, and other prosocial interactions) states. When children feel the safety of connection with a trusted caregiver, their parasympathetic nervous systems are more dominant, allowing higher cortical areas of the brain (e.g., prefrontal cortex) to more fully engage and mid-brain structures responsible for memory consolidation (e.g., substantia nigra/ventral tegmental area and the hippocampus) to translate learning into long-term memory storage (Gruber, Gelman, & Ranganath, 2014).

Furthermore, connection is one of seven essential mental hygiene practices that support neuroplasticity and optimal mental functioning throughout the lifespan (Rock, Siegel, Poelmans, & Payne, 2012). The other six essential practices include sufficient sleep, regular exercise, focus time, time-in, playtime, and downtime. According to Rock et al. (2012), connection is the sense of "feeling felt" and being seen and known by another person. The "Be-With" Attitudes in CPRT (e.g., I am here, I hear you, I understand, I care) provide the kind of presence and acceptance necessary for neuroplasticity-enhancing connection. Similar to Porges's polyvagal theory described above, these experiences foster a sense of openness and curiosity, promoting embodied learning.

CPRT also teaches parents how to facilitate experiences with their children that allow them to learn and *practice* critical skills. The practice component is essential for promoting neuroplasticity. Children are allowed to explore and struggle with developing responsibility, self-efficacy, and self-control. For example, parents learn how to return responsibility to the child. The Rule of Thumb: Don't do for the child what the child can do for him- or herself illustrates this point. Parents' responses, such as "*that is something you can do*" or "*we can work on that problem together*" allow the child to gain a felt sense of overcoming a challenge and of achievement.

Parents are also taught the difference between praise versus encouragement. CPRT emphasizes "encouraging the effort rather than praising the product" so that children can engage in self-appraisal and move towards looking inside themselves for evaluating worth. I can almost see the neurons firing as children experience the feeling of being prized for their efforts and being allowed to determine the value of their products. Neural connections link the positive sensations of creativity and mastery with the sense of being cherished and accepted.

Finally, the CPRT process of limit setting provides an opportunity for children to bring themselves under control and to gain a sense of safety (e.g., "where there are no limits, there is no security"). Through an accepting yet firm response to certain behaviors (e.g., "*I know you really want to hit me with the sword, but I am not for hitting. You can choose to hit the bop bag or the floor*"), children are allowed the time and space to regulate their impulses. They are able to experience what it feels like in their bodies to want to do something but choose not to do it. They learn other acceptable outlets for particular desires.

The repetition of these internalized felt sense experiences build neural nets of positive feelings, thoughts, and behaviors. The more these experiences occur, the stronger and more automatic they will become in the brain. Although the neural connections will not be fully myelinated until adolescence and early adulthood, a strong foundation is laid that will guide future development of these capacities.

Neuroanatomy of Memory and Emotion

Implicit Memory

Within neuroscience, memory is often referred to as explicit (declarative) or implicit (non-declarative) (Kandel, 2009; Siegel, 2012). Explicit memories are episodic (e.g., remembering a specific event, such as eating strawberry ice cream on your eighth birthday) or factual (e.g., remembering a specific piece of knowledge, such as recalling an article that recommended children sleep 10–12 hours a night). Implicit memories do not carry with them a conscious sense of remembering. Rather, they are interwoven in the mind and body in such a way that they filter the outside world and influence perceptions, emotions, behavioral impulses, and bodily sensations. Implicit memories are the only kinds of memories individuals can form until about 18 months of age and remain primary throughout much of early childhood. Implicit memories play a critical role in the brain's job of anticipating, predicting, and reacting to environmental stimuli in an efficient and effective manner.

The attachment system, and the styles individuals develop to meet attachment needs, are considered a type of implicit memory (Badenoch & Cox, 2010; Schore, 2012; Siegel, 2012). Siegel (2012) defined the attachment system as an "inborn system in the brain that evolves in ways that influence and organize motivational, emotional, and memory processes with respect to significant caregiving figures" (p. 91). Broadly speaking, individuals develop attachment styles along a continuum of secure to insecure. The more secure individuals are, the more likely they are able to rely on significant relational figures to help regulate stress. They are also more likely to be curious about the world around them and seek out novelty and growth. Secure individuals have an internalized sense of "I am worthy and loveable. Although people are not perfect, I can usually trust others to help me when needed. The world is full of interesting people, places, and things and I want to go out and explore it." Individuals who have more insecure attachments tend to struggle with self-regulation and have more negative views of self, others, and the world.

Implicit memories, especially mental models of attachment, can play an important role in work with parents (Siegel & Hartzell, 2003). All individuals carry with them implicit memories of their own childhoods and ways of being and relating in the context of family relationships. Badenoch and Cox (2010) noted that implicit memories can tell "us about our value and what we can expect in relationships" (p. 466). Sometimes implicit memories filter present moment experience in a negative way and begin to interfere with the parent-child relationship. Implicit memories may inhibit parents' abilities to be emotionally present for their children and to respond in empathic and intentional ways. Recognizing when reactions or responses are the result of implicit biases versus present moment realities is often the first step in creating more choice and change (Siegel & Hartzell, 2003). Although neuroscience research regarding implicit memories is still emerging, one of the best known ways to integrate and transform problematic implicit memories is through disconfirming relational experiences and mindfulness-based exercises that promote greater bodily awareness and acceptance of present moment experiences (Badenoch, 2008; Siegel, 2012). CPRT can help facilitate both new relational experiences and mindful parenting practices.

A relevant CPRT Rule of Thumb to the concept of implicit memory is You can't give away that which you don't possess. Parents can only provide as much emotional presence and acceptance as they are willing to experience and develop within themselves. These abilities are often linked to implicit attachment styles (Schore, 2012). The nature of instruction and group process in CPRT increases the likelihood that implicit memories will be triggered, and thus identified and worked through. Parents are often unaware of the roots of their emotional reactions to their children or even their children's emotional reactions to them and others. In my experience facilitating CPRT groups, discussions related to implicit memories have helped parents decrease self-blame and begin to transform implicit memories into more coherent and integrated ways of being. Badenoch and Cox (2010) noted that "when implicit neural networks are activated in group, the group, supported by the therapist, can amplify the sense of attunement and, consequently, potentiate the possible repair" (p. 468). The group can serve as a source of regulation and act as disconfirming experiences that can help transform automatic reacting into reflective responding.

Parents are also taught in CPRT that "what's most important may not be what you do, but what you do after what you have done." This concept aligns with the implicit attachment notion of repair (Siegel & Hartzell, 2003; Siegel, 2012) and can help parents foster a secure attachment with their children. Parents do not have to respond perfectly to their children all the time to promote secure attachment. In fact, parents who foster both secure and insecure attachments only "get it right" about one third of the time (Badenoch, 2008). The difference between the two parenting styles is that parents who foster secure attachments recognize when they have "gotten it wrong" and loop back around to try it again (i.e., repair). This process of rupture and repair is believed to build resilience in the brain. Parents learn this important brain-building skill in CPRT.

Emotions

Understanding the role emotions play in brain functioning is essential to work with parents and children. In recent decades, significant emphasis in mental health treatment has been on cognitive theories of change. According to many of these models, emotional and behavioral change results from identifying and disputing maladaptive thoughts (Hofmann, Asnaani, Vonk, Sawyer, & Fang, 2012). These models do not necessarily reflect how our brains and bodies are designed to respond, especially when individuals perceive threat or are under high levels of stress (Field, Beeson, & Jones, 2015; Gaskill & Perry, 2014; Siegel & Hartzell, 2003). Scholars have used a number of terms to describe the way the brain processes and responds to such stimuli (e.g., low road/high road, fast thinking/slow thinking, and bottom-up/top-down). Individuals who have underdeveloped higher cortical brain structures (e.g., children, individuals who have unresolved traumas) are more likely to rely on bottom-up processing that is quick, largely automatic, and non-conscious. Such processing is motivated by primitive emotional states and activates physiological responding that assists with survival (Panksepp & Biven, 2012).

The cortex, dominant in self-reflection, perspective taking, and thinking about long-term consequences, is largely bypassed in bottom-up processing (Field et al., 2015; Gaskill & Perry, 2014). The ability to learn new information, problem solve, and express empathy is temporarily impaired in such instances. Gaskill and Perry (2014) noted that "reflection on behavior is impossible for the child in an alarm state, and cognitive strategies to modify behavior (even if previously internalized and mastered) cannot be recruited in an efficient way because the cortex is relatively inaccessible under threat" (p. 185). Age, life history, and current stressors all impact whether a person operates out of bottom-up or top-down processing. In general, emotional regulation through more top-down neural processing is a skill initially learned in early childhood through relationships with caregivers and then refined throughout the lifespan.

Play has an important role in the development of emotional regulation (Kestly, 2016; Pankseep, 2009). The Broca's area of the brain, dominate in language development, grows throughout childhood, allowing children to become increasingly capable of verbal expression (Sprenger, 2008). Despite this development, however, play continues to be the most appropriate means of communicating emotional information. Through play, children are allowed to express their inner lives and learn the boundaries of their emotional expression. Play within the context of safe, connected relationships is believed to activate aspects of the parasympathetic and sympathetic nervous systems that allow processing of real-life scenarios and struggles (Kestly, 2016). Perry, Hogan, and Marlin (2000) also noted that play tends to mirror other aspects of physical, cognitive, and social-emotional development. In this manner, playing with a child can provide a window into their neural developmental functioning.

The CPRT approach is consistent with neurobiological understandings of emotions. Parents are taught that play is a more natural way for children to communicate emotions. Parents are provided with the instructions and support for setting up special playtimes that allow that natural communication to occur. Parents are also taught skills to help respond and cope with emotions outside of the special playtime. One of the first skills taught to parents in

CPRT is reflective responding. CPRT facilitators support parents in being able to understand and communicate that understanding to their children. This skill alone can help soothe emotional overwhelm. Siegel (2012) refers to the phrase "name it to tame it" when talking about the effect identifying and labeling emotions has on calming the nervous system.

The CPRT Rule of Thumb: When a child is drowning, don't try to teach her to swim is an excellent example of the approach honoring emotions. Parents are taught that moments of emotional overwhelm (e.g., tantrums, meltdowns) are not times to teach lessons or have children reflect on their behavior. Rather, parents are encouraged to find ways to connect with and soothe the child. Siegel and Hartzell (2003) referred to these incidences as "limbic override" and noted the importance of connection before correction.

Neuroscience of Adult Learning

One of the most exciting findings to come out of neuroscience fields in the last few decades is the notion that the brain can change throughout the lifespan (i.e., adult brain plasticity). Although learning does not occur as easily or efficiently as it does in early childhood and adolescence, counselors can join with parents to create real structural changes (Bavelier, Levi, Li, Dan, & Hensch, 2010). Cozolino and Sprokay (2006) outlined five principles of adult learning that enhance neuroplasticity (p. 12):

1. A safe and trusting relationship with an attuned other
2. Maintenance of a moderate level of arousal
3. Activation of both thinking and feeling
4. A language of self-reflection
5. Co-construction of a narrative that reflects a positive and optimistic self

The first principle, creating a safe and trusting relationship with an attuned other, relates to the social nature of the brain (Cozolino & Sprokay, 2006; Sprenger, 2008). Sprenger (2008) noted that "brains learn best with other brains" (p. 3). As has already been noted in earlier sections, plasticity is enhanced within the contexts of safe relationships. The brain's sympathetic nervous system, which focuses more on here-and-now survival, is able to relax, allowing parts of the brain responsible for long-term learning and planning to take the lead.

The second principle, maintenance of a moderate level of arousal, reflects research on the role of motivation, rewards, and stress on learning (Cozolino & Sprokay, 2006; Gruber et al., 2014). Neural activity in largely automatic areas of the brain, including the amygdala, hippocampus, and the orbitofrontal cortex, play an important role in translating new information into long-term memory storage (Gruber et al., 2014; Siegel, 2012). Too little arousal, and the brain perceives the information as unimportant for storing. Too much arousal, and the brain is inhibited by other stress response functions in the brain, and memories can become largely implicit and fragmented (Elzinga, Bakker, & Bremner, 2005). Arousal can be regulated through a balance of challenge and support and making sure the information is meaningful and relevant to the learner.

The third principle, activation of both thinking and feeling, reflects the increased understanding of the role emotions play in cognitive learning (Immordino-Yang & Damasio, 2007; Rose, Gilbert, & Smith, 2013; Siegel, 2012; Sprenger, 2008). Emotional centers of the brain play an important role in filtering incoming information for memory salience, as well as in generalizing skills learned in an academic setting to real-life situations. Executive functioning relies heavily on the connection between the orbitofrontal and ventromedial prefrontal cortex and the emotion-producing limbic region (Cozolino & Sprokay, 2006). The Latin root of the word e-mot-ion is e (prefix)-mot (move). Without integration of these brain regions, individuals fail to adequately apply judgment and take appropriate action (i.e., move). Increasingly, state-dependence is emphasized in teaching and learning (Jovasevic et al., 2015). State-dependent learning generally refers to the notion that individuals' memory retrieval is enhanced when the context of learning and the context of application match. For example, parents learning to reflect their child's feelings should practice that skill under circumstances similar to those with which they will actually be reflecting the child's feelings. Ways to promote state-dependent learning include role-plays, true-to-life application exercises, and in vivo experimentation that activate both thinking and feeling.

The final two principles, a language of self-reflection and co-construction of a positive and optimistic self-narrative, also relate to research on how information is organized and stored in the brain for later retrieval (Cozolino & Sprokay, 2006). Cozolino and Sprokay (2006) noted that "because narratives require the participation of multiple memory networks, these stories serve as ways of enhancing memory through linked associations" (p. 16). Information learned through rote memorization relies heavily on prefrontal cortex functioning, an area of the brain most susceptible to suboptimal functioning when under stress (e.g., insufficient sleep, hunger, emotional overwhelm). Information learned through embodied experiences and incorporated into the narrative of the self, however, is believed to be stored in subcortical, as well as cortical, parts of the brain and is more resilient to stress and overwhelm. The tone and focus of self-reflections (e.g., focus on strengths versus focus on deficits) are also critical in the neuroscience of adult learning. The stories individuals tell themselves about their adequacy and competence as a parent have important implications for behavior. Positive self-narratives beget more positive parenting behaviors.

The CPRT process aligns quite nicely with these neuroscience-informed principles of adult learning. The approach is designed as a group experience, allowing for the development of safe, supportive relationships and as a place to acknowledge emotions and rewrite parenting self-narratives. Counselors facilitating CPRT acknowledge strengths (e.g., positive parenting behaviors, successes) and empower parents through active affirmation. This idea is particularly illustrated in the Rule of Thumb: It is difficult to believe in yourself if no one believes in you. Parents' struggles are normalized within the group, and they are able to both give and receive support, enhancing relevance and meaning.

Furthermore, in CPRT counselors utilize a number of strategies that evoke thinking and feeling, as well as further foster development of positive self-narratives. The CPRT Treatment Manual, 2nd Edition, includes a number of stories and analogies (e.g., the struggle to become a butterfly, oxygen mask on an airplane), and participants are encouraged to share examples and areas of concern. Throughout the group experience, participants engage in state-dependent learning through conducting their own play sessions, engaging in role-plays (e.g., practice limit setting, choice giving, self-esteem-building responses), and completing homework assignments (e.g., Feeling Responses, skill tracking, Sandwich Hug/Kiss, positive character quality notes).

Conclusion

Neuroscience research is increasingly relevant in counseling. Some scholars have referred to neuroscience as the fifth force in the counseling profession (McHenry, Sikorski, & McHenry, 2014). Fortunately, this shift in the field does not necessarily mean counselors have to completely rethink their approaches. As has been presented in this chapter, much of what counselors already do align with neuroscience principles. CPRT is a good example of this notion. CPRT is consistent with principles of brain development, neuroanatomy of emotions and memory, and neuroscience of adult learning.

As counselors learn more about neuroscience principles that underlie their work, they can begin sharing this knowledge with clients. Excellent resources exist for counselors interested in sharing neuroscience principles with parents, including an article I wrote in a recent edition of *The Journal of Mental Health Counseling* (Miller, 2016), as well as multiple texts by Dan Siegel and various co-authors (for a complete list of books, visit www.drdansiegel.com). Additional information to share can be found through reputable online websites (e.g., Center on the Developing Child at developingchild.harvard.edu).

References

Andersen, S. L., Tomada, A., Vincow, E. S., Valente, E., Polcari, A., & Teicher, M. H. (2008). Preliminary evidence for sensitive periods in the effect of childhood sexual abuse on regional brain development. *Journal of Neuropsychiatry and Clinical Neurosciences, 20*, 292–301. doi:10.1176/appi.neuropsych.20.3.292

Badenoch, B. (2008). *Being a brain-wise therapist: A practical guide to interpersonal neurobiology*. New York, NY: W. W. Norton.

Badenoch, B., & Cox, P. (2010). Integrating interpersonal neurobiology with group psychotherapy. *International Journal of Group Psychotherapy, 60*(4), 463–481. doi:10.1521/ijgp.2010.60.4.462

Bavelier, D., Levi, D. M., Li, R. W., Dan, Y., & Hensch, T. K. (2010). Removing breaks on adult brain plasticity: From molecular to behavioral interventions. *The Journal of Neuroscience, 30*, 14964–14971. doi:10.1523/JNEUROSCI.4812-10.2010

Cornett, N., & Bratton, S. C. (2013). Examining the impact of child parent relationship therapy (CPRT) on family functioning. *Journal of Marital & Family Therapy, 40*(3), 302–218. doi:10.1111/jmft.12014

Cozolino, L. (2010). *The neuroscience of psychotherapy: Building and rebuilding the human brain* (2nd ed). New York, NY: W. W. Norton.

Cozolino, L., & Sprokay, S. (2006). Neuroscience and adult learning. *New Directions for Adult and Continuing Education, 110*, 11–19. doi:10.1002/ace.214

Elzinga, B. M., Bakker, A., & Bremmer, J. D. (2005). Stress-induced cortisol elevations are associated with impaired delayed, but not immediate recall. *Psychiatry Research, 134*, 211–223. doi:10.1016/j.psychres.2004.11.007

Field, T. A., Beeson, E. T., & Jones, L. K. (2015). The new ABCs: A practitioner's guide to neuroscience-informed cognitive-behavior therapy. *Journal of Mental Health Counseling, 37*, 206–220. doi:10.1774/mehc.37.3.02

Gaskill, R. L., & Perry, B. D. (2014). The neurobiological power of play: Using the neurosequential developmental model of therapeutics to guide play in the healing process. In C. A. Malchiodi & D. A. Crenshaw (Eds.), *Creative arts and play therapy for attachment problems* (pp. 178–194). New York, NY: Guilford Press.

Gruber, M. J., Gelman, B. D., & Ranganath, C. (2014). States of curiosity modulate hippocampus-dependent learning via the dopaminergic circuit. *Neuron, 84*, 486–496. doi:10.1016/j.neuron.2014.08.060

Hofmann, S. G., Asnaani, A., Vonk, I. J. J., Sawyer, A. T., & Fang, A. (2012). The efficacy of cognitive behavioral therapy: A review of meta-analyses. *Cognitive Therapy Research, 36*, 427–440. doi:10.1007/s10608-012-9476-1

Immordino-Yang, M. H., & Damasio, A. (2007). We feel therefore we learn: The relevance of affective and social neuroscience to education. *Mind, Brain, and Education, 1*, 3–10. doi:10.1111/j.1751-228X.2007.00004

Jovasevic, V., Corcoran, K. A., Leaderbrand, K., Yamawaki, N., Guedea, A. L., Chen, H. J., . . . Radulovic, J. (2015). GABAergic mechanisms regulated by miR-33 encode state-dependent fear. *Nature Neuroscience, 18*, 1265–1271. doi:10.1038/nn.4084

Kandel, E. R. (2009). The biology of memory. *The Journal of Neuroscience, 29*, 12748–12756. doi:10.1523/JNEUROSCI.3958-09

Kestly, T. A. (2016). Presence and play: Why mindfulness matters. *International Journal of Play Therapy, 25*, 14–23. doi:10.1037/pla0000019

Kleim, J. A., & Jones, T. A. (2008). Principles of experience-dependent neural plasticity: Implications for rehabilitation after brain damage.

Journal of Speech, Language, and Hearing Research, *51*, 225–239. doi:10.1044/1092-4388(2008/018)

Landreth, G. L., & Bratton, S. C. (2019). *Child-Parent Relationship Therapy (CPRT): An Evidence-Based 10-session filial therapy model* (2nd ed). New York, NY: Routledge.

McHenry, B., Sikorski, A. M., & McHenry, J. (2014). *A counselor's introduction to neuroscience*. New York, NY: Routledge.

Miller, R. M. (2016). Neuroeducation: Integrating brain-based psychoeducation into clinical practice. *Journal of Mental Health Counseling*, *38*, 103–115. doi:10.17744/mehc.38.2.02

Miller, R. M., & Barrio Minton, C. A. (2016). Experiences learning interpersonal neurobiology: An interpretative phenomenological analysis. *Journal of Mental Health Counseling*, *38*, 47–61. doi:10.17744/mehc.38.1.04

Pankseep, J. (2009). Brain emotional systems and qualities of mental life: From animal models of affect to implications for psychotherapeutics. In D. Fosha, D. Siegel, & M. Solomon (Eds.), *The healing power of emotion: Affective neuroscience, development, and clinical practice* (pp. 1–26). New York, NY: W. W. Norton.

Panksepp, J., & Biven, L. (2012). *The archaeology of mind: Neuroevolutionary origins of human emotions*. New York, NY: W. W. Norton.

Perry, B. D. (2009). Examining child maltreatment through a neurodevelopmental lens: Clinical applications of the neurosequential model of therapeutics. *Journal of Loss and Trauma*, *14*, 240–255. doi:10.1080/15325020903004350

Perry, B. D., Hogan, L., & Marlin, S. J. (2000). Curiosity, pleasure, and play: A neurodevelopmental perspective. *HAAEYC Advocate*. Retrieved from www.childtrauma.org

Porges, S. W. (2009). The polyvagal theory: New insights into adaptive reactions of the autonomic nervous system. *Cleveland Clinic Journal of Medicine*, *76*, S86–S90. doi:10.3949/ccjm.76.s2.17

Rock, D., Siegel, D. J., Poelmans, S. A. Y., & Payne, J. (2012). The healthy mind platter. *NeuroLeadership Journal*, *4*, 1–23.

Rose, J., Gilbert, L., & Smith, H. (2013). Affective teaching and the affective dimensions of learning. In S. Ward (Ed.), *A student's guide to education studies* (pp. 178–188). New York, NY: Routledge.

Schore, A. N. (2012). *Affect regulation and the origin of the self: The neurobiology of emotional development*. New York, NY: Taylor & Francis.

Siegel, D. J. (2012). *The developing mind: How relationships and the brain interact to shape who we are* (2nd ed). New York, NY: Guilford Press.

Siegel, D. J., & Hartzell, M. (2003). *Parenting from the inside out: How a deeper self-understanding can help you raise children who thrive.* New York, NY: Penguin Group.

Sprenger, M. (2008). *The developing brain: Birth to age eight.* Thousand Oaks, CA: Corwin Press.

CHAPTER 3

UNIQUE FEATURES OF CPRT

There are many significant and dynamic features of CPRT that set this model apart from other parent training programs. The following parent-child dimensions and training dimensions make CPRT a unique form of parent training.

Parent-Child Dimensions

Parent-Child Relationship

The primary focus of CPRT is on enhancing and strengthening the parent-child relationship by equipping parents with basic Child-Centered Play Therapy skills that have been proven to be necessary and effective dimensions in facilitating the development of secure attachment relationships. Most other parent training programs focus primarily on teaching specific techniques or problem-solving skills to be utilized in the correction or extinguishing of specific child-related behaviors. CPRT is based on the rationale that the relationship between parent and child is the essential and curative therapeutic dimension for improving and correcting children's problems and preventing the development of future problems.

Communication Is Play Based

Unlike other parent training models that rely on verbal skills stressing family discussions or parent-child discussions to resolve problems, **CPRT and other forms of filial therapy rely on the child's natural means of communication—play—as the primary medium for communicating the child's feelings, needs, wants, wishes, fantasies, experiences, and thoughts.** In filial therapy, play is the communication medium for understanding the child and building the parent-child relationship. Children are comfortable with the medium of play and can, therefore, more easily lead the play experience/relationship to focus on dimensions important to them. The child's communication through play is, thus, less restricted.

Symbolic Expression

Since play is the child's natural medium of expression and CPRT is play based, it is the only parent training model that allows children to express their emotions fully through the safety of symbolic expression and within the context of child-directed play. Toys are not merely used as a way to get the child to talk or to provide parents a means to apply discipline strategies. Parents are taught that children's play behavior has meaning, and demonstrations with toys are used to convey examples of how a child's self-directed play with the selected toys may relate to events, fears, etc., in the child's life. Parents are taught to be sensitive to possible meanings in their child's play. However, they are not expected to figure out or understand symbolic meaning in a child's play, only to be sensitive to the importance of the play and the therapeutic value of play. The important factor is that the child has an opportunity to play out potentially significant messages. The playing out is more important than whether or not the parent understands the symbolic meaning.

Child Takes the Lead

In the special playtimes, the child is allowed to lead. The parent does not initiate topics of conversation, content of play, or how the time will be spent or offer suggestions for solutions to problems. The child leads throughout the 30-minute special playtime, and the parent follows. The focus of the time together is determined by the child, regardless of previous child behaviors that may concern the parent. In most other parent training programs, content and direction of parent-child interactions are determined by the parent. Allowing the child to lead provides the child with opportunities to experience what responsibility feels like.

Acceptance Rather Than Correction

In CPRT, there is no emphasis on correcting a child's behavior. The focus of the training is on developing skills to be utilized during a special 30-minute playtime. For 30 minutes, the parent is to be accepting of the child and the child's decisions within appropriate boundaries or limits. The child is allowed to make decisions related to the playtime, what the child will play with, how the child will play, etc., and the parent accepts those decisions. The parent does not correct the child, except in situations where limits are needed, does not wish the child were different, and allows the child to make mistakes without interfering or offering suggestions. For 30 minutes, the child is in charge and is accepted as she is.

Training Dimensions

Group Process/Group Therapy

The process or group therapy component of CPRT is unique and vital to the success of CPRT, because parents often have strong reactions to their children and feelings about themselves and their family members that they need to process in order to be fully present and emotionally available to learn what is being taught in the CPRT training sessions. This process is described in the following self-critique of a graduate student in a supervised filial therapy practicum experience.

> I recognized that Ashley and her husband had an argument on the way to the filial session, and it was obvious that she was going to have a hard time listening until she was able to process how she was feeling right then; so I put my training agenda aside to help her process her feelings. I learned that this kind of flexibility is crucial to filial training. Taking the time to allow Ashley to express her feelings and be heard before I asked her to listen to my training points facilitated the development of rapport

> and trust in our relationship in addition to clearing her system so she could listen. Allowing her to explore her feelings facilitated not only the expression of her feelings but also a greater awareness of her own needs. I believe this will help her to have more effective play sessions with her son because she will better understand the power and process of reflection which I modeled. On a personal note, once again I learned the power of reflection. I did not try to help her come to a resolution in her argument with her husband, but I simply reflected and followed her lead. My reflections facilitated some interesting insights. At the end of the session, she reported feeling much better.

Parents' strong reactions to their children and feelings about themselves and their family members also need to be processed in CPRT training so parents can be fully present and emotionally available to their children as is called for in the special play sessions. One mother described the necessity of processing as "I grew up in a highly dysfunctional family, and I'm experiencing some really strong gut reaction feelings about my parents that are probably preventing me from hearing the emotional messages communicated by my child in our playtimes." The didactic/therapeutic dimensions of filial therapy training sessions and the processing of the parents' special play sessions with their children often reminds parents of emotional wounds and issues with their own parents that have been pushed aside over the years. These issues are explored in the context of their interference with the parents' role of relating to their children as therapeutic agents of change, not in the context of "There is something wrong with you that you need to change," or as personality issues that need to be corrected. Therefore, this component of filial therapy is referred to as group process or as a group therapy type component.

Parents are not in CPRT to receive group therapy. They need training and development of relationship skills. But they also need to develop insight into personal issues that interfere with their relating to their children as change agents, and the processing of personal issues facilitates the inner growth required to enable parents to incorporate the new skills and apply the new behaviors required.

During a CPRT training session focused on developing the skill of reflecting children's feelings, Angela seemed particularly resistant and adamantly questioned the importance of reflecting her child's feelings. In a later training session, she shared:

> I've been thinking about reflecting a child's feelings, and I now understand why it is important. As a child, I would tell my mom I didn't want to stay home with my father when she went out shopping. My mom ignored my pleadings, and my father sexually abused me. I grew up not trusting my feelings and not trusting myself because my mother didn't listen to my feelings. I now realize that when you validate children's feelings, you teach them to trust themselves.

Processing her childhood experience and current feelings in the filial group freed Angela to identify, emotionally relate to, and validate her child's feelings. Angela's sharing her insight also reinforced the leader's emphasis on the importance of reflecting children's feelings and provided added impetus for the other parents to invest energy in validating their children's feelings.

Hearing other parents' experiences breaks down barriers of defensiveness and isolation. Therefore, the leader is active in facilitating interaction among parents and helping them to feel included in the group. The power of the group was summed up by Emily in the last training session as she described what had impacted her in the CPRT training:

> Dr. Landreth could sit there and tell us all day that there are other parents like us who are struggling, to try to make us feel better, but knowing that there are other people we can see, hear, and touch makes a big difference. It helped me so much to hear you-all describe your problems and struggles with your children.

The critical importance of the group process/group therapy component of filial therapy was supported in Eardley's (1978) research. A model of filial therapy structured exclusively around didactic training components coupled with the utilization of demonstrations and required parent-child play sessions with supervision feedback was found to be less effective than a model of filial therapy incorporating a combination of didactic training components and group process components. The effectiveness of filial therapy training is dependent on parents actively processing personal issues related to themselves, their children, the play sessions, and their family.

Future Focused

CPRT training is future focused. Most other parent training models are grounded in past relationships and happenings with an emphasis on correcting the way the child has been. CPRT is focused on what the child is capable of being or becoming, not what the child has done. Therefore, minimal time is spent on parents recounting their children's behaviors. Responding to children based on past behaviors restricts children to continue to be the way they have been.

If significant adults in children's lives perceive them as being incapable of change, then children are bound to their past. It is not possible for a child to become what the child is capable of becoming until a significant adult in the child's life believes the child is capable and responds to the child as though the child were capable. CPRT is based on a belief in the child's capacity for positive self-directed change and, therefore, focuses on the child's potential rather than the child's problem.

Experientially Based

CPRT is primarily experientially based, relying on the principle of learning by doing. Most other parent training models use a lecture–discussion format to teach principles and procedures considered to be important. The experiential approach engages parents more quickly, maintains a high level of parent interest and involvement, and provides opportunities for the trainer to supervise the development of skills. The experiential approach also engages or draws out parents who are hesitant, quiet, or somewhat reserved about talking in a group. This process can be seen in the following description in a filial therapist's report.

> Maria has really surprised me. At first, she was quiet and did not participate in the group discussion. She seemed to become more comfortable in the third session, and then really seemed to explode with excitement once she began the play sessions with Adam. Wow, the excitement and enjoyment she had was exciting to me! She was faithful in bringing her video-recording each week. On the video-recording, it was evident that she understood the skills we taught and was applying them. In fact,

> I was surprised at the pace at which she really learned the skills. By the fifth training session, Maria began to share her feelings about the playtimes and began asking how she should respond in specific situations outside the play session.
>
> She also began sharing what she was learning with her husband and even video-recorded him in a play session with Adam, then brought the video, with her husband's permission, for us to view. As we viewed the video of his play session, Maria pointed out how he should have responded and in general took on the supervisor role. She reported that the play sessions were fun for her and for Adam, that Adam was treating his sister better and was much more obedient and cooperative at home. Adam's teacher reported that his behavior in the classroom was much more positive, he was more socially interactive and more cooperative at school.

Practicing new skills in a role-playing format in the training sessions prior to implementation of the special play sessions increases the confidence level of parents and helps ensure the new skills will be used correctly in parent-child interactions in the required at-home special play sessions. One filial therapist observed:

> It is not enough for a parent to tell you she understands limit setting. I am sure Margaret did understand. However, it is different when the parent is put in the position of actually setting a limit without having had enough rote memorization of how to state the limit. Margaret did set a limit in her play session, but it was set in the way that she would have done it in the past because she couldn't remember how to actually state the limit in the new way. I can really see the value of role-playing and how beneficial it is to practice in a group where a parent can observe others doing it, too.

The most dynamic part of experiential learning occurs in the required parent-child special playtimes as parents implement their new role of therapeutic agent with their child. These special play sessions are usually times of exciting discovery for parents about themselves and their children and are often reinforcing times for parents as they successfully implement new skills.

The experiential approach of role-playing during training sessions and then having special play sessions that are viewed by other parents in the group allows parents to engage in the process of giving supportive feedback and encouragement. Peer group support is more powerful in influencing parental behavior than comments made by the CPRT trainer. These dimensions are vital in building parents' confidence in trying new ways of responding to their children.

Building a Relationship Rather Than Correcting a Problem

The focus of CPRT training is on equipping parents with the skills necessary to develop a therapeutic relationship with their children. There is no emphasis on correcting a specific problem a child may have. The rationale for this approach to parent training is that improving the parent's relationship with a child will positively impact the underlying causes of the problematic behavior, which will in turn result in positive changes in the behavior of concern. The person of the child and the parent's relationship with the child is always more important than the problem the child may have. Therefore, CPRT training sessions focus on developing therapeutic relationship skills rather than on techniques or methodology for correcting problems.

Changing the Child's Perception

A central objective of CPRT training is to change the child's perception of the parent and the parent-child relationship rather than to change the child's behavior. Behavior is viewed as a function of perception. Therefore, a change in perception will result in a change in behavior. In CPRT, parents learn how to establish an understanding, accepting, and empathic play session environment in which the parent comes to be viewed by the child as an ally, because for 30 minutes the parent gives up any attempt to correct or change the child. Parents learn how to look through their child's eyes, to assume their child's perceptual frame of reference.

Focus on Parental Efficacy vs. Changing the Child

Parents who come for filial therapy often feel out of control, believing what they need to learn is a method to control their child. While most parent training models prescribe strategies for changing the child, that is not the objective in CPRT training. Rather, this approach focuses on changing the parent through increased parental efficacy. Parents who feel more confident in their ability to respond appropriately to their children feel more in control.

How parents feel about themselves, their sense of adequacy as a person and a parent, significantly affects their interaction with their children and thus their children's development. Parenting is at best a difficult, stressful, and often frustrating process for even the most skillful and dedicated parent. When difficulty occurs in the parent-child relationship and things just are not going well, parents are susceptible to self-blame and doubt their adequacy as a parent. Research has shown that parental efficacy can have a profound impact on any number of the dimensions of children's development. Rohner (1986) reported that the children of parents who were warm, accepting, and nurturing exhibited more positive social skills. Children who were experiencing difficulties with social skills had parents who were rigid, authoritarian, and cold. Other studies concluded that parents scoring high in internal locus of control appear to influence their children's development in positive ways (Schaefer, 1981; Swick & Graves, 1986). Swick, Gladstone, and Hayes (1988) noted that parent interventions designed specifically to increase parents' sense of control resulted in improvements in children's behavior.

The dynamics of the relationship between parent and child most assuredly affect children's development, and a major factor in this relationship is the parent's attitude and perception of self, as related to parental locus of control. Parent's perception of self affects their locus of control, which in turn influences the direction and extent of parental guidance and involvement in their children's lives. Generally, when a child experiences some developmental difficulty or parents experience prolonged difficulty in their interpersonal relationships with their children, parents feel out of control, they believe they can do nothing, and they feel inadequate. Therefore, a major objective in CPRT is supporting and encouraging parents. The sensitive therapist will convey faith in the parent's ability to grow in understanding and acceptance of the child and to have a positive impact on the child's development. Parents need assistance in learning skills that encourage the development of positive parent-child relationships. To assume that most parents already know what these skills are and how to utilize them is incorrect, because relatively little effort has been put forth in our society to teach parents how to interact with their children in effective ways.

As parents learn the basic Child-Centered Play Therapy skills of reflective responding and therapeutic limit setting, they gradually begin to perceive themselves as being capable because they have new tools to utilize in their interactions with their children. As a result, parents feel empowered and their self-perception is improved. Changes in self-perception result in changes in parental behavior. As parents feel more confident and in control in their role as a parent, they are able to shift their focus from controlling their child to accepting their child as being capable of positive self-directed change. This change in perception on the part of the parent is a powerful therapeutic dimension that frees the child from defending a rigid perception of self, thus enabling the child to change. Thus, a major focus in CPRT is helping parents develop a more realistic and tolerant view of their children.

Understanding the Relationship vs. Purpose of Behavior

In CPRT training, the emphasis is not on understanding the purpose of behavior, but rather on understanding the child, the child's emotional needs, and the importance of the relationship with the child. It is not necessary to understand the why of behavior. It is always important to understand the child and the child's needs. Parents are often more concerned about understanding why their children behave as they do rather than understanding their child as a person. This need to have an answer seems to be motivated by a belief that if the parent can just find an answer to why her child behaves the way he does, that will solve the problem. This solution-focused approach reinforces a need for control and overlooks the importance of the person of the child.

Internal Locus of Control vs. External Locus of Control

CPRT and other forms of filial therapy are unique in emphasizing the importance of responding to children in ways that develop an internal locus of control. The accomplishment of this objective is facilitated in developing a relationship with the child in which the parent's responses communicate a belief in the child's ability to respond responsibly by returning responsibility for decisions in the special playtime to the child. This belief in the child is grounded in developmentally appropriate boundaries that are established in such a way as to allow the child to develop inner control. This is not a completely permissive relationship. There are limits on behavior. However, the behavior being expressed by the child is viewed in the context of the relationship, and understanding the child is more important than stopping the behavior.

Understanding the child means responding to the intrinsic variables related to the child's motivation, perception of self, independence, and need for acceptance. In the CPRT relationship, the objective is not to stop a child's behavior. Statements such as "Stop that, don't do that" and "You can't do that" promote the development of an external locus of control. The focus in the CPRT approach is on understanding the unique perspective of the child, the child's feelings, what the child wants, and what the child is trying to communicate. Therefore, rather than trying to stop the behavior, the objective is to communicate understanding of the child—"*You would like to pull that doll's head off*," "*You're angry at me*"—and to respond to the child in such a way as to allow the child to stop himself: "*The doll's head is not for pulling off*," "*I'm not for hitting*," "*The playdough is for playing with on the cookie sheet*." These responses allow the child to say "No" to self and they facilitate the development of an internal locus of control in the child. Significant change comes from within the child, and this belief is modeled by the parent responding in ways that empower the child.

Required Laboratory Sessions

CPRT training is very systematic and follows a structure that involves parents in an ongoing learning experience that does not leave the acquisition or practice of skills to chance. CPRT is the only parent training model of its kind that requires a structured laboratory experience. Unlike other parent training models that wait for an opportune time, usually initiated by a child's behavior, to utilize a new technique or skill, parents in filial therapy are required to have a scheduled 30-minute special playtime with their child of focus (the child identified by the parent as needing help) once a week in their home or other designated location. During this special playtime, parents are to practice Child-Centered Play Therapy skills learned in the training sessions.

Specific Set of Play Materials

Parent-child special play sessions utilize a specific set of play materials that have been found to facilitate a wide range of children's play behaviors and emotional expressions. In the special playtimes, play materials are used by children in the act of play to communicate their personal world. Since the toys and materials selected for the play sessions are a significant therapeutic variable, parents are not allowed to introduce other toys into the playtimes unless they have been approved. All play materials do not automatically encourage the expression of children's needs, feelings, and experiences.

Skills Are Required to Be Practiced Only During Special Playtimes

The general expectation in parent training programs is that skills learned will be practiced by parents 24 hours a day, 7 days a week. Such expectations build in failure experiences, because even the best-intentioned parent is not able to always put into practice new techniques or acquired skills 24 hours a day. Parents get caught up in emotional experiences, they become overly stressed, or their lives become so hectic that they simply forget to try to apply new procedures, and then they feel guilty because they failed. CPRT is structured to promote success by requiring parents to utilize skills learned only during the designated 30-minute special playtimes. This time-limited requirement helps elicit cooperation from even the most resistive parents. As one parent put it, "I can do almost anything for just 30 minutes once a week, but all day every day is an impossibility for me."

Skills Are Generalized

Since the skills learned are not problem/correction focused, they can be generalized to situations outside the special playtimes. Even though parents are required to use the skills only during the special playtimes, parents quite readily begin to spontaneously respond to their children at other times in a manner similar to the way they have been responding during the special playtimes. This transfer of new parent behaviors outside the special playtimes occurs naturally and is an indication that the new behaviors have been incorporated into the parents' natural way of responding. Parents in CPRT training often report they even find themselves responding empathically or giving choices in their work experience encounters.

Supervision

A critical component of CPRT training is the structure and provision of supervision experiences. CPRT training is a very structured approach to learning. Nothing is left to chance. There is no guesswork about whether parents have learned the skills or are able to appropriately utilize the skills. Parents are required to video-record their special playtimes and present the video to be viewed during training sessions, or parents bring their child to the training setting and the training group observes special playtimes through a two-way mirror. When these options are not available, parents have a special playtime in the training setting and the training group sits in the room and observes.

It is essential that the filial therapist know whether parents have learned the skills. Parents' descriptions of how they have utilized the skills during special playtimes are often incomplete and perceptually biased, especially during the early stages of training. Parents simply are not aware of many of their negative communication behaviors. There is no substitute for direct observational supervision or seeing oneself on video. It should be pointed out that the primary focus of supervisory feedback, even in cases similar to the session described in the next paragraph, is always on positive behaviors parents have exhibited during the special playtimes.

The importance of supervision in the learning process and the necessity of insisting that this part of the training model not go overlooked for any parent can be seen in the following report of a filial therapist in our training program.

> Jeanie didn't bring a video-recording of her play sessions with her child until our final training session. Until then, her reports sounded like she was utilizing the skills she was learning. After viewing her video, however, it was obvious she just didn't understand the principles and didn't know how to apply the skills. There were no reflection of feelings, virtually no tracking responses, almost all verbal interchanges were in the form of questions, and she maintained control during the entire play session. I wish I had seen this video in one of the earlier training sessions so I could have worked with her on developing her skills. She would have benefited from some intensive one-on-one role-playing. If she continues having the play sessions the way she is now responding, I'm not sure there would be any point. It was really disheartening to see this kind of play session at the end of the training, especially since she really seems to want to do the best she can for her children and thinks she is doing things the correct way. I really hope she will take another filial therapy class!

The inclusion of a structured approach to supervision in the CPRT training model is unique among parent training programs.

Applicable to a Wide Range of Parents

CPRT has been demonstrated through rigorous scientific studies to be effective with a wide range of parents and problematic behaviors of children (see Chapter 26 for a review of research findings). Parents from all rungs of the socioeconomic scale have been able to learn and effectively utilize the skills taught in CPRT. CPRT has been shown to be effective with a wide range of parental populations such as incarcerated parents, immigrant parents, parents of emotionally disturbed children, adoptive and foster parents, Native American parents living on a reservation, parents residing in a domestic violence shelter, nonoffending parents of sexually abused children, parents of chronically ill children, parents of children with speech problems, single parents, parents of children with learning difficulties, and other populations. Research results have been so robustly positive with a wide range of parents and in severe training circumstances that there can be no doubt as to the efficacy of CPRT with most parent populations.

Trainer Qualifications

Filial therapists generally have a master's degree in a mental health field such as counseling, psychology, or social work; specific training and supervision in Child-Centered Play Therapy; and advanced clinical experience in play therapy, as well as group therapy. Filial therapists are expected to be able to train parents to use the Child-Centered Play Therapy skills while at the same time attending to and facilitating group dynamics. Other parent training models may only require a few hours of training for a nonprofessional person to be considered qualified to train parents.

References

Eardley, D. (1978). *An initial investigation of a didactic version of filial therapy dealing with self-concept increase and problematic behavior decrease.* Unpublished doctoral dissertation, The Pennsylvania State University, University Park.

Rohner, R. (1986). *The warmth dimension: Foundations of parental acceptance/rejection theory.* Newbury Park, CA: Sage.

Schaefer, E. (1981). Development of adaptive behavior: Conceptual models and family correlates. In M. Begab, H. Haywood, & H. Garber (Eds.), *Psychological influences on retarded development: Vol. 1. Issues and theories in development.* Baltimore, MD: University Park Press.

Swick, K., Gladstone, D., & Hayes, J. (1988). *In search of themselves: Special needs children in a preschool setting.* Unpublished report on the Special Needs Learner Project, University of South Carolina's Children's Center, College of Education, University of South Carolina, Columbia.

Swick, K., & Graves, S. (1986). Locus of control and interpersonal support as related to parenting. *Childhood Education, 62*, 26–31.

CHAPTER 4

TRAINING AND SUPERVISION OF CPRT FILIAL THERAPISTS

The field of play therapy is still a developing area in the mental health profession, and filial therapy is an even more recent, innovative and unique modality within the field of play therapy. Only a handful of university counseling, psychology, or social work programs offer graduate training in filial therapy. This chapter presents some guidelines for training in the CPRT model, essential personal characteristics of filial therapists, and important variables in facilitating a CPRT group.

Training Experiences

Training and supervised experience in Child-Centered Play Therapy are prerequisites for becoming a filial therapist. This is a logical sequence, because filial therapists must be able to teach Child-Centered Play Therapy skills to parents and supervise parent-child play sessions. In our counseling program at the University of North Texas, graduate students in filial therapy training are required to complete a 3-hour graduate credit course in Child-Centered Play

Therapy that has a supervised mini-practicum component. They are also required to complete a 3-hour graduate credit course in Group Play Therapy, which includes a practicum component, prior to enrolling in a 3-hour graduate credit course in Filial Therapy, which includes a 10-session filial therapy supervised practicum component. As a part of the supervision experience for the filial therapy course, graduate students watch videos of their filial therapy sessions and write a weekly self-critique paper focusing on topics such as what went well, areas for improvement, and what I learned about myself. A goal of this experience is that the process of self-observation and self-evaluation will continue after the graduate student is no longer in a formal educational experience. All practicing therapists should be engaged in a process of continually learning about self in the therapeutic relationship. This exploration is not likely to occur if the process has not been initiated and experienced in a training setting.

Some graduate students colead filial therapy groups in our training program and others lead filial groups by themselves. The criteria for placement in a coleading experience is based on the graduate student's knowledge, clinical experience, self-confidence, attitude, insight into self, and general professional maturity. There are distinct **advantages to coleading a filial therapy group**, as is evident in the following graduate student's self-critique[1]:

> I enjoyed the experience of working with a coleader. It made leading the group easier by **taking some of the pressure off each of us**. If I forgot a point, my co-leader was able to cover it. I felt more confident because I wasn't always "on the spot" or the focus of attention. I could pull some of my thoughts together while my coleader was running the show. An unexpected learning was **how important communication between the two of us was** between sessions, not only for processing the experience, formulating assessments of individual parent needs, and planning for the next training session, but also to keep our relationship open and honest about our reactions to each other, and what we noticed in each other during the sessions. I benefited greatly from our different styles of leadership, and I learned a great deal from the way she responded to parents and the way she picked up on cues that I had missed. **An important learning for both of us**

> **was how to read each other** so we would know when to take the lead without interrupting or monopolizing.

A caution about coleading a filial therapy group is that **one of the leaders may assume a role that is not active enough**, as is evident in a graduate student's self-critique:

> I learned that I have difficulty asserting myself. I have to continually work on this. My coleader did the majority of the speaking/leading in this first session, and I did not assert myself. As a result, I feel like the group members did not fully understand what my role was; whether I was a coleader or simply there to "aid" the group leader. This was frustrating to me because I wanted our roles to appear equal. My coleader and I have designed a more structured outline for the second session in order to prevent this from becoming the rule rather than the exception.

Regular supervisory sessions are needed to work on these and other issues inherent in coleading a filial therapy group. Differences in style of leadership can also present a problem:

> I am learning that it can be difficult to colead a group because of difference in styles. I like to let the group process "happen" and Stacey enjoys the "teaching" aspect of working with a group. We are open with each other about this issue and taking steps to reconcile these differences in the form of a compromise so we both get our needs met.

Supervised Experience

In addition to completing the introduction to play therapy, group play therapy, and filial therapy courses, graduate students are required to complete a supervised Practicum in Play Therapy in the Center for Play Therapy and an internship where they can continue clinical experiences in play therapy and filial therapy. Even though most supervisors would agree that the general purpose of supervision is to facilitate the filial therapist's personal and professional development, the personal dimension is often only minimally focused on in supervisory relationships. Too often, supervision is a cognitive process focused on instructing and educating the therapist, questioning his decisions, identifying mistakes, providing information, interpreting parents' motivation, and offering suggested ways to respond to parents. Since the filial therapist's own inner struggles and conflicts can inhibit the progress of a filial therapy group, the filial therapist should engage in a process of learning about self. Learning what skills to teach in CPRT is not nearly as important as developing an awareness of the dynamics of the process of teaching those skills and how to utilize one's self in facilitating the learning process of parents. We propose that it is more important to focus the supervision experience on the attitudes of the filial therapist rather than techniques, on feelings rather than content, on the relationship rather than specific responses, and on accepting rather than evaluating. Supervision is a critical element in training filial therapists, especially in the areas of therapist reactions, feelings, and attitudes; insight into self; pacing in presenting material; facilitation of the group process; and gaining insight into parents' emotional needs. Beginning filial therapists need assistance in understanding themselves and the underlying inner motivations and dynamics of parents.

It is the person of the therapist that is the most significant factor in determining the effectiveness of the CPRT experience. The therapist's understanding of self is more important than what the therapist knows, some intellectual knowledge, for it is the person of the therapist and how the therapist uses herself in the context of the CPRT group that parents react to most. A goal of supervision is that the therapist will develop self-understanding and self-acceptance so the therapist will be able to spontaneously incorporate the person she is into the training experience with parents. To do this, the therapist must engage in a process of learning about self.

The therapist's emotional reactions to resistive parents, the process of teaching, and the pressure of the amount of material to be taught can inhibit the therapist's natural use of self and, therefore, should be processed in the supervisory relationship. It is the dynamics of the inner person of the therapist that largely determine whether the experience with parents is therapeutic. Therefore, the supervisory relationship must be therapeutically oriented in order to deal with the dynamics of the emotional issues of the filial therapist in training.

The self-critique of a filial therapist in training illustrates the importance of supervision in dealing with some of these personal dimensions.

> I experienced a range of emotions about parents missing training sessions, including anger, disappointment, and sadness. I also ran a gamut of feelings about some parents' fear of doing something different with their children, and these feelings progressed to impatience with the parents' obvious reluctance to hold special playtimes or be observed on video. A particularly growth-promoting experience for me in this filial therapy class was the continuous exploration of my feelings and thoughts in supervision. I came to realize that these parents were no different from anyone else who was trying to break an ingrained habit, and parenting behaviors may well be some of the most difficult to alter. I came to realize that, just as we try to help parents view the world from their children's eyes, I, too, must step outside my perspective and view the parents' world from their perspective in order to be of help to them.
>
> Eventually, as I worked through my intense feelings toward the parents, I reached the core of my feelings: my anger at parents for their shortcomings went directly back to my own guilt for not having done with my own child all the things I know today. This awareness will hopefully prevent my own baggage from interfering with the process of training.

Development of this kind of insight into self is essential for the filial therapist to be able to put personal reactions aside, understand the needs of parents, and facilitate an understanding and accepting atmosphere in the CPRT group. A resistive or overtly rejecting and hostile parent can cause an inexperienced filial therapist to experience feelings of frustration and anger, as indicated in the following self-critique by a graduate student:

> I feel frustrated and irritated at parents in the group who don't contribute or volunteer information to the group. I know that it is my job to include these particular parents

> and seek feedback from them, yet I find myself feeling agitated when they are not actively contributing to the group.

Another graduate student wrote:

> Towards the end of this session, I was feeling very frustrated with a particular parent. It appeared that he was challenging me and trying to "prove me wrong." I was feeling very upset and irritated at him. Looking back on the experience, I think I was wanting him to agree with me on the specific topic. I need to be more comfortable with parents not agreeing with what I am teaching them.

CPRT training groups may stimulate a wide range of emotional reactions in inexperienced filial therapists, and therefore they will need an opportunity to process those reactions in a supervisory relationship.

Essential Personal Characteristics of Filial Therapists

The characteristics essential for an effective filial therapist are basically the same characteristics considered to be necessary for effective play therapists. The development of these characteristics is a function of the training and supervision the filial therapist receives that facilitates insight into self and an understanding of and sensitivity to the inner dynamics of children and parents. **Filial therapists need self-understanding and insight** into their own motivations, needs, blind spots, biases, personal conflicts, and areas of emotional difficulty, as well as personal strengths. Therapists should not assume they can keep their own values and needs compartmentalized and separate from their relationships with parents. Personal needs and values are a part of the person of the therapist and thus become a part of the relationship with parents. Therefore, training and supervision of filial therapists must incorporate a process of self-exploration that will promote self-understanding, thus minimizing the potential impact of the therapist's motivations and needs.

A focus of the supervision relationship should be on developing **therapist qualities that facilitate the learning environment** in the filial therapy relationship. **Warmth and caring** must be integral parts of the filial therapist's personality and readily experienced by parents as warmth, kindness, and friendliness. Warmth and caring increase parents' confidence and encourage open expressions of emotions and thoughts. The ability to warmly accept parents is predicated on the therapist's ability to understand and accept himself.

The **attitude of the therapist is the key to the learning environment** in CPRT because it is the therapist's attitude that sets the tone in the CPRT group and quickly permeates the entire training experience. Parents are impacted much more by the person of the therapist than by the knowledge of the therapist. Effective filial therapists appreciate their own uniqueness and are therefore able to accept the uniqueness of parents. The filial therapist is **intentional about creating an atmosphere** with parents that optimizes learning opportunities.

The effective filial therapist is relatively **free of threat and anxiety** and is thus **open to receiving parents as they are**, as they present themselves in the filial therapy group. The therapist is able to turn loose of his world of reality and to experience the parent's world of reality. This open-minded dimension allows the therapist to receive fully and with accuracy the meanings communicated by parents verbally and nonverbally in their interactions in the group. Many parents are fearful of rejection of the person they are or rejection of the kind of parent they are when they enter CPRT training. Experiencing **acceptance** helps them to lower their defenses and consider the possibility of incorporating new parenting skills into their relationships with their children. Acceptance means prizing the unique person of the parent and does not imply approval of all of the parent's behaviors.

Because parents are always in a process of becoming, the therapist should project a **future-mindedness** in relating to parents by not restricting them to the past through attitude or verbal responses. This means not restricting parents to ways they have previously described themselves as being, but being open to perceiving ways in which parents have changed. Therefore, the therapist is always engaged in a process of trying to catch up to where the parent is this week. This future-mindedness does not project or lead the parent into the future, but is an attitude of receptivity to the parent being in a continuous process of becoming.

The effective filial therapist acts and responds out of **personal courage** by admitting mistakes, by being vulnerable at times, and by admitting inaccuracies in personal perceptions. Personal courage is needed to take risks and to act on intuitive feelings in response to parents' sharing. Personal courage based on inner confidence may be required when a parent is angry, resistive, or defensive. Therapists who have low tolerance for these behaviors and lack self-understanding may respond inappropriately by being defensive or by rejecting the parent. Such situations call for a high degree of **patience**. The therapist is able to be patient with parents because of her willingness to accept her own imperfections and to forgive herself for not being perfect; that is, to accept her own humanness. Therefore, no need exists to have the parent be perfect. The effective filial therapist is **personally secure** and thus recognizes and accepts personal limitations without any sense of threat to her feelings of adequacy. A supportive supervising relationship is essential to help beginning filial therapists feel personally secure.

Being real means being vulnerable enough to admit, "I don't have solutions to all the problems parents describe with their children." Being real is dependent on a high degree of self-understanding and self-acceptance, which implies having insight into self: being aware of and accepting one's own feelings and reactions with insight into the accompanying motivations. A therapist who lacks self-understanding of her own motivations may inappropriately project rejection to the parents whose experiences and value systems are different. This struggle can be seen in the self-critique of a filial therapist in training:

> This was my fifth filial therapy session, and **I am still struggling with being judgmental of parents**, expecting more from them than I should. I have difficulty accepting that people are doing the best they can versus making improvements to do it "better." I have a tendency to think that people should always be working on themselves, their issues, and their relationships. This expectation of people often impedes my ability to really hear them, to be supportive and to provide helpful interventions.

Filial therapists should work through such issues in supervisory relationships.

Realness is an attitude of willingness to allow parents to experience the many parts of the person of the therapist, not just the professional self. Beginning filial therapists often experience difficulty allowing the uniqueness of their person to be seen:

> Observing myself on video reminded me of how task-oriented I can be, and how I often have a difficult time **focusing on the current moment**. I can be so worried about the future that I am not present in the present. I learned how my driven behavior affects every area of my life. I was reminded of how I desire to be seen as intelligent and professional. I have a tendency to become too distant and disconnected as the informative group leader. I will attempt to **balance the professionalism with sincerity and vulnerability**.

CPRT training can really be fun and exciting, and the therapist should be comfortable enough with herself to relax and enjoy the process. The humorous part of the therapist should be readily interjected into the training experiences with parents. A **sense of humor** helps parents to relax, puts them at ease, and helps them to share personal dimensions of their lives. Well-placed **humor can make learning fun** for parents and can be used to help get points across to parents that might be difficult for them to accept, as in the following filial therapy interaction.

Pat: (a single mom) Things are really hectic at my house in the mornings. I'm trying to get to my university classes on time, and Josh is in the front room in his pajamas watching TV. I take his breakfast in to him and feed him while he's watching TV.

Dr. L.: (interrupts) Excuse me, Pat. How old is Josh? (This fact was already know by Dr. L.)

Pat: He's 5, and that's not all. After I feed him, I dress him, and I'm still late getting to my classes.

Dr. L.: (looking at his notes) Pat, I don't remember you telling us Josh has both arms broken.

Pat: They're not.

Dr. L.: Are his legs broken?

Pat: No.

Dr. L.: Is he in a full body cast? (group laughs)

Pat: Not yet! (group laughs) (silence as Pat thinks) OK, I get the message. He's old enough to feed himself and dress himself. I've known I should do that, but just haven't done it. I just need to give him the responsibility for doing so. OK! Tomorrow I will do it!

Dr. L.: So you haven't done what you knew was the best thing to do, but I hear your commitment now. Next week, I'll check on you to find out how it went.

As in play therapy, the effectiveness of the filial therapist is largely dependent on the relationship the therapist creates with parents in the training setting and the extent to which the therapist is able to facilitate the creation of a therapeutic relationship between parents and their children in specially structured play sessions. It is the parent-child relationship that is created in the play sessions that makes the experience unique, not the toys or the setting, for most parents already play with their children.

Learning How to Lead a CPRT Group

Part of graduate students' supervision experience in our program is the requirement that they engage in a process of self-critique and self-analysis related to their experiences in leading CPRT training groups. The following excerpts, selected from lengthy self-critiques because they represent diverse reactions, provide insight into beginning filial therapists' experiences, some points of learning about themselves, and their discovery of important variables in facilitating a CPRT group that merit attention by most filial therapists. A striking dimension in these critiques is the depth of insight into self these inexperienced filial therapists developed.

Mike: If I can touch parents where their needs are, I have done well. Filial therapy is about enriching the relationship between parent and child to enhance the healthy growth of the child. I have found that while doing that, the parent's self-esteem goes up, their effectiveness goes up, and, therefore, their level of health and well-being also increases. I really enjoy filial therapy.

I have also learned that **when I move too quickly through the material, the parents do not learn** what I think they learn. I must take the time to get feedback from the parents and not move so rapidly next time. If what I am teaching them sparks new thinking, they will be involved in their own thought process. If I do not wait for them to do all of their processing, they will draw inaccurate conclusions from the other snatches that they catch on the way. They will get lost while I jump too quickly to another subject.

Valerie: I need to **improve my ability to respond to parents' nonverbal communications, reflect their feelings more often, and model the skills I am teaching them to use**. I often felt clueless when the opportunities to respond arose. **My need to be liked and looked on as an authority interferes** with my willingness to observe and respond to nonverbal cues. I feel silly admitting that I know the material, believe in it, and use it myself, but can't even see how to model these behaviors for parents! This fear of not being liked by the parents, coupled with my fear of not having answers to parents' questions, places undue stress on me to perform rather than lead and guide. Sometimes on the videos of my filial group, I sounded "preachy." I believe this is the result of my need to be an expert.

Margaret: I need to **improve my skill in redirecting parents and keeping them on track** when they are relating information. Occasionally, we ran out of time because we had spent too much time allowing parents to share too many details about problems at home. On numerous occasions, I recognized after the fact that I should have gently interrupted a parent, summarized the topic, and generalized the point to other parents. Secondly, I need to **utilize more insightful questions when processing information from parents**. Instead of merely accepting a report about a play session or a homework assignment, I need to challenge parents more by asking what they learned from these experiences, what they recognized about their child that they hadn't known before, what they learned about themselves, etc.

Mary: There is a fine line between being a therapist and a teacher. The therapist in me wanted to be understanding and empathetic when a parent missed a training session or did not have a playtime one week. However, the teacher in me was disappointed when either situation occurred. I had one parent who did not have her playtime two weeks in a row. I should have been **firmer with her when she reported that she did not have a play session** those weeks. I did not want the parent to get mad and not come back to class, so I was hesitant in how to handle this situation. (Supervisor comment: Ask the parent, "Can I get a commitment from you that you will have a session this week?")

Kay: I recognized that I was not as comfortable in the teaching role as I am in a counselor role. Partially, this is due to my lack of experience in this role and with this material, but I felt that I was not as genuine while teaching as I normally am. **It was obvious on my videos when I felt uncomfortable** by watching my body language and listening to my tone of voice. I spoke faster, looked down at my notes a lot, used excessive hand gestures, and my tone of voice was higher pitched than usual while teaching the filial group. I will need to continue to be aware of this and, hopefully, with more experience I will become more comfortable. I also learned that **when I lack confidence in myself, my level of genuineness tends to decrease and is evident through my nonverbal cues**.

Karen: I feel positive about the improvement that I have made in my ability to **keep the parents on track**. During the early training sessions, I had to focus on keeping the parents on task during role-playing sessions, and on **returning responsibility to answer questions back to the parents** instead of providing them with the answers. As the training sessions progressed, I improved in using nonverbal cues, such as handing out papers, as a means of indicating that we were ready to begin the next topic. I also improved in being able to use what the parents said to focus the conversation back on the topic at hand and then continue with the next topic for discussion. In addition, I am improving at being more direct, at being **able to redirect off-task conversations in an inconspicuous manner, and at providing more structure in guiding the length of conversations**.

Matt: My most significant learning from leading a filial therapy group is: **Never underestimate the power of filial therapy**, even three or four sessions. I met with Greta and watched a video of her play session with her daughter. She did an exceptional job setting limits in the play session. She reported that she has been giving choices outside the playtimes, and they are working. Her daughter is now going to sleep an hour earlier and sleeping much better through the night. Greta is also using the limit setting and choices successfully at work. She reported feeling more in control of herself with her daughter and stated that her daughter feels more secure. During the supervision time, Greta brought up some personal issues, and I asked if she would consider individual counseling to help her with these issues. She said that she would and planned to call the counseling center.

Randy: In this first filial therapy session, one area for improvement that I noted is my overuse of verbalization. Filial therapy has a teaching aspect, and in that vein, I can really "get into it." I have a hard time not talking. **I need to learn to be quiet sometimes**. I think this happens because I do enjoy teaching and being in charge. I also can be prone to having some lack of faith in myself, which means I might tend to overdo the talking in an effort to ensure I am making my point.

Janet: Looking back on the first session, I recognize several areas for improvement. If I could go back and redo the session, I would definitely **talk more slowly**. Mallorie and I raced through the material, as if we were trying to "cram in" as much information as possible. Sometimes I talked so fast that I could not understand myself! The quizzical looks on the parents' faces should have been my clue to slow down. Every once in a while, I paused momentarily and asked "Any questions?" Of course, none of the parents replied. They were probably shell-shocked! Instead of asking for questions, I should have said, "Tell me what you understand." This statement focuses on what they know, rather than pointing out what they do not understand. I need to **pay more attention to group dynamics**. I felt as if I was teaching a class rather than facilitating a group. I know I missed several opportunities to get in touch with the parents. I especially want to **look for reactions of group members while one of the parents is speaking**. Often, a parent in the group may have experienced the same problem and could identify with the parent that is sharing. Focusing on these dynamics would strengthen the cohesiveness of the group.

Shelly: One area, which needed improvement in this third session, was more involvement from the parents. I think Janet and I felt so rushed that **we did not stop and involve the parents enough**. We needed to do more role-playing. During the next session, we are going to focus on role-playing and helping the parents to get involved. We also need to do a better job of **relating to Tasha, who appears not to believe a lot of what we say. We need to help her to become more directly involved and interactive with the other parents**. I think I am scared that she will ask me a question, and I will not know the answer! This is compounded by my reaction that a question means the parent has doubts.

I need to let the parents develop their own answers at times.

Gail: I was uptight about presenting information to my filial therapy group due to my perfectionism. I always feel that I have to do it right even though I know intellectually that there is no specific right way. **I did tend to get into a lecture mode in this first session, instead of keeping the interaction more casual.** I do have a need to be in control, to make sure something is being accomplished.

I became more relaxed in the second session after I began to focus more on the material and information and less on me, and this resulted in a better flow. In the fourth session, I became **aware of just how important role-playing is helping these new ways of responding to become second nature** to these parents.

Justin: I have learned that **parents change when they are ready** and often in ways which I least expect, but they do change. In almost every case, I learned the lesson of **trusting the process**. I also learned that by sharing my experiences with other counselors in supervision, we can maintain enthusiasm and hope, even when we are experiencing difficulties.

I have learned in leading my filial group that I have a great opportunity to be creative and to **put my own unique spin on the process**. It reminds me of my brother, a jazz musician. He took tons of theory classes, but when it came to improvisation, he said he had to put all the theories and techniques and exercises on the shelf, and **play from his heart**. The same holds true for me as I attempt to integrate what I have learned.

Note

1 Emphasis (in extracts) has been added to the student critiques to highlight critical insights.

CHAPTER 5

CRITICAL COMPONENTS IN FACILITATING THE PROCESS OF CPRT

The CPRT process is characterized by **two key components: a didactic component and a group process component in the context of a safe, reassuring, supportive, nonthreatening environment** that encourages parents to explore feelings, attitudes, and perceptions about themselves, their children, and parenting. This safe, accepting environment also facilitates risk taking that leads to behavioral change. In her ethnographic study of the process of the CPRT 10-session filial therapy model as facilitated by Dr. Landreth, Lahti (1992) concluded that the careful, skilled balancing of the didactic element of CPRT filial therapy with a group process/therapy element is a unique aspect of CPRT filial therapy's nature and may be the primary key to the manner in which CPRT filial therapy effectively facilitates change.

Group Process Component

The supportive format in a CPRT group often resembles group therapy as the leader responds empathically to parents' issues and emotional reactions related to their family or their role as parents. Likening the emotional exploring and supportive component of

CPRT to group therapy does not imply that the objective is to provide group therapy, only that some aspects of the group interaction and process take on the nature of group therapy for short periods of time as parents explore their feelings about themselves, their children, and their families. When Mary complains that she can never do enough for her daughter, the leader responds, "*You're feeling frustrated and helpless, sometimes.*" The transition from this empathic group therapy type element of exploring an emotional issue to the didactic element can be accomplished by limiting the group therapy exploration to a few minutes of interaction, making an empathic reflection that summarizes the parent's feeling, and then making a teaching point that is related to the content of the parent's sharing:

> Mary, that was a very frustrating experience for you. Group, just as you need someone to understand your frustration, when your child is frustrated, your child needs to know you understand, and understanding is communicated by reflecting your child's feeling. For example, "*That is really frustrating to you when the pieces won't stick together.*" Let's work on reflecting feelings now.

The struggle to maintain an effective balance between the didactic and process dimensions of CPRT was expressed by a filial therapist in training:

> The area I need to make the most improvement in is related to balancing teaching with counseling. I am more comfortable teaching the information related to filial therapy and less comfortable addressing the emotional needs of parents as they arise in the group. Although I recognize these needs, I struggle with how I should address them, how often and how in-depth I should go. I believe I am currently missing many opportunities to quickly address emotional needs of parents which would allow them to better focus, and I am missing many opportunities to role-model how reflecting feelings and communicating understanding can be impactful, the very skills I am training them to use with their children.

The implementation of this kind of insight will make CPRT groups more dynamic and effective.

In CPRT training, it is common that the discussion of relationship skills elicits in parents current and/or long-standing intense feelings and reactions about their children. Parents need time to process these feelings in order to clear their cognitive and emotional systems before they can incorporate and integrate the new concepts, principles, and skills being taught. **Processing parents' reactions and feelings about their children promotes the beginning of change in parents' perceptions about their children.** The filial therapist must maintain a delicate balance between the didactic and process dimensions without being rigid in covering the scheduled training material or allowing the group to become bogged down in the group therapy dimensions of the process. A filial therapist in our training program described the process as:

> The crunch of trying to get in all of the training agenda in each training session nagged at me in every session, and I sometimes felt myself become annoyed when parents would go into a drawn-out story about their children. About halfway through the 10 training sessions, I learned how to loosen my grip on the agenda of the sessions in order to meet more of the personal, emotional needs of the parents. As the weeks went on, I became more relaxed about this, realizing that parents occasionally need to vent their feelings in order to clear their systems so they can concentrate and really learn the content of the training. I also became much better at redirecting a parent when it was time to move on. I have been taught my whole life not to interrupt people, so this task took some effort.

It is imperative that the leader intersperse the teaching component of CPRT with building **group cohesiveness**, especially in the first two or three training sessions. This is accomplished when the therapist generalizes parent disclosures to help parents identify with each other by asking questions such as "*Does this sound familiar to anyone else?*" or "*Anyone else ever yell at your child?*" and "*What was that like for you?*" when a parent responds affirmatively. When parents nod their heads understandingly as a parent describes a problem, the leader can comment, "*So the rest of you know what that is like.*" This **linking of parents** helps breaks down barriers of isolation and the feeling "I'm the only one who feels this way" or "I'm the only one who ever yells at her child."

If a parent describes a point of difficulty in a play session, the leader can ask, "*Group, what Rule of Thumb applies here?*" The leader can also encourage group interaction by inviting parents to respond to each other's questions: "*Linda, how would you suggest Erika respond when her son wants to paint her glasses?*" This question not only facilitates interaction but also decreases parents' dependence on the leader for solutions by inviting parents to contribute their ideas. If a parent seems to be thoughtful about something, the leader can invite sharing: "*Angela, what are you thinking?*" The guiding principle for the leader is careful adherence to the **Rule of Thumb: The leader is a facilitator of interaction, not just a trainer**. An objective is that as the training progresses, the interaction among the parents will increase, and they will be more actively supportive of and offer suggestions to each other.

The development of group interaction and group cohesiveness is described in the following filial therapist's report:

> The family that has struggled with the father's severe medical problems has seen a sharp increase in angry outbursts from their 3-year-old daughter, Melissa. As the group discussed ways to facilitate healthy expression of feelings, Melissa's mother had a sudden flash of insight and burst out, "We're not validating her anger!" Melissa's parents stopped trying to distract her and started reflecting her feelings and had extremely positive results. Another very positive experience in the filial therapy group has been the parents' dedication to the group and support of each other. The father with health problems became wheelchair-bound for about 2 weeks during the training, and yet he continued to come to the group and even did his play sessions from his wheelchair. This same couple brought a book to help a child adjust to the birth of a new baby and gave it to the parents who are expecting. Another group member was obviously struggling with the filial skills, and when he showed his video, the other group members worked very hard to find and reflect his strengths. It was really wonderful to see these parents trust us as leaders and trust each other enough to

allow themselves to be very vulnerable in the process of learning new ways to relate to their children. These parents felt safe enough to struggle openly with self-doubt and feelings of inadequacy in the parent role and were genuinely supportive of each other in these struggles.

The group process components that are facilitative to the process of CPRT are highlighted in the following transcriptions of dialogues between Dr. Landreth and parents who participated in one of his 10-session CPRT training groups. The group process components illustrated by selected transcriptions are

- normalizing and generalizing individual parental concerns and fears to the group;
- encouraging a parent to explore thoughts and feelings more fully; and
- building group cohesion to encourage or teach members.

Normalizing and Generalizing Individual Parental Concerns and Fears to the Group

Scenario 1: One parent may disclose information to the group about her child or herself that may feel shameful or embarrassing. Hearing similar happenings or reactions from other parents normalizes the disclosure and creates a safe environment for all parents, encouraging them to reveal their own similar experiences so the disclosing parent realizes she is not alone in her feelings or experience.

Debbie: I think my daughter is of average intelligence, and strong willed. I am rejecting her as a person because I am having so many problems with her.

Dr. L.: So she is demanding and bossy. How do you react to her when she is bossy?

Debbie: Honestly? Extremely loud.

Dr. L.: I gather from the way you say that that you get really angry sometimes. Any of the rest of you get angry with your children?

Kim: Yes, absolutely.

Scenario 2: Sometimes generalizing to the group opens up an opportunity for another parent to discuss more fully her own concerns associated with those revealed by the first parent.

Sonya: His dad has always been the one who disciplines him. There have been problems at school, but since his dad moved out of the house, he has gotten better at school. I am just losing patience.

Dr. L.: Anyone else lose your patience when reacting to you children?

Nita: Yes, I do.

Dr. L.: What is that like for you?

Nita: I get angry and say things that I wish I had not said.

Encouraging a Parent to Explore Thoughts and Feelings More Fully

Scenario 1: When a parent has made an emotionally laden comment, the parent is encouraged to talk more, so that the parent may put words to the thoughts and feelings that often huddle beneath the surface of a first response.

Dr. L.: Let's see what the video of your play session looks like, Laura.

Laura: The play sessions are more about just allowing me to appreciate my son more than anything else.

Dr. L.: Laura, add to that.

Laura: We were having a really hard time, and I didn't like a lot of his behavior. Being a single parent, I feel so much that I'm always the one who has to discipline him, and that I forget to just enjoy and play with my children. So the play sessions have allowed me to do that, with joy.

Scenario 2: Encouraging a parent to elaborate allows the parent to describe specific events or situations that are troublesome, which in turn allows the therapist to teach the group about filial therapy skills that will benefit the entire group.

Dr. L.: Well, how were your playtimes this week?

Kathy: Ours started a little bit late Thursday night because we went out to eat, but we had the session right after we ate.

Dr. L.: You did have it.

Kathy: Yes, we had a pretty good one.

Dr. L.: Tell us some specifics. What happened in the playtime?

Kathy: He wanted to play with some different games this time. He really didn't ask me to do anything with him. So I just sat there and watched him. And sometimes when I told him that I saw what he was doing, he'd say, "Mom, I know that already. I know what I'm doing already."

Dr. L.: Let's work on that. Say to him, "Well, I'm just really interested in what you're doing, and I want to let you know that I see what you're doing. I don't know any other way to say it."

Emily: Very good, because I had the same problem with my child. She would tell me she didn't want me to tell her what she was doing. She got really agitated with me for doing it.

Dr. L.: It may also be that your children feel that you're tracking them a little too closely.

Building Group Cohesion to Encourage or Teach Members

Scenario 1: Asking parents to explain skills or teaching points to parents who were absent not only builds group cohesion, but also secures parents' commitment to the process and abets accountability. Knowing that they may be called on to describe a skill or explain a rationale to the group increases parents' attention and understanding.

Dr. L.: Well, we need to do some review of last week's session. Last week we worked on limit setting. What I'd like to do, Sonya and Kim, is let you all do a little bit of review about limit setting for the others who weren't here.

Sonya: Oh yes, I remember.

Dr. L.: If you would tell everyone what you remember about limit setting, that would help them learn it.

Sonya: How about telling them about ACT?

Dr. L.: OK.

Sonya: Dr. Landreth gave us an acronym, ACT. "A" means acknowledge the feeling or the want of the child, such as, "I know you want to stay up later," or "I know you want to hit me or your sister," or "I know you feel angry." Then "C" is for communicate the limit, such as "It's time to go to bed," or "It's bedtime," or "It's not OK to hit me," whatever you need to say to communicate the limit. "T" is for targeting the choices. All together, you would say something like, "I know you feel angry, but it's not OK to hit me. You may hit your stuffed animals." Then Dr. Landreth gave us an assignment to write down two times when we used ACT setting limits.

Scenario 2: Rather than teach and provide all the answers in the group, the leader allows parents to apply their newly learned skills and abilities and become a part of the solution in which all group members learn.

Dr. L.: Your son is too subtle. If he picked up a hammer, you'd know he was going to hit the mirror, but he does a lot of things that are on the borderline, doesn't he?

Nita: Yes, a lot, and it's hard to know whether or not to set a limit.

Dr. L.: So what would you all like to suggest? Laura, what would you suggest?

Scenario 3: Use group management skills to involve all parents, and encourage parents to direct comments to each other to obtain the most power from parents' observations.

Dr. L.: My, such patience, Laura. Not once in your playtime did I hear you say, "Now hurry up. You've been washing your hands there a long time now. Now hurry up." Group, I want you all to give Laura some feedback. What did you see and what did you hear?

Debbie: (looking at Dr. L.) She stayed right with him.

Dr. L.: You all tell Laura. Don't tell me, tell Laura.

Nita: I agree. You didn't overtrack.

Sonya: You didn't overtrack. You stayed right there. You look relaxed, real comfortable, real calm. You look like you've done this for years.

Kathy: I liked your facial expressions.

Kim: You varied your responses. He knew you were interested.

Teaching Components

Presenting the information to be learned in **simple one-item teaching points** is the key to parents learning and assimilating new information. Giving parents too much information in one training session or presenting complex information is overwhelming to parents. One parent noted, "There was a lot of information, but it wasn't overwhelming because it was presented one step at a time."

An essential strategy to insure parents' success in learning and applying the CPRT skills is adherence to the **3 Ds: Describe, Demonstrate, and Do**. We first *describe* the skill, then *demonstrate* the skill through video and live example, followed by having parents *do* in partner role-plays what they saw in the demonstration. If parents do not feel they can quickly implement a new skill, they are not very likely to attempt to use the new skill.

Simple homework assignments and concise informational handouts are provided to reinforce teaching points made in the training sessions. A parent commented:

> I'm amazed at how simple the homework is. It makes me aware of how I respond to my child. The homework

> makes a real difference in the effectiveness of this class. Sometimes it takes a direct assignment to make me stop the busy work and learn to relate to my child.

The simplicity of the homework and presenting this new approach to parenting in small incremental steps reduces parents' anxiety about trying something new and motivates them to attempt the assignments.

An overriding objective in CPRT is to **empower parents**. This is accomplished by creating a safe, supportive, nonthreatening atmosphere in the group and by being understanding of parents' difficulties, accepting of their weaknesses and mistakes, encouraging of their efforts, supportive of their struggles to try new behaviors, and actively communicating a belief in their capability. This last dimension is perhaps the most crucial. **Rule of Thumb: It is difficult to believe in yourself if no one believes in you.** This attitude of belief in the parent frees the parent to risk being imperfect and reduces parents' dependence on the leader. Focusing on parents' positive behaviors, successes, and effectiveness and accentuating parents' progress inspires confidence, reduces defensiveness, and engenders the courage to change. **Active affirmation** of parents' efforts is considered to be a critical key to the effectiveness of CPRT.

Employing a variety of teaching tools such as **stories, analogies, and metaphors to emphasize teaching points** helps to maintain a high level of parent interest and facilitates the learning process. Parents may have difficulty recalling a teaching point in isolation, but when the point is attached to a short, interest-catching story, **parents will remember the story and then the teaching point**. Such stories are most effective when they are inserted during parents' disclosures to clarify or support parents' efforts or to teach a new principle. This seems to make the stories personally meaningful.

Catchy "Rules of Thumb" also help make teaching points easier for parents to remember. When teaching major principles, the rule of the day is **repetition, repetition, repetition**. For example, the four therapeutic messages "I am here," "I hear you," "I understand," and "I care" are reviewed at a pertinent point in each training session.

Modeling by the therapist is a key component of the teaching process. The **therapist's responses to parents should**

consistently model basic Child-Centered Play Therapy principles and skills, thus enabling parents to personally experience the impact of skills they are being asked to use with their children. Modeling allows parents to learn these principles and skills by experiencing. This learning can be emphasized by the therapist first reflecting a parent's feelings and then asking the group, "*What did I just do*?" The therapist may have to identify for the group what he did and then elicit help from the parent whose feelings he reflected to explain the impact of the reflection. One parent's reaction at the end of the first CPRT training session was, "I've taken lots of parenting classes, but I already see a difference in filial training. I will experience it!"

The therapist can use **self-disclosure** about his efforts and mistakes as a parent to illustrate teaching points and to model permission to make mistakes. Hopefully, the therapist will also be secure enough to point out the mistakes he makes in videos or live demonstration play sessions. Such disclosures create a more relaxed atmosphere in the group and seem to remove parents' self-imposed pressure to be perfect.

Modeling is also utilized by **showing videos of the therapist's play sessions** or by the therapist conducting a live play session to demonstrate the kind of responses hoped for by parents in their play sessions. When viewing a video, the video should be stopped frequently to point out skills and specific responses that have been emphasized in the training sessions. A parent commented on the benefits of viewing videos of the therapist's play sessions:

> Watching Dr. Landreth's videos was an added dimension that we've never gotten in other parenting classes. Seeing how he responded made learning the skills come alive. You can't get that from a book or from someone just telling you how to do it.

When **viewing the video of a parent's play session**, the video should be stopped frequently to validate and affirm the parent's efforts. **The focus is on what the parents are doing correctly** rather than focusing on mistakes. The therapist's focus on providing positive feedback models for parents how they are to give feedback to each other. The therapist can help parents to begin thinking about the meaning of their children's play by making comments such as "*He did a lot of nurturing and taking care of you during the medical kit play.*" It is also helpful to call attention to patterns or themes in the play sessions and to infer children's needs and motives based on their play behavior. This provides insight and encourages parents to move to a higher skill level. After watching herself in a play session with her child, a mother said, "That was a real growth experience for me. I wasn't aware of my behaviors until I saw myself in the video."

The teaching components that are facilitative to the process of CPRT are highlighted in the following transcriptions of dialogues between Dr. Landreth and parents who participated in one of his 10-session CPRT training groups. The teaching components illustrated by selected transcriptions are

- Modeling acceptance, reflective listening, and focused attention
- Fallibility of therapist (as expert)
- Encouraging parental strengths
- Utilizing specific instruction
- Providing concrete examples
- Imparting expert knowledge
- Using analogies to increase parent awareness
- Encouraging role-play and practice of skills
- Making suggestions for improvement
- Identifying what is learned from events in special playtimes
- Identifying shifts or changes in behavior (in child or in parent)
- Facilitating insight and
- Clarifying

Modeling Acceptance, Reflective Listening, and Focused Attention

Acceptance

Scenario 1: A critical aspect of CPRT is the parent's acceptance of the child, practiced through many different skills in special playtimes. The therapist models acceptance in sessions with parents, so that parents may experience what that type of acceptance feels like; parents can, in turn, practice acceptance of their children in the playtimes.

Laura: My special playtime is supposed to be on Tuesday afternoon, but Tuesday was a really hectic day, and I forgot the playtime. Then Thursday I finally remembered and had the playtime just before his bedtime. I can remember to go to my university class, but I forget my son.

Dr. L.: Your life gets really hectic sometimes, and you feel guilty about forgetting your special playtime, but the important thing is that you did have it. **The Rule of Thumb that applies here is the most important thing may not be what you do, but what you do after what you have done.** You love your son and made a special time for him. That's an important message.

Scenario 2: The therapist should take every opportunity to acknowledge and label parents' acceptance of their children's feelings during training sessions with parents.

Emily: I reflected what he was doing. I didn't say, "You're stabbing them in their private areas." I just simply stated, "Oh, you're stabbing the baby, and now you're stabbing the mom."

Dr. L.: That was enough.

Emily: And then he started slashing furniture with the rubber knife. He was just a little animal. At that point, I said, "You look really angry." That's when he threw the knife down and crawled up in my arms, and that was it.

Dr. L.: The important thing is that your child got to express his feelings, and he felt understood. His feelings were accepted, not necessarily the act, but the feelings were accepted.

Reflective Listening

Scenario 1: The therapist models reflective listening skills, in addition to teaching parents these skills, so that parents experience being heard and practice the same reflective listening with their children.

Sonya: I have two children, both are girls. I am a single parent, divorce pending, and it is harder than I thought it would be. Right now, I think my older daughter is trying to tell me something.

Dr. L.: And you are not quite sure what it is.

Sonya: Sometimes she shows me with her anger that she is scared. Since my husband and I separated, there is no consistency with visitation. She loves her daddy, and he is just not there; he never was. I try to open up the arena to talk about stuff, but I sense that she feels it is not OK to talk. She has started doing some things that I am confused about.

Dr. L.: I hear two things: that you are trying to be all things to her and that is not quite possible. The other thing is you want so much to understand what your daughter is saying to you, but she can't sit down and say it. That's one of the things that I am going to work on: to help you become a keen observer of your child's play and to learn as much as you possibly can from your child's play.

Scenario 2: Parents' descriptions of their interactions with their children provide occasions for the therapist to model reflecting feelings.

Kathy: This playtime was NOT an enjoyable experience for me at all. He was violent the whole time. He was attacking me.

Dr. L.: He was trying to hurt you, and the whole experience wasn't very satisfying for you.

Kathy: Yeah. He hit me with the plastic reflex hammer while he was playing doctor, and I said, "You may play with the hammer, but you can't hurt me."

Dr. L.: So you were able to set a limit.

Kathy: Yeah, but I was exhausted. By the time the playtime was over, I was really glad to stop.

Dr. L.: So you were able to set a limit, but it sounds like the playtime was an emotionally draining experience for you.

Kathy: Yes. We come from an abusive situation, and when I see him act like that, I can see his father. I just get kinda petrified.

Dr. L.: You were really frightened and wanted out of there.

Focused Attention

Scenario 1: CPRT training emphasizes teaching parents to focus attention on their children. The therapist points out occasions when parents give their undivided attention to their children and makes sure parents recognize the positive impact of this kind of attention.

Dr. L.: This segment of your video is an example of when your facial expression says a lot more than any words can ever say. You reflect his feelings with your face. Watch your face. No words. Everything about your face says, "I'm here with you, I hear you. I understand. I care." I hear your message in your face. You're excited about that. It's fun for you. You say no words, and yet you conveyed everything you needed to convey to him.

Laura: I don't think he ever looked at me.

Sonya: I think so. Yes, he's checking.

Dr. L.: Watch this. (plays video) He did see you—right there. (stops video) Children don't miss a thing. This is a delightful scene right here, clearly enjoyed by both of you.

Scenario 2: During a training session, the therapist models focused attention, often recognizing a parent's nonverbal behavior and asking the parent to comment so that other parents have the opportunity to experience the benefits of focused attention.

Debbie: That's the thing that I'm still having trouble with—being in the middle of the crisis, and being able to step back out of the crisis.

Dr. L.: And be objective.

Debbie: And be objective from it, and know that it's OK, too. That I don't have to react, that I can step back and get in control of my own emotions, and then decide what to do.

Dr. L.: Laura, you were reacting to that, when Debbie said she can step back.

Laura: When my son does these things, the first thing I do now is just tell myself that he is not really doing this just to get me. I used to feel, "You are doing this on purpose to get me." But when I take myself out of it, then I handle the whole situation a lot better, and I'm a lot happier, and he's a lot happier.

Fallibility of Therapist (As Expert)

Scenario 1: If parents believe their filial therapist is an infallible expert in child behavior, they may feel intimidated and inadequate, leading to possible reluctance to participate or unwillingness to demonstrate newly learned skills and techniques. The therapist can weave personal commentary on his own mistakes in parenting into his groups, as well as oversights he has made while in playtimes with children. These disclosures help parents realize there is no standard of perfection, and no one is capable of doing everything right at all times with children.

Dr. L.: Let's check some more of this video of my session with this little girl. (Video is played.) Do you realize what I just missed?

Sonya: That she was happy.

Dr. L.: Yes. You would think that after doing this for 25 years that I would have caught that. But I'm just like you all are. I'm not perfect either. I slip up lots of times, Sonya. I still don't know why I didn't respond to her feeling. It's so obvious she's delighted with that. I think I got too caught up in what she was doing with her hands, just tracked that, and I missed her feeling. So if I miss her feeling after all these years of experience, surely it must be OK if you miss your child's feelings now and then.

Debbie: Is it OK if we follow up after missing a feeling?

Dr. L.: Yes, I get a chance to come back to it. (Video is played.) Just a little slow, but I finally got around to saying, "That surprised you."

Scenario 2: By relating his parenting mistakes with his own children or in play sessions, the therapist reduces parents' fears that he will judge them as a parenting expert incapable of erring.

Dr. L.: When my oldest daughter was three years of age, we were visiting in my parents' home in another state. It was 9:30 at night. Out of the kitchen came my 3-year-old daughter. By the way, I just told you something really important about me. It's 9:30 at night, and my 3-year-old daughter . . .

Debbie: Is still awake.

Dr. L.: Yes, she is still awake. So what does that tell you, Debbie? I'm just like the rest of you. I didn't always put her to bed at the time she should have been in bed. I'm like the rest of you. I don't always do what I should all the time as a parent.

Encouraging Parental Strengths

Scenario 1: Teaching parents new and different skills is a basic part of CPRT. The therapist can employ modeling as one method of demonstrating to parents the impact of allowing their children the freedom to decide in play sessions.

Dr. L.: These toys on the list can only be played with for 30 minutes once a week.

Emily: What if my son already has a bottle that he uses once or twice a week; I'll open the playroom door and it's in his mouth, and he's saying, "goo-goo-ga-ga," because he was never nurtured as an infant, and so he still wants to play that way. Do I now take that bottle he's had for the last year in our home away, and tell him this is only for this special playtime? How do I handle that?

Dr. L.: You can decide that. It can be OK either way.

Scenario 2: Parents can learn that the therapist will not provide all the answers for them. Parents learn to trust their children's abilities.

Dr. L.: Nita, how was your session?

Nita: It was great.

Dr. L.: What made it great?

Nita: He played with the toys he never even picked up before. He had never even opened the Tinkertoys box. He opened the box.

Dr. L.: He finally opened the Tinkertoys.

Nita: I was going to ask you something. If he names things wrong during the special playtime, I can't tell him he's wrong, right? You know, parents are supposed to label things correctly.

Dr. L.: What do you think my answer is?

Nita: Your answer would be "No." But in the play session, I thought, "I can't let him get away with thinking that's what that is." But I didn't say anything. It's like he was waiting for me to tell him that he was wrong. And I just sat there.

Dr. L.: So you passed the test.

Scenario 3: The therapist recognizes parents' successes in giving their children the lead.

Kim: He wanted me to tell him if it was the right color when he did the color drawing. He had two different colors of sun. He knew the right answer. He was waiting for me to tell him, to see if I'm listening, I guess. I didn't tell him.

Dr. L.: So you let him be in charge.

Utilizing Specific Instruction

Scenario 1: Highly didactic methods can be used to teach parents specific information, such as how to build their children's' self-esteem.

Dr. L.: I want to show you two minutes of a video of a 4½-year-old child with me in the playroom. I want you to focus on how many times you hear me make a self-esteem-building response. This will just be a review of what we've talked about many times before. A self-esteem-building response is when you give your child credit for knowing or doing something, such as "You stacked those just as high as you wanted." Count how many times you hear a self-esteem-building response. (Video is played.)

Dr. L.: How many did you hear?

Kim: I got eight.

Sonya: I got 12.

Scenario 2: Homework assignments tasking parents with practicing very specific exercises are given to hone parents' skills.

Dr. L.: I'd like you to specifically work on building up your child's self-esteem in the 30-minute session this week. That will be one of your assignments: to give your child credit. "*You figured out how to make that work,*" or "*You can count all the way to three!*" Give your child credit for all the little things they do in the 30-minute play session.

Providing Concrete Examples

Scenario 1: The therapist utilizes his own experience in play sessions to teach parents.

Dr. L.: At this point in the video, the child and I just walked into the room. I'm going over to be closer to the child, so he'll know I'm interested. Now, let's talk about what you saw me do.

Sonya: You gave him space when he came into the room, which gave him his freedom, or space.

Dr. L.: I let the child move away and settle in, and then I went over to the sandbox. What else did you see me do?

Sonya: You let him pick what he wanted to do.

Dr. L.: Yes, I let him choose. He's in the lead. This is his time to play with any of the toys that he chooses to play with.

Scenario 2: Setting therapeutic limits is a crucial aspect of CPRT, and one in which most parents have no training and limited skills. Therefore, the therapist uses didactic methods and provides specific examples to help parents master the new language.

Dr. L.: I'm going to ask you to pick a special place that these playtimes will occur. If the kitchen is not a private place, and there are other people in the house, and you can't have a private time, then you may need to choose a place like your bedroom. If there is a carpet, then you'll have a big beach-type towel, or a big piece of cardboard, and when the child pulls the playdough out, you say, "The playdough is for playing on the towel," a new way to set a limit.

Scenario 3: Parents often need help in making an appropriate response that is specific.

Dr. L.: (Group has been watching a video of a parent's playtime.) He's asking you to do something that you really don't want to do.

Kathy: That's right.

Dr. L.: He's asking you to use a word that you don't want to use. So, what would you like to say to him?

Kathy: "I don't want to say that."

Dr. L.: Sounds great to me.

Kathy: OK, but I thought I was supposed to do what he wants me to do through this whole playtime.

Dr. L.: There are limits.

Emily: Well, if he wants to mark on the wall, you're not going to let him mark on the wall.

Kathy: No, that's true, I'm not.

Dr. L.: There are limits. This is not a completely free or completely permissive relationship.

Imparting Expert Knowledge

Scenario 1: The therapist, while acknowledging lack of perfection, is nonetheless a mental health professional trained in knowledge of children's behavior. There are opportunities during group sessions for the therapist to impart knowledge to parents.

Dr. L.: When you say, "You're just so angry at me because you don't want to go to bed," your goal at that moment is that tomorrow night or the next week your child will say "I'm angry" instead of saying "I hate you." When your child says, "I hate you," my suggestion is that you not take it personally, because you're not a "hateable" person. I suggest that you wonder, "What is my child trying to say to me?" and then respond.

Scenario 2: The therapist can reframe parents' pejorative descriptions of their children's behaviors into an interpretation of the behavior that is either more positive or more developmentally aligned with the children's ages. Often, parents are assisted in recognizing the part they play in the difficulty.

Dr. L.: In this video of your play session, your son surely is doing lots of exploring. I don't know how you all view that, but when your child is curious and does lots of exploring, that is a very positive thing. It is helpful to be able to look at such behavior and say, "Oh, I'm so thankful my child is interested in things," rather than, "Oh goodness, he gets into things all the time." You wouldn't want the opposite of that: a child who never gets into anything, is never interested in anything. That would not be a very creative, spontaneous, outgoing sort of child. So it's a very positive thing when your child does lots of exploring.

Laura: But we try to conform them to the other way.

Dr. L.: Oh, yes. It's called lack of tolerance on our part. But for 30 minutes in these play sessions, your child gets your full tolerance and patience, Laura.

Using Analogies to Increase Parent Awareness

Scenario 1: Some teaching points may elude even the most earnest parent. Analogies can be used as another tool to explain points to parents.

Dr. L.: I hear you saying that maybe she was feeling both ways.

Debbie: Well, she was probably, yes. I would say she was angry.

Dr. L.: Then respond to that more.

Debbie: But I feel like, in that particular thing, she's manipulative.

Dr. L.: Oh, so you know what she is doing.

Debbie: Right, but validating her feelings at bedtime doesn't change the fact that it's bedtime.

Dr. L.: And it's not expected to.

Debbie: OK, well that's maybe in my mind.

Dr. L.: These responses work even when they seem not to be working. Let me explain. Have you ever cut your finger? You put medicine on it, and you put a bandage on it, and 30 minutes later you take the bandage off; the cut is still almost exactly like it was, so you wipe the medicine off and throw the bandage away. Have you ever done that?

Debbie: No.

Dr. L.: You leave the medicine on. Why?

Kim: So it will slowly heal it.

Dr. L.: You assume it will eventually begin to be helpful.

Scenario 2: Parents are often more capable of understanding teaching points when the essence is portrayed in an everyday situation.

Dr. L.: Have you ever gone to the doctor when you have had a really sore throat, and he said, "Take this twice a day for seven days?" You take it for one day, wake up the next morning and your throat's still sore, so you throw the pills away? No, you don't do that. Why?

Debbie: You know you have to give it time.

Dr. L.: You assume that it's going to work, and it is working. You just don't see an immediate result. And with these responses, you won't always see immediate results. Over time, your child comes to realize that you understand, and so she doesn't have to push so hard to get her message over to you.

Encouraging Role-Play and Practice of Skills

Scenario 1: Role-playing and practice are essential to learning the new skills taught in CPRT.

Dr. L.: Let's do some quick role-playing. You two can be partners, you two are partners, and you two are partners. The person closest to me in each pair is the child first. Let's work on two things. Limit setting: those of you who are the children, do some things like threaten, "I'm going to paint on the wall," or "I'm going to cut this," or "I'm going to break this," and let your "parent" set a limit. And also, just play. Those of you who are the parents, practice what you saw in the video we just watched; make tracking and self-esteem-building responses and set limits. (Group role-plays.)

Dr. L.: Children, give some feedback to your parents. Tell them how they did, be specific. No generic praise. (Group gives feedback in pairs.)

Dr. L.: Now let's change roles. Children, you're now the parent, so switch roles. (Group role-plays.)

Dr. L.: OK, children, you can stop and give your parents some feedback. Tell them how they did. (Group gives feedback in pairs.)

Scenario 2: The therapist encourages parents to think through situations and come up with responses in advance of being faced with the dilemma, to give the parents a greater sense of agency over the new skill or technique.

Dr. L.: Let's just see how it will work, if you practice that response ahead of time so that you already have it. If he should start to shoot you with the dart gun, you say, "I'm not for shooting." Then you go to the next step, "I'm not for shooting. You can pretend the Bobo is me and shoot the Bobo," and you point to the Bobo.

Sonya: Can you set the limit that "I'm not for shooting," and if the child persists, say, "If you insist on shooting me, then

I will have to remove the gun from the playroom." Can you set that kind of limit?

Dr. L.: That will work. You figured it out.

Making Suggestions for Improvement

Scenario 1: Parents are sensitive to criticism of their parenting skills, so care must be given to the means and methods of making suggestions for improvement. The therapist gives parents the opportunity to search for alternatives and assists them in crafting responses that will enhance the parents' relationships with their children.

Debbie: My daughter insists on having other toys. She's just disinterested in the play session. She just wants to go play with her friends.

Dr. L.: So what might you say to her, if you were reflecting her feelings?

Debbie: I did the 5-minute thing. I said, let's play for 5 more minutes. And then in exactly 5 more minutes, she asked again.

Dr. L.: Be sure to reflect her feelings. "Oh, if you can't have other toys, then you just don't want to play at all. It doesn't seem as much fun to you if you can't have the toys you want." That might be the beginning of her expressing her anger. And you open the door by being understanding. That may open the door for her to stick it out. Let us know next week how it works out.

Scenario 2: Instead of telling parents they said or did something incorrectly, the therapist often frames his alternatives as suggestions or variations.

Dr. L.: There could be a variation on that response. Instead of saying, "That can be whatever you want it to be." When he said "What's this?" and then almost immediately banged it on top of his head, you said "I think that's what that's for." I think that is a very appropriate response. One of the things I hope you all begin to do is vary some of the things that we've worked on here so that your response becomes more "you." It doesn't have to always be said just the way we might work on it here.

Scenario 3: A specific suggestion may need to be made to counter a parent's natural instincts to teach and show.

Kathy: I told him I hoped we got the handcuffs off. He wanted to take them off and I didn't know he could. So I took them off.

Dr. L.: I heard you say also, "I don't think you can."

Kathy: Maybe I shouldn't have done that.

Dr. L.: Did you know he couldn't?

Kathy: No, I didn't know for sure that he couldn't, but . . .

Dr. L.: Therefore, you let the child try. And then it's his decision about whether or not he figures out that he can't take them off. You give him credit. In that way, he gets to feel powerful in a more positive way, because it seems to me he wants to feel powerful, to push you around, make you say things. Maybe that's not so good. He can feel powerful by doing something constructive. He figures out how to take the handcuffs off, and then he hears a self-esteem-building response from you, and he feels powerful in a more positive way.

Identifying What Is Learned from Events in Special Playtimes

Scenario 1: While interpretation is not emphasized in CPRT, parents are assisted in recognizing their children's feelings and often unspoken notions.

Dr. L.: If you put yourself in your son's spot, and your mom likes being in this session with you, looks forward to it, has fun while you're together, how would your son feel? How would that make him feel?

Kim: Pretty special.

Dr. L.: Yes, special.

Kim: Loved.

Dr. L.: Loved. Yes. And that he's important. "I'm important because she wants to be with me." That's a special gift you're giving.

Scenario 2: The therapist encourages parents by letting them know how effective even the smallest change in a parent's behavior has been on a child's outlook.

Sonya: A lot of times, my daughter just wants me to acknowledge her feelings on something. Like the time when she said, "I don't like you. You're not my friend anymore." I haven't been feeding into that. I just kind of check in that she is angry or frustrated. Usually, she's angry. I just say, "Sounds like you're very angry because I won't do what you want me to do," and it works great.

Dr. L.: At that moment then, your child knows that her message has been received by you. "Mom understands." They hear the labeling coming back that touches their feelings. And at that moment, too, you get a chance to teach your child an appropriate label: this is anger; it's not that I hate you.

Identifying Shifts or Changes in Behavior (in Child or in Parent)

Scenario 1: The therapist helps parents recognize shifts in their own behavior and/or their children's behavior after the playtimes.

Emily: The last time he did this it ended up a full-scale temper tantrum where his caseworker had to sit physically in front of her door to keep him in the room. It's different now because he'll just talk very calmly. There's no temper tantrum, there's no arguing.

Dr. L.: At home he's really different and has been consistently different with you in the way he reacts.

Emily: Yes, he is.

Dr. L.: So something has really changed.

Emily: Yes.

Scenario 2: Parents can discover new aspects of their relationship with their children and new aspects of themselves about which they may have been unaware.

Dr. L.: It's almost as though, Nita, you're saying, "I've rediscovered how to be a loving mother."

Nita: Yes, I used to think that everything has to be in control, and perfect, and that makes for a perfect love. Now, I've found that I can leave everything scattered around me, and I can take care of myself, too.

Dr. L.: So, your life is different.

Nita: He knows he can do other things. He knows he can hit the pillow. He laughed because Mom did it—I did it. He watched me hit the pillow, as something he could do.

Dr. L.: As I listen to you, Nita, one of the things that occurs to me is that it's almost as though you're saying, "I'm more free now."

Nita: Yes, I was in "the mommy" trip.

Dr. L.: And this is a different place.

Nita: Yes.

Facilitating Insight

Scenario 1: Parents are often surprised that just a few playtimes will result in a change in their children's behavior.

Kim: I was shocked to see him clean each brush and put it back. I was concerned that he was going to mix them, but he put them back in the right places. And he washed each one of them, cleaned them up, and cleaned the whole sink after all that.

Dr. L.: Why is it that your children will take this kind of responsibility in this 30-minute playtime?

Kim: This is his choice. It wasn't because Momma was standing there telling him to do it. And he wasn't standing there saying, "I'm not going to do it just because you're telling me to."

Dr. L.: No struggle.

Debbie: No battles.

Dr. L.: And when your children are free to make some of these kinds of decisions, they naturally move toward taking care of themselves and the situation without a lot of hassle. What an important discovery! How could we discover that unless there is a free time for your child to play when you're not the teacher, you're not the boss, and you're not correcting. Your child's self-direction just comes forward. The only way you could have discovered that is in this kind of free time. This works!

Scenario 2: Parents are given tools to help their children begin to learn the skills the children will need as they grow up and become responsible members of society.

Nita: I might say, "I can see you're very angry with me, but I'm not for kicking and hitting and calling names. You may tell me you're angry with me, or you can hit the Bobo or the floor."

Dr. L.: Sounds great. You got all the steps in there, and now he has a choice. He can say it or he can act it out. Could it be that your children, lots of times, just didn't think of any other way of doing it?

Sonya: You know, what's real interesting is that we adults go through life trying to find out what our choices are, in buying a car, in doing all these things. The more choices we get, the more freedom we feel like we have to choose what is best for us.

Dr. L.: It's important for children to find out what their choices are, and learn how to make decisions. When you make a decision, what happens? Where's the responsibility? On the person who makes the decision. So you're helping your child learn what it feels like to be responsible.

Clarifying

Scenario 1: Parents are taught how to help their children stop their own behavior. Choice giving is integral to this process.

Dr. L.: In limit setting, it's really important that you point to what the acceptable item is when you give a choice. You always point to the acceptable choice. In this approach, we don't grab hold of the child, literally or figuratively, and stop them. The objective is to help them to learn inside themselves to say "No" to self. They start to do something and we say, "*The wall is not for marking on, the paper is for marking on.*" Now, if the child chooses not to mark on the wall, and go mark on the paper, the child has stopped himself. He has said "No" to self. Where we're headed with this is when your child is 13 or 15, and they're out somewhere else, not under your thumb, they need to stop themselves because someone else may not stop them. They'll need to say "No" to themselves, and they need to know what that feels like.

Scenario 2: Parents learn that it is not their responsibility, but their children's, to stop the children's behavior. Children *are* able to learn how to do this.

Emily: Having the play sessions has brought a different dimension to my son and me, and things are much better. We had started some of the limit setting before the play sessions, but we didn't always follow through. Now, we're not about to do that. A lot of times, I would just stop the behavior, and now I've watched him so many times: he'll clinch his fist, and he'll hold it like this, but he doesn't act with it.

Dr. L.: So, he's stopping himself.

Conclusion

A variety of group process elements and teaching points have been presented as critical components of the 10-session CPRT model.

Clearly, this listing of excerpts from actual group dialogues does not represent a complete array of skills and methodologies that help create the environment for change in the CPRT approach. Nonetheless, these excerpts serve to illuminate the breadth of topics and skills that this model incorporates.

Reference

Lahti, S. (1992). *An ethnographic study of the filial therapy process.* Unpublished doctoral dissertation, University of North Texas, Denton.

CHAPTER 6

CPRT SKILLS, CONCEPTS, AND ATTITUDES TO BE TAUGHT

The Child-Centered Play Therapy skills, concepts, and attitudes taught in CPRT are presented in this chapter in greater detail to provide the filial therapist with a theoretical framework and a deeper understanding of these principles and procedures. Experienced play therapists who are well grounded in the child-centered theoretical approach are likely already familiar with these basic skills and concepts. For these play therapists, this information can serve as a review of the necessary skills and concepts to be taught in the 10-session CPRT model.

The material in this chapter is taken extensively from Landreth's book *Play Therapy: The Art of the Relationship* (2012) and some limited use is made of the material in Giordano, Landreth, and Jones's book *A Practical Handbook for Building the Play Therapy Relationship* (2005).

Objectives of the Parent-Child Playtime

The focus is on the child and all that the child is capable of becoming. The relationship is viewed as the vehicle for the process of change.

Therefore, the overall aim is for the parent to relate to the child in ways that will release the child's inner-directed capacity for constructive forward-moving growth. With this in mind, the filial therapist helps parents focus on the following objectives for the special playtime:

1. **Establishing an atmosphere of consistency and predictability for the child.** The child cannot feel safe or secure in a relationship that contains no limits. A feeling of security and predictability is promoted by the consistency of the parents' responses and behavior in the playroom.
2. **Understanding and accepting the child's world.** Acceptance of the child's world is conveyed by being eagerly and genuinely interested in whatever the child chooses to do in the playtime. Acceptance also means being patient with the pace of the child's play. Understanding is accomplished by relinquishing adult reality and seeing things from the child's perspective.
3. **Encouraging the expression of the child's emotional world.** Although the play materials are important, they are secondary to the expression of feelings by the child, which they facilitate. In the playtime, there is an absence of evaluation of feelings. Whatever the child feels is accepted without judgment.
4. **Establishing a feeling of freedom.** An important aspect of the special playtime is that the child feels or senses the greater freedom available in this setting to express his thoughts, feelings, and needs in ways that may not be permissible at other times. However, this is not a totally permissive relationship; parents learn to allow their child more freedom within secure limits. Allowing the child to make choices also creates a feeling of permissiveness.
5. **Facilitating decision making by the child.** This is accomplished largely by refraining from being an answer source for the child. The opportunity to choose which toy to play with, how to play with it, what color to use, or how something will turn out creates decision-making opportunities that, in turn, promote self-responsibility.
6. **Providing the child with an opportunity to assume responsibility and to develop a feeling of control.** Actually being in control of one's environment may not always be

possible. The significant variable, though, is that children feel in control. Children are responsible for what they do for themselves in the 30-minute playtime. When parents do for children what they can do for themselves, children are deprived of the opportunity to experience what self-responsibility feels like. *Feeling in control* is a powerful variable and helps children develop positive self-esteem.

Structuring the Special Playtime

Structuring is a very important skill and means more than simply planning ahead and setting up the toys. The word *structuring* is used in this instance to mean helping the child understand the nature of the play session. It involves verbally letting the child know such things as "*During our special playtime, you can play with the toys in lots of the ways you want to*" or "*You can decide . . . that's up to you.*" These statements are freeing in that they convey to the child responsibility for direction. Words should be chosen carefully to communicate to the child freedom, self-direction, and the parameters of the relationship. Boundaries on freedom are conveyed by the words "*in a lot of the ways*," which in effect communicates limits on behavior. This is a key phrase. The words "*any way you want*" are avoided because this is not a time of complete freedom. Parents sometimes introduce a child to the playtime with "This is our playtime, and this is a place where you can play with the toys *any way* you wish," only to have to withdraw their absolute approval as they are about to be shot with the dart gun or as the child throws the airplane at the lamp.

More important than words are the ways the parent nonverbally communicates the specialness of the playtime in the first play session. The parent is encouraged to enter the play session with eager anticipation. Since this is the child's time, the parent should sit down, preferably on the floor or at the child's level, further communicating to the child interest and willingness to allow the child to lead. Remaining standing may result in the parent towering over the child and conveys that the parent is in charge or is about to do something else, so the child waits expectantly. The parent should move closer to her child when the child is intent and focused on her play, and join in when invited. It is important for the parent to be comfortable, not detached, during her play sessions with her child.

The parent can also be involved in and be a part of the child's activity without physically following the child around the room. The parent can be quite active by shifting body posture or by leaning forward to be closer to the child's activity to convey interest and involvement.

In supervising parents, we have often observed parents turning their head 90 degrees to track children with their eyes while the rest of their body remained motionless and projected away from the child, communicating only minimal involvement with the child. When the parent's whole body turns toward the child, and the parent conveys genuine interest and full attention, the child feels the parent's presence.

RULE OF THUMB:

The parent's toes should follow his/her nose.

Helping Parents Enter the Child's World

Although parents occupy time and space with their children, many do not *know* or *understand* their children. Children need time for emotional sharing with their parents. A major goal for the parent-child play session is to help parents learn how to facilitate this kind of relationship with their children. The process begins by helping the parent become more sensitive to and understanding of their child's emotional world by entering into the child's world of play. Hopefully, the uppermost thought in the parent's mind at such times is "I want to know my child better." The parent is taught to wonder, "Does the love, the warmth I feel for my child show in my face? Does my tone of voice reveal kindness? Does my child know that I think he is important, the most important person in the world at this moment? Do my eyes show that? Is my caring about how my child feels inside being communicated? Do my words convey that caring?"

RULE OF THUMB:

Be sensitive to the child's world.

Through the process of accepting the child's attitudes, feelings, and thoughts, the parent enters the child's world. In this way, the child feels understood and accepted by the parent, and a deeper parent-child bond begins to develop.

A New Kind of Language: Communicating "Being With"

The typical approach in parent-child interactions is characterized by an attitude of evaluation of the child based on what is known about the child and previous circumstances. Seldom does a parent strive to understand the immediate internal frame of reference of the child, the child's subjective world, to genuinely "*be with*" the child. Sensitive understanding of the child occurs to the extent the parent is able to put aside personal experiences and expectations and appreciate the personhood of the child, as well as the child's activities, experiences, feelings, and thoughts. Children are not free to explore, to test boundaries, to share frightening parts of their lives, or to change until they experience a relationship in which their subjective experiential world is understood and accepted. The attitude of the parents is essential in "*being with*" their child in such a way that the child feels understood and accepted. This depth and dimension of understanding means remaining free of a stylized role and participating deeply and meaningfully in the work of understanding the child. This means putting aside the tendency to evaluate and judge, and to see from the viewpoint of the child.

Responding to children in a way that communicates sensitivity, understanding, and acceptance and conveys freedom and responsibility is for many parents like learning a foreign language and requires a drastic shift in attitude and a restructuring of words used in responses. From this new perspective, children are viewed as being capable, creative, resilient, and responsible. The objective of CPRT is to help parents develop an attitude of genuinely believing **their children are capable** of figuring things out for themselves, within the boundaries of their developmental capabilities, and communicating this attitude through responses to their children in the play session.

The parent communicates "*being with*" by being a verbally responsive participant in his child's play. The child may often be engrossed in play and not talkative about what is being played out, and no feelings are evident or sensed by the parent. At such times, the parent can respond to the child's nonverbal play by what is being observed. "*You're using lots of colors to make that.*" "*Now, you're putting her in the bed.*" "*That one just crashed right into the other one.*" These responses, which are referred to as "tracking responses," communicate the parent's involvement, interest, and understanding. Parents are taught to avoid lengthy responses that disrupt the child's focus, resulting in the child being caught up in using energy to try to understand what the parent is saying, which tends to change the direction of the child's expression. **Responses should be short and interactive**, much like a conversation.

The parent also communicates his understanding of his child through accurate reflection of the child's level of affect. The parent should avoid getting overly excited beyond the child's level of affect about little happenings such as, "*Oh, my! Isn't that wonderful! You found a colored rock in the box!*" This kind of excitement may cause the child to feel something is wrong or to distrust her own reaction because she does not feel equally excited. Expressing affect beyond the level expressed by the child is structuring and will lead the child into expressing affect and behaviors beyond what the child is genuinely feeling. For example, this can be seen when David hits the bop bag with minimum effort and the parent responds with, "*Wow! You really socked him that time*!" Then, David proceeds to hit the bop bag with more force and looks at the parent for approval.

Another typical parent response that prevents the parent from fully "*being with*" the child is questioning. Questions place the parent in a leading, controlling position. Generally, **if the parent has enough information on which to base a question, enough**

information is available on which to make a statement. Generally, questions imply a lack of understanding. "*Did that make you angry?*" communicates the parent's lack of understanding, yet the parent does sense the child feels angry or he would not ask the question. The parent should trust what has emerged in his own intuitive system and make a statement, "*You feel angry about that.*" Empathic statements go into the child's heart and soul. Questions go to the mind to be processed and evaluated.

- **Conveying an Understanding of the Child's World: The "Be-With" Attitudes**

Only when the child begins to become accustomed to the special playtime and the new verbal language of the parent will the child begin to express and explore the emotionally meaningful experiences that have been experienced. The parent must wait for this development. It cannot be rushed or made to happen. This is the child's time, and the child's readiness or lack of readiness to play, talk, or explore must be respected.

When the child experiences the freedom and permissiveness of directing his own play in the context of an empathic and caring relationship with his parent, the child develops self-discipline and perseverance that comes from the sustained effort required to carry out or complete a self-selected activity or project. The process of independently choosing an activity, directing the action, and relying on self for the outcome enhances self and develops self-reliance.

The parent's responsibility in the relationship can be summed up in the following four healing messages, referred to in CPRT training as the **"Be-With" Attitudes**. The parent works hard to communicate to the child at all times, not just in words, but with his total person.

1. **I am here.** Nothing will distract me. I will be fully present physically, mentally, and emotionally. I want to be so fully present that there will be no distance between myself and my child. I want to enter fully into my child's world, to move about freely in my child's world, to sense what my child senses, feel what my child feels. Once I have achieved this kind of knowing contact, it is easy to know when I am not in

touch with my child. Can I enter so fully into my child's world that I have no need to evaluate or judge my child?

2. **I hear you.** I will listen fully with my ears and eyes to everything about my child, what is expressed and what is not expressed. I want to hear my child completely. Can I experience, hear, my child as she is? To accomplish this kind of hearing, I must be secure enough within myself to allow my child to be separate from me.
3. **I understand.** I want my child to know I understand what she is communicating, feeling, experiencing, and playing, and so will work hard to communicate that understanding to my child. I want to understand the inner depth and meaning of my child's experience and feelings. The crucial dimension in special playtimes is the communication of this kind of understanding and acceptance to the child.
4. **I care.** I really do care about my child and want my child to know that. If the parent is successful in communicating fully the first three messages, the parent will not be perceived as a threat, and the child will allow the parent into his world. Then, the child will know the parent cares. This kind of caring releases the dynamic potential that already exists in children.

• Conveying Acceptance: A Necessary Dimension of "Being With"

Acceptance grows out of a genuine and sincere interest in one's child, a belief that he can assume responsibility for himself. Children who experience such an atmosphere of acceptance in their special play session with their parents learn that they can depend on others for support while developing their own sense of adequacy and independence. Acceptance is communicated through the parent's patience and willingness to trust the process. Patience allows the parent to see things from the child's perspective. The parent's acceptance is reflected in refraining from offering advice, suggestions, or explanations, and in not questioning or interrupting the child. The parent's empathic responses communicate understanding and acceptance to the child, thus freeing the child to be more creative and expressive.

By empathically reflecting happenings and feelings, the parent expresses respect for the child and affirms the child's right to have feelings and to express herself through actions. Even when the parent must set limits on the child's behavior, the parent conveys acceptance of *the child*. Acceptance, then, occurs in conjunction with permissiveness, but does not necessarily imply approval of what the child is doing.

The parent's attitude and expression of acceptance encourages a child to explore thoughts and feelings further. When a child's feelings are expressed and accepted by the parent, they are experienced with less intensity by the child. The child then is more fully able to integrate and deal with feelings by expressing positive and negative emotions in a more focused and specific way. Focusing on the child's feelings validates the person of the child rather than the importance of the problem.

Allowing the Child to Lead to Facilitate Self-Direction and Responsibility

Parents are usually in the position of being "the expert." Children look to parents for direction, permission, and answers. During the play session, the parent is not the teacher or a person who corrects children's responses. During play sessions, a child is able to call a "giraffe" a "horse" without being corrected.

The child can add five plus one and get an answer of seven. In addition, the child can choose to spell any way the child decides. This is an accepting and permissive environment. The child can learn spelling and addition outside the play session.

• Returning Responsibility to a Child and Facilitating Decision Making

The child leads and the parent follows. The child decides what toys to play with and how to play with the toys, within appropriate boundaries. The child is allowed to solve problems. The parent has no solutions. During the 30-minute playtime, the parent has no information the child needs. The child directs the drama.

• What Is Meant by Returning Responsibility and Facilitating Decision Making?

When children ask questions or seek assistance, the parent will make a response that returns the responsibility to the child. These responses encourage children to make their own decisions and to take responsibility for a current concern. For example:

Child: What should I play with first?

Parent: In here, you can decide what you want to play with first.

- **Why Facilitate Responsibility and Decision Making in the Child?**

Children can learn how to make decisions and take responsibility for themselves at a young age. These skills are developed throughout childhood and will prepare children to make decisions during the teen years and into adulthood. Children who are provided opportunities to learn decision making and self-responsibility become self-directed, self-motivated, and feel a sense of control in their lives.

Responsibility is learned through experience. When parents make decisions for children that children are capable of making themselves, children are deprived of a learning opportunity. Instead of developing self-responsibility, children learn to become dependent upon the parent.

Allowing a child the freedom to engage in the process of decision making provides opportunities for the child to project his own personal meaning onto the item or material. This inner experience of making decisions strengthens the child's self-concept and provides the child with experiences that can become incorporated into a changed perceptual view of self. This is a growth process that will enable the child to respond emotionally to future problems and situations in a more effective way. Therefore, the parent refuses to accept responsibility for making decisions for the child during the playtime, no matter how insignificant the decision may seem to be. To the child's question, "*What color is the moon*?" the parent replies, "*The moon can be any color you want the moon to be.*" Thus, the child is encouraged to accept responsibility for self and, in the process, discovers personal strengths.

Therapeutically facilitative responses return responsibility to the child, thus helping her to feel in control and to become intrinsically motivated. The parent conveys a belief in the child, by allowing the child to make decisions, and is committed to providing opportunities for self-direction by avoiding interfering with the process.

At the beginning of the first playtime, a child often wants the parent to identify what to do, what things are used for, and how to "undo" difficult things. The child may hold up a toy that the child obviously knows the name for and ask, "*What's this?*" This is a moment when the parent does not know for sure the motivation behind the question. To name the item may inhibit the child's creativity, structure the child's expression, or keep responsibility in the hands of the parent. Responsibility could be returned to the child by responding, "*That can be whatever you want it to be.*" Similar responses, depending on the child's request, might be "*You can decide*" or "*That's something you can do.*" If the child needs help to complete a task she is not capable of completing without assistance, the parent can respond, "*Show me what you want done.*" These responses allow a child to assume responsibility and to make a decision and, typically, by the end of the session the child is stating what things are without asking for the parent's decision.

Children will often answer many of their questions if the parent simply will not be so quick to reply. A thoughtful "Hmmmm" by the parent may be all that is needed.

- **Example Parent Responses That Return Responsibility**

1. Child: (picks up handcuffs and asks) What are these for?
   Parent: In here, you can decide what those are for.
2. Child: (picks up baby bottle and asks) What is this?
   Parent: That can be whatever you want it to be.
3. Child: What color are elephants?
   Parent: You can paint elephants any color you want them to be.
4. Child: (struggling to get glue bottle open)
   Parent: Hmm, you are really working hard to get that open.
   Child: Here, open this for me. Please.
   Parent: Show me what you want done.
5. Child: How do you spell happy?
   Parent: You can spell happy any way you want.

- **Example Parent Responses That Facilitate Decision Making**

Child: (Enters the play and looks around the room. Parent-child play session was in a clinic.) What should I do?

Parent: In here, you can decide what you want to play.

Child: (Walks toward the arts and crafts table and pulls out a piece of paper.) I know what I can do.

Parent: You figured out what you want to do.

Child: I am gonna make a picture for my teacher.

Parent: You've got a plan and know just what you want to do.

Child: (Begins to pick out colors from the markers/crayons and starts drawing.) I'm gonna make a rainbow.

Parent: You know just what you want to do and how to make it.

Child: Yeah . . . what colors should I put in my rainbow?

Parent: You can decide what colors to use.

Child: I think I'll use blue and red because they are my favorite colors.

Parent: You figured out a way to decide what colors to use.

Reflecting a Child's Nonverbal Play Behavior (Tracking)

- **What Is Acknowledging Nonverbal Behavior?**

The parent responds to the child's actions and nonverbal play. The parent describes what the parent sees, hears, and observes the child doing. For example:

> You are pushing *that* (car) right through *there* (tunnel).
> You are putting lots of sand in that (bucket).
> Note: The parent does not identify the item until the child does.

- **Why Acknowledge Nonverbal Behavior?**

When children provide little to no verbal content to respond to and are not expressing any particular emotion, acknowledging children's behavior helps children feel the parent is interested in their world, cares about their world, and that the parent is striving to understand their world.

- **Rationale for Not Labeling Toys**

Toys used during the playtime should not be identified or labeled until the child has verbalized an identifying label for the item. Labeling a toy anchors the child to reality and interferes with the child's creativity and fantasy. Once the parent has identified the item as a truck, it can no longer be a school bus or an ambulance. Referring to a toy as "it," "that," "her," or "him" allows the child to decide what she wants the toy to be. When the child picks up the car and puts it into the box, the parent responds, "*You just put that right in there.*" The child is now free to continue with her original intent that the car is a giant bug. This response also communicates to the child that the parent is *with her*. When the parent labels toys and behaviors according to an adult perspective, inaccurate assumptions and responses may be made. If a child is pushing a block into the sand and the parent responds by stating, "*You are pushing that block deep into the sand.*" The child could be pretending that the block is a bulldozer, a spaceship, or an animal. A response that avoids labeling would be **"You're pushing that into the sand."** When a parent inaccurately labels a toy, some children will correct the parent and some will not. Children may feel restricted and less understood by a parent if the toy is inaccurately labeled. Not labeling toys creates a freer environment that encourages the child to be creative and to use toys in other ways than in a conventional manner.

- **Guidelines for Responding to Nonverbal Play Behavior**

1. **Responding infrequently:** If the parent is silent during the child's play, the child will begin to feel watched or that the parent is uninterested in the child. Instead, the parent wants the child to feel as though the parent is a part of the play. This is similar to being in a conversation with an adult. Adults

know that a person cares and hears them when the person listens and verbally responds. In a like manner, the parent listens with ears and eyes and verbalizes what she hears and sees.

2. **Responding too frequently:** If the parent acknowledges nonverbal behavior too frequently, the parent may sound like a sports commentator providing play-by-play action. This type of commentary does not sound genuine and conversational. The child may experience the comments as intrusive. The goal is for responses to be genuine and conversational, interactive—a genuine attempt to convey the "Be-With" Attitudes: I'm here, I hear you, I understand, and I care.
3. **Acknowledging nonverbal behavior/Personalizing the response:** Begin the response with "You're" or "You are." This personalizes the message and places the focus on the child instead of the toy. It also promotes a feeling of the child being in control. For example, the child is playing with a car, which he has previously identified as a car, and is driving it around in large circles. ***"You're driving that car around and around"*** (focus is on the child; helps the child feel empowered). **"That car is going around and around"** (focus is on the toy; depersonalized message, does not help the child feel important or empowered). During the first play therapy session, the parent may be more talkative and acknowledge nonverbal behavior more frequently to help alleviate the child's uneasiness. If the child is absorbed in play, fewer responses may be needed.

- **Example Parent Responses That Acknowledge Nonverbal Behavior**

Child: (Pushes a truck across the carpet.) Vrrmm.

Parent: You're pushing that right across there.

Child: (Gets up and begins looking around the room.)

Parent: Looking around for something else.

Child: (Puts the plastic soldiers on the carpet and begins to set up a scene using all the toys he has brought over.)

Parent: You've got all you want for now and you are putting them the way you want them.

Child: (Puts the plastic soldiers in a straight line, then begins to build a wall around them.)

Parent: You're lining them up and making a wall around them.

Child: (Begins to enact a battle with the plastic soldiers.) Pow, bang, boom.

Parent: Sounds like they are really fighting.

Reflecting a Child's Verbalization (Content)

- **What Is Reflecting Content?**

The parent repeats in slightly different words something that the child has said. For example, the child is working in the corner and states, "*There is going to be a big earthquake soon. No one can keep it from happening; not even Superman.*" Parent responds, **"No one can help stop the earthquake."** The child places the dishes on the floor and states, "*It's time for dinner, everyone come to dinner this very minute.*" Parent responds, **"You're letting everyone know that dinner is ready to *eat*."**

- **Why Reflect Content?**

Reflecting content helps the child know that you hear and understand the content of her message. It also provides the child with the opportunity to hear the message so that she can hear what she has said. This helps validate her perspective and clarify her understanding of self. When presented with a choice to reflect feeling or content, respond to the child's feeling or combine a feeling and content response. If a child's feelings are not obvious, listen to the tone of voice the child uses to help discern the feeling within the message.

- **Example Parent Responses That Reflect Content**

Child: An earthquake is happening.

Parent: Here comes an earthquake.

Child: Batman and Robin are here! (Child drops figures on the earthquake.)

Parent: Batman and Robin dropped some things on the earthquake.

Child: But they can't stop it.

Parent: No matter what they do, it's not enough to stop that earthquake.

Reflecting a Child's Feelings/Wants/Wishes

Because most parents' life experiences have not taught them to value and express emotions, the most difficult filial skill to teach is helping parents identify and reflect their children's feelings, wants, and wishes. Parents need to be aware of feelings that they avoid or are uncomfortable dealing with in their lives. Sometimes these same feelings are difficult to acknowledge in the child. Examples of responses that recognize the child's feelings, wants, and wishes are *"You seem frustrated that . . .," "You look happy . . .," "You're angry that . . .," "You're confused . . .," "You look excited . . .," "You are sad . . .," "You really like . . .," "You don't like . . .," "You really want . . .," "You wish. . . ."*

• Why Reflect Feelings/Wants/Wishes?

Reflecting feelings communicates understanding and acceptance of children's feelings and needs. It also shows children that you are interested and that you want to understand them. This process helps children understand, accept, label, and communicate. If a feeling, desire, or need is expressed and goes unrecognized, children may think that the feeling or expression is not acceptable.

• Guidelines for Reflecting Feelings/Wants/Wishes

1. Look into the child's eyes for clues to feelings.
2. After you've decided what the child is feeling, put the feeling word into a short response, personalize the message by beginning the reflection with "you." For example, "*You seem sad,*" "*You're really mad at me right now.*"
3. At the beginning of reflections, avoid repetitive use of phrases such as "sounds like."

- **Example Parent Responses That Reflect Feelings**

Child: I like to go to school because I get to play with my friend.

Parent: You like school and have fun with your friend.

Child: (Goes to the paper and begins to draw.) Yeah, but sometimes we have to read.

Parent: Sounds like you don't like to have to read at school.

Child: (Begins to play with the dart gun.) I like this.

Parent: You found something else you like.

Child: Yeah! I can use this to shoot things!

Parent: You are really excited about what you can do with that.

Child: Yeah—look how far I can shoot it!

Parent: You are really proud of yourself.

Self-Esteem Building and Encouragement

One goal of filial therapy is for the child to build esteem by internalizing her own positive statements about herself. Praise is defined as nondescriptive evaluative statements containing words such as wonderful, good, great, and beautiful. These words evaluate the child or the child's product (a painting, block tower, etc.). The evaluator holds the power and the child learns to need additional praise in order to feel good about herself. This type of praise does not make a positive long-term impact on the child because it lacks description. If the child relies on external praise and evaluations, her peers, family members, and other adults' comments define what she thinks and how she feels about herself.

On the other hand, comments that acknowledge time, effort, and hard work describe the process of creating a picture or block tower. This type of message can be internalized. "I worked hard to make this tower." Thus, the parent's recognition of efforts and hard work can be integrated into the child's self-concept and beliefs about herself. The child learns to acknowledge her own personal qualities, commitment, and effort.

Responses should always be personalized and address the presence of the child. Responding to David, who is busy banging on the Bobo, by saying "*David really likes hitting that Bobo*" causes the child to feel talked about as a non-person. *"You really like hitting that Bobo"* addresses the child personally. "*You*" gives the child credit and recognizes ownership.

Some parents are prone to inappropriately include themselves in the interaction. Beth talks about playing soccer and how much she wanted to win but her team lost. The parent responds with, "*Sometimes it feels bad when we lose and want to win.*" The parent was not a part of the happening, and the use of "we" shifts the focus away from the child. (Additional information about self-esteem and specific examples of responses are included in Chapter 14 of this volume and in "Self-Esteem Building" in Session 7 of the Therapist Notebook in the CPRT Treatment Manual, 2nd Edition.)

- **Encouragement vs. Praise**

Praise judges a child's abilities and self-worth. It tells the child what *you* think about his or her abilities. Praise teaches the child to value "self" based upon other's positive and negative comments and, as such, facilitates an external locus of control. The child learns to allow others' ideas and beliefs to direct his or her life. Examples of praise include such statements as, "*Great job*!" "*What a beautiful picture*," "*You're such a good boy*," "*That looks awesome*," "*You're good at that*," and "*What a fantastic tower.*"

Conversely, encouragement acknowledges the child's *effort*. It helps a child develop an internal locus of control and to become self-directed and self-responsible. Children who are intrinsically motivated do not need others' praise and comments to determine self-worth. They are able to applaud their own efforts and accomplishments. Encouraging responses include such statements as, "*You are making it just the way you want," "You did it," "You got it," "You are trying hard," "You worked hard," "You really like your [picture]," "You know just how you want it to go," "You are proud of [your tower]," "Sounds like you know a lot about [dinosaurs],"* and *"You know how to count [feed the baby, build the blocks, write your name, etc.]*." The statement *"you know how to"* reflects ability instead of making a judgment as to the child's ability (*"You're good at counting"*).

Scenario 1: Child draws a picture, then asks, "Look mommy, do you like my picture?"

Example of Praise: **"That's a beautiful picture!"** This type of response reinforces the child's need for a positive external locus of evaluation. If a child can make a beautiful picture, she can also make a picture that displeases the parent.

Example of Encouragement: **"You worked hard on that picture."** This type of response helps a child learn to give credit to him or herself and to appreciate his or her own abilities. The child will learn to be proud of self and will not formulate ideas about self-concept solely based upon other's evaluation.

Scenario 2: Child cooks dinner and hands the parent a plate with a pretend chicken leg on it, then asks, "How do you like it?"

Example of Praise: **"This dinner is delicious!"** This response evaluates and judges the cook's performance. This encourages the child to be motivated by your comments and praise.

Example of Encouragement: **"You worked hard making this dinner just for me."** (Show admiration in tone of voice.) This response focuses on the child's work and effort. It encourages the child to develop internal motivation. The child will become self-motivated instead of relying on praise from others.

- **Example Parent Responses That Facilitate Encouragement and Esteem Building**

Child: (Child builds a very tall tower out of blocks.) Look at this. Isn't it awesome?

Parent: You really like the way it turned out.

Child: Yeah. But what do you think of the tower?

Parent: You put a lot of time into making it and you look proud of your work.

Child: I am proud of my tower. (Walks over to the construction paper and begins to write multiplication problems on the paper.) I know how to do multiplication.

Parent: You know how to multiply numbers.

Child: (Child multiplies the numbers 20 times 20. Writes the answer 400 under the problem.) Look at this! (Pride in voice.)

Parent: You're excited and proud of your ability to do multiplication.

Child: (Writes another multiplication problem and the answer.) I had to do so many worksheets for homework before I could do this.

Parent: You put a lot of work and effort into learning how to do multiplication.

- **Encouraging a Child Who Needs Help Completing a Task**

1. When you see a child struggling to complete a task, don't jump in to help. Wait until the child asks for help. Encourage the child while he or she is working on the task: **"You are really working hard to get that done." "You are figuring out a way to get that open."** Every time you do something for a child without allowing her to struggle with figuring it out for herself, you rob her of the opportunity to feel competent and capable.
2. Encourage the child to complete age-appropriate tasks on his own. For example, a 3-year-old child may have difficulty taking off a lid that has been tightly put on a plastic jar. It is appropriate to work together as a team to open the jar lid. While working on the task together, encourage the child: **"You are working hard."**
3. Don't complete a task for a child who has not made an attempt at the task and asks for help.
4. If a child (a) tries to accomplish the task, (b) asks you for help, and (c) the task seems challenging for someone his or her age, respond, **"Show me what you want done."** This response encourages the child to make decisions about how

he would like you to help. This approach also helps the child focus on what specifically needs to be done to accomplish the task. (Additional information about encouragement and examples of responses are included in Chapter 15 of this text and in Session 8 of the Therapist Notebook in the CPRT Treatment Manual, 2nd Edition.)

Therapeutic Limit Setting

The CCPT skill of limit setting is foundational to the effectiveness of the CPRT parent-child play sessions. Therefore, it is essential that Chapter 11, "Therapeutic Limit Setting," in Landreth's, 2012 text Play Therapy: The Art of the Relationship be studied carefully. The material on limit setting in this CPRT text is only a summary of that chapter.

Limit setting is one of the most important aspects of parent-child play sessions and is also the most problematic for most parents. Consistent limits provide structure and security for children and are critical to a healthy parent-child relationship. Parents often feel insecure about trying to limit their children's behavior in a new way and they may be slow to apply limits. Sometimes the parent is reluctant or inconsistent in setting limits because of a desire to be liked by the child.

• Basic Guidelines in Limit Setting

Permissiveness in the special playtime does not mean the acceptance of all behaviors. Limits provide children with an opportunity to learn self-control, that they have choices, what making choices feels like, and how responsibility feels. Therefore, when limits should be set and are not, children are deprived of an opportunity to learn something important about themselves. In therapeutic limit setting, children are given the opportunity to choose. They therefore become responsible for themselves and their own well-being in the special playtime.

The parent's belief that children will choose positive cooperative behavior is a significant and impactful variable in the play process. Children are more likely to comply with limits when they experience respect for themselves and acceptance for their feelings and behaviors—both positive and negative. Therefore, the parent will be most helpful by focusing on the child's unexpressed need for defiance, for example, while continuing to express fundamental understanding, support, valuing of the child, and a genuine belief in the child.

In therapeutic limit setting, **the focus and emphasis is always on the child in order to clearly convey where the responsibility lies.** A response such as "*We don't draw pictures on the wall*" is inappropriate because the parent has not the least inclination to draw pictures on the wall. Yet the use of "we" and "our" implies the parent is a part of the process.

- **When and How to Present Limits**

Providing a long list of limits at the beginning of the first playtime is not necessary. This tends to set a negative tone and interferes with the objective of establishing a climate of freedom of expression. Since the special playtime is a learning experience for children, the best time to learn is when the limit issue arises. Self-control cannot be learned until an opportunity to exercise self-control occurs.

RULE OF THUMB:

Limits are not needed until they are needed.

The establishment of total limits rather than conditional limits seems to work best. Total limits are less confusing to children and help the parent to feel more secure. "*You may put a little paint on the table*" leaves the issue wide open as to how much paint. A total limit would be *"The table is not for painting on."* The child now knows exactly what is not permissible. Conditional limits, such as "*You can't kick the door hard*," can become the basis for arguments. What the parent thinks is hard may not be perceived by the child as hard.

The need for consistency and follow-through in applying limits cannot be overstated. Parents who do not follow through harm their relationship with their child by sending the message "You cannot count on me to do what I say."

- **Rationale for Therapeutic Limits**

All feelings, desires, and wishes of the child are accepted, but not all behaviors. Destructive behaviors cannot be accepted, but the child can be granted permission to express herself symbolically without fear of reprimand or rejection. The therapeutic rationale for limit setting during the 30-minute play session is contained in the following six statements and accompanying discussions.

1. **Limits provide physical and emotional security and safety for children.** Basic commonsense health and safety limits prevail in the playtime. A child may not stick a pencil up his nose or cut himself with the scissors. Likewise, the child may need to be protected from potential guilt, as in the case when a child wants to draw with markers on the parent's face, pour glue on the parent's clothes, or shoot the parent with the dart gun. Although a child may express a desire to hit the parent, break a toy, or damage furniture, such behaviors are limited in order to prevent accompanying feelings of guilt and anxiety. In responding to situations described here, the parent always maintains an accepting attitude of the child's feelings and desires.

   When children discover where the boundaries are in the playtime relationship and experience those boundaries being adhered to consistently, they feel secure because there is predictability in the relationship and setting.
2. **Limits protect the physical well-being of the parent and facilitate acceptance of the child.** The inherent growth potential in children is facilitated by the parent's acceptance and warm caring, and it is limit setting that allows the parent to remain empathic and accepting of the child throughout the playtime. For the parent to maintain a warm, caring, accepting attitude toward a child who is hitting the parent in the face with a toy sword is virtually impossible. In this situation, the parent will very likely experience feelings of resentment and rejection, which will in turn be communicated to the child at some level. **Any form of direct aggressive physical acting out or attack on the parent should be prohibited**. Such behaviors are not to be tolerated under any circumstances

because they will interfere with the parent's empathic acceptance of the child.

3. **Limits facilitate the development of decision making, self-control, and self-responsibility of children.** In the midst of experiencing the welling up of intense emotion, children are often unaware of their behavior and so are equally devoid of feelings of responsibility. Limit setting addresses the immediate reality of the situation and indirectly calls attention to the child's behavior through statements such as "*The wall is not for painting on.*" How can children develop a feeling of responsibility if they are unaware of what they are doing? And how can they experience a feeling of self-control if they are too defensive to change their behavior? Rather than focusing on what the child is doing that is unacceptable, the parent focuses on the child's feelings or desires and matter-of-factly states the rule. This can be seen clearly in the statement "*You would like to play with the playdough on the carpet, but the carpet is not for putting playdough on,*" as opposed to "*Billy, don't put that on the carpet.*"

   Responsibility is further communicated by providing acceptable alternatives, such as "*You can play with the playdough on the tray*" (pointing to the tray). No attempt is made to stop the expression of the feeling or the need. Such a statement clearly indicates to the child a permissible way to express herself. Now the child is confronted with a choice: to act on the original impulse or to express herself through the alternative behavior. The choice is the child's and the parent allows the child to choose. **The decision is the child's and responsibility accompanies decision making**. If the child chooses to play with playdough on the tray, it will be because the child decided to and exercised self-control, not because the parent made the child.

4. **Limits anchor the playtime to reality.** When the parent verbalizes a limit, the experience is quickly changed from fantasy to the reality of a relationship with an adult where certain behaviors are unacceptable, as is true in the world outside the playtime, except that in the playtime substantially fewer limitations are established on behavior. When the parent interjects, "*You would really like to dump that playdough on the carpet, but the playdough is not for dumping on the*

carpet. You can dump the playdough on the tray," the child is confronted with the reality of having crossed an unacceptable boundary, has been presented the opportunity to choose what will be done next, and experiences the accompanying responsibility.

5. **Limits promote consistency.** Some homes are characterized by inconsistency in behavior on the part of adults who have difficulty maintaining rules. In these homes, what was prohibited today may or may not be prohibited tomorrow.

   One of the ways the parent establishes a consistent environment in the playtime is through the introduction and use of consistent limits. Limits are presented in a consistently nonthreatening manner, and the parent is consistent in seeing that the limits are adhered to—not in a rigid manner, but in a consistent manner. **Limits, therefore, help to provide the structure for a consistent environment**. What was prohibited last time is prohibited in this playtime. Thus, the playtimes have predictability. Without consistency, there can be no predictability, and without predictability, there can be no security.

6. **Limits protect the playtime materials and room.** Allowing random destruction of toys could become an expensive process and at the same time would not be helpful to the emotional growth of the child. Therefore, "*Bobo is for hitting, not stabbing with the scissors.*" Although it might be great fun for the child to jump on the dollhouse and smash it to pieces, it would probably not be repairable and should be protected with "*The dollhouse is not for jumping on.*" Less expensive items also are not for breaking or smashing. These are opportunities for limit setting, and thus opportunities for the child to learn something valuable: how to bring self under control. The playtime is not a place of limitless freedom where the child can do anything.

   An important consideration, however, is that children have an opportunity to appropriately express their feelings through acceptable items. Just limiting the behavior is not sufficient. Therefore, every playtime box should have some inexpensive items that are for smashing, breaking, or throwing. Egg cartons seem to fit this purpose quite well. They can be stacked and kicked over, jumped on and smashed, broken apart, thrown, and painted. Playdough can also be suggested as an acceptable substitute for smashing.

Actually, the number of limits set during a playtime is minimal and involves setting limits on behaviors in the following areas: (a) harmful or dangerous behavior to the child and parent, (b) behavior that disrupts the routine or process (continually leaving the room, wanting to play after time is up), (c) destruction of room or materials, (d) taking toys from playtime, and (e) socially unacceptable behavior.

- **Procedures in Therapeutic Limit Setting**

The process of setting limits is a carefully thought out procedure designed to convey understanding, acceptance, and responsibility to the child. The objective of the parent is not to stop the behavior but rather to facilitate the expression of the motivating feeling, want, or need in a more acceptable manner. **The parent is a facilitator of expression rather than a prohibitor of action.**

Rather than attempting to stop behaviors, the parent's objective is to respond to the child in such a way that the child is left with the responsibility for changing her behavior. If the parent tells the child what to do, then the parent is responsible. When the parent trusts the child's capacity to respond responsibly and communicates, "*The lamp is not for throwing at. The bop bag is for throwing at*," the child is then free to decide what to do next and is thus responsible.

A different message is obviously communicated in each of the following statements to a child who is about to draw on the wall.

1. It's probably not a good idea to draw on the wall.
2. You can't draw on the wall.
3. Maybe you could draw on something else other than the wall.
4. The rule is you can't draw on the wall.
5. The wall is not for drawing on.

- **Steps in the Therapeutic Limit Setting Process**

Parents are taught the three-step A-C-T method of limit setting to facilitate the process of communicating understanding and acceptance of the child's motives, to make the limit clear, and to provide acceptable alternative actions and behaviors. When limit setting is needed, the parent can remember to **ACT** in instituting the steps in the process sequence.

A—Acknowledge the child's feelings, wishes, and wants.
C—Communicate the limit.
T—Target acceptable alternatives.

STEP 1. Acknowledge the child's feelings, wishes, and wants. Verbalizing understanding of the child's feeling or want conveys acceptance of the child's motivation. Simply setting the limit without acknowledging the feeling might indicate to the child that his feelings are not important. Verbalizing an empathic understanding of the feeling often helps to defuse the intensity of the feeling. This is especially true in the case of anger and is often all that is needed for the child to begin modifying his behavior. Acceptance of the feeling or desire often satisfies the child, and a need for the act no longer exists. **Feelings should be reflected just as soon as they are recognized:** "*You're angry at me.*" Once the block of wood is in flight across the room, acceptance of the feeling can no longer be a deterrent.

STEP 2. Communicate the limit. Limits should be specific and should clearly delineate exactly what is being limited. Limits that are "fuzzy" or unclear interfere with the child's ability to accept responsibility and to act responsibly.

The parent may not always be able to follow these steps in sequence. The urgency of the situation—the child is about to throw the truck at the window—may necessitate stating the limit first, "*The window is not for throwing things at,*" and then reflecting, "*You want to throw the truck at the window, but the window is not for throwing at.*" In this example, no feelings are evident, so the child's desire is reflected.

STEP 3. Target acceptable alternatives. The child may not be aware of any other way to express what is being felt. At that moment, the child can only think of one way to express himself. At this step in the process of limit setting, the parent provides alternatives to the child for the expression of the action. This can involve pointing out different alternatives to the child. *"The dollhouse is not for standing on. You may choose to stand on the chair."* A different surface may be needed to draw on: *"The wall is not for drawing on. You may choose to draw on the paper or the egg carton."* A substitute may need to be selected to replace the parent as the recipient of aggressive behavior: *"Ellen, I'm not for hitting. The Bobo is for hitting."* A nonverbal cue pointing toward the alternative(s), in conjunction with the verbalized alternatives, is especially helpful in diverting the child's attention from the original source of focus and facilitating the process of choice making. Using the child's name helps to get the child's attention.

The following interaction shows how the A-C-T model is applied when 6-year-old Robert is just as angry as he can be at his parent, picks up the dart gun, and glares at his parent as he begins to load the dart gun.

Parent: Robert, I can see you are really angry at me.

Robert: Yes! And I'm going to shoot you good!

Parent: You are just so angry at me you would like to shoot me. (Robert now has the gun loaded and begins to take aim at the parent.) But I'm not for shooting. (Robert interrupts before the parent can go on with the limit.)

Robert: You can't stop me. Nobody can! (points the gun at the parent)

Parent: You're so powerful no one can stop you. But I'm not for shooting. You can pretend the Bobo is me (parent points toward the Bobo) and shoot the Bobo.

Robert: (Swings the gun around, takes aim at the Bobo, and yells) Take that! (as he shoots Bobo)

The important consideration here is that the feeling is expressed and the child has assumed responsibility for both feelings and controlling behavior. This is a significant step in the therapeutic process of learning self-control and self-direction, and that feelings are acceptable.

- **When Limits Are Broken**

When a child is reluctant to abide by the limit and pushes the boundary, the parent does not threaten the child or extend a consequence to the next playtime. Choices and consequences should apply only to the current play session. Each play session should be an opportunity for a new beginning for a child.

When a child persists in expressing or pursuing the original behavior and continues to break an established limit, verbalizing an additional step to the limit setting sequence may be necessary. Before explaining this step, a caution is in order. Too often parents become overly involved in trying to force the acceptance of the limit and move much too quickly to implement this final step. **Patience is the rule of the day**. In most instances, the first three steps should be gone through in sequence at least two or three times before verbalizing the final step. This final step should rarely be used.

STEP 4. State final choice. At this point, an ultimate or final choice is presented to the child. The parent either indicates the child can choose by his behavior to have the item placed off limits for the rest of the playtime or presents leaving the playtime as the ultimate choice. This step must be carefully stated so the child clearly understands he has a choice and that whatever happens will be the result of his choice. "*If you choose to shoot me again, you choose [not to play with the gun anymore today] [to end our playtime].*" Limits presented in this manner are neither punishment nor rejection of the child. If the child shoots the parent one more time, the child has clearly indicated by action the choice to leave the playtime or to stop playing with the gun, depending on which choice was presented. In this process, leaving the playtime or having the gun removed is not the parent's choice. Therefore, the child is not rejected.

Children need to realize they have a choice and that consequences are related to their behavior. Therefore, once this final choice has been presented, and the child has indicated the choice by his behavior (either stops shooting or shoots one more time), the parent must follow through and see that the child's choice is carried out. Therefore, if the child chooses to break the limit again, the parent stands up and says, "*I see you have chosen to end our special playtime for today.*"

- **Situational Limits**

Taking Toys or Materials from the Playtime
This experience can really tug at the parent's emotions when a child begs ever so pitifully, "*Can I please just take this little car to play with? I really want it to play with my truck and police car.*" The parent's first reaction may be "Sure, why not? There are lots of other toys here and even another one just like that one." There are two basic reasons for not allowing toys to be taken out of the special playtime box. Limiting the use of the toys to the special playtime enhances the specialness of the playtime and facilitates the development of learning how to delay the need for gratification.

To a child's request to take a toy out of the playtime box, the parent could respond: "*Having that car to play with would be fun, but the toys are for staying in the playtime box so they will be here next time for our special playtime.*" This response generalizes to all the toys, thus preventing the necessity for restating the limit on the next 10 items the child wants to take out of the playtime box and shows great respect for the child with "*so they will be here next time for our special playtime.*"

Leaving the Playtime
Allowing a child to go in and out of the playtime at random during the session is not permitted. The 30-minute play session is a consistent structure the parent provides for the child each week. Children need to learn that they cannot run away from the responsibility of seeing things through and that commitment to a relationship means staying and working things out, especially when a limit has been set or the child has just expressed some angry or frightening feelings. Allowing children to leave the room and return at will can turn the experience into little more than a game. After the child has gone out and in a couple of times, the parent can inform a child that if the child chooses to leave, he chooses for the special playtime to be over for that day.

In most cases, the preferable procedure is not to allow a child to leave the playtime until the scheduled time is up, except to get a drink or to go to the bathroom. Usually a rule of one trip out for a drink and one trip out to the bathroom is sufficient. However, this cannot be adhered to rigidly because some children may genuinely need to go to the bathroom more than once. To help avoid this problem, parents should take the child to the bathroom prior to each playtime. A small pitcher of water or juice and a small cup or two for sharing can be brought into the playtime to be used for baby bottle, tea party, etc.

Time Limits

A 30-minute playtime is sufficient, and whatever time span has been communicated to the child should be adhered to. The parent should remind the child when 5 minutes are left in the session. Young children who do not have a clear conception of time and children who are completely immersed in their play may need an additional one-minute time "alert." These reminders help children to get ready to end the experience and give them an opportunity to complete the task at hand or to move quickly to something else they had planned to do. This latter behavior is typical of many children and speaks of their planning ahead in their play.

References

Giordano, M., Landreth, G., & Jones, L. (2005). *A practical handbook for building the play therapy relationship*. Lanham, MD: Aronson.

Landreth, G. (2012). *Play therapy: The art of the relationship*. New York, NY: Routledge.

CHAPTER 7

THE 10-SESSION CPRT TRAINING PROCESS

Utilizing a small group format, parents are trained in basic Child-Centered Play Therapy (CCPT) principles and skills. As in CCPT, CPRT is not focused on solving specific problems or a "quick fix," but rather is structured to enhance the relationship, in this case between the parent and child, with the parent serving as the therapeutic agent of change. Play is the primary way children express themselves and work through issues. Therefore, CPRT utilizes play as the means to facilitate interaction and enhance the relationship between parent and child. Parents practice these new skills with their child in weekly 30-minute special play sessions and report their experiences to the group.

The combination of didactic instruction coupled with required parent-child play sessions and supervision in a supportive atmosphere provides a dynamic process that sets filial therapy training apart from most parent training programs, the majority of which are exclusively educational in nature. These key training components are critical to the successful CPRT training process and cannot be overstated. The filial therapist's greatest challenge throughout the 10-session training—and it is a challenge even for the most experienced therapist—is balancing the parents' need for support and encouragement with the need to cover the training curriculum in order that parents learn the attitudes and skills necessary to conduct successful home play sessions with their children.

Weekly Parent-Child Play Session

The importance of the weekly 30-minute parent-child play session cannot be overstated; it is the essential element in the success of CPRT. The parent's weekly application of play sessions provides the structure for all learning and change. Parents are trained in the use of Child-Centered Play Therapy procedures in order to create an accepting and nonjudgmental play session environment in which their children can freely express their thoughts, feelings, and behaviors, within certain limits. The basic principles for the filial play sessions include:

1. The child should be completely free to determine how he will use the time. The child leads and the parent follows without making suggestions or asking questions.
2. The parent's major task is to empathize with the child, to understand the intent of his actions, and to understand his thoughts and feelings.
3. The parent's next task is to communicate this understanding to the child by appropriate comments, particularly, whenever possible, by verbalizing the feelings that the child is actively experiencing.
4. The parent is to be clear and firm about the few "limits" that are placed on the child. Limits to be set are time limits, not breaking specified toys, and not physically hurting the parent.

Because the parent's major task is to empathize with the child, the parent develops a new perceptual awareness of the child and her potentialities. Moreover, because the parent is taught to follow the child's lead, the child is free to express fully her own developing creativity and resourcefulness, and, in turn, experience the accompanying responsibility. For 30 minutes, the child is free, within appropriate boundaries set by the parent, to direct one's self, to be creative, to be bossy, to be silly, to be somber, to be serious, and to just enjoy the fullness of being alive at that moment without any fear of parental rejection. Within this potent context, change occurs within both parent and child, and the parent-child relationship is enhanced.

Although there are situations when parent-child play sessions may be conducted at the therapist's office/playroom, the emphasis is on helping parents learn to conduct these special play sessions at home with their child. Therefore, time is spent during training helping parents select the necessary toys and choosing a location for play sessions. The location should be one that allows for movement and a degree of messiness without the need for excessive limits. The therapist must emphasize the importance of establishing a consistent time and place to conduct playtimes. Our experience is that most parents have a great deal of difficulty with providing consistency in their children's lives, and finding a time to hold play sessions is no exception. Parents are asked to treat the filial play session "appointment" time the same as an important meeting with their employer—one that they would not dare miss! Since parents are expected to demonstrate the skills they have been taught **only** during the limited time of the scheduled once-a-week 30-minute play sessions, they are not threatened by the magnitude of having to completely change their approach to parenting. Chapters 9 and 10 of this volume provide more suggestions regarding helping parents plan for and successfully conduct the weekly play session.

Child of Focus

Parents are asked to select one child between the ages of 2 and 10 years that they will focus on during the 10-session training period. Because the focus is on the parent-child relationship, special playtimes are always conducted with *one* child and *one* parent. The therapist helps the parent decide which child would likely benefit the most from the weekly play sessions. In some cases, the child who needs the parent the most may not be the child exhibiting the most behavioral difficulties. Parents with more than one child often have difficulty choosing. The therapist addresses parents' concerns that invariably arise about other children in the family not having a special playtime and suggests "special" activities for the other children to be involved in while the parent conducts a play session with the "child of focus" (e.g., a relative taking other children to the park or for an ice cream cone). If both parents or caregivers attend the training, each one selects a different child of focus (assuming there is more than one child in the family) to conduct weekly play sessions with for the duration of CPRT training. In the case of an only child and both parents participating, the child receives a play session with each parent each week.

Although CPRT is typically utilized with children ages 2 to 10, the basic child-centered principles and skills can be adapted for infants and preadolescents. For older children, instead of a "play" time, more developmentally appropriate activities, such as baking, pumpkin carving, building a birdhouse, crafts, model airplane project, etc., are substituted, with the focus remaining on allowing the child to lead or choose the activity.

Training Structure: Balancing Didactic and Group Dynamic Components

CPRT is a blending of didactic elements with timely exploration of feelings and emotional reactions in the group as parents interactively share feelings about themselves and their children. *The expression of these feelings and exploration of their underlying dynamics in the group setting helps parents to develop insight and prevents emotions from building up and being acted out at home.* Therefore, skill and experience in facilitating group therapy, as well as expertise in play therapy, is essential for the professional contemplating employing CPRT. Filial therapists must have sufficient training and supervised experience in play therapy to develop the self-confidence necessary to effectively model and demonstrate specific play therapy skills for parents. Inexperienced filial therapists often have a tendency to be caught up in exploring parents' feelings to the exclusion of providing the necessary training. Maintaining a sensitive balance between teaching specific skills and exploring emotional experiences is essential. Exclusive group therapy is not the order of the day. Parents also need to learn new skills of parenting.

Filial therapists who lack training and experience in group facilitation often make the mistake of allowing a parent to dominate group discussions, resulting in the other group members feeling left out and unimportant. All parents need the opportunity to share. The group format and the time-limited structure of the 10-week model requires a skilled therapist to balance the didactic and dynamic components of the CPRT training. There are specific skills that must be taught, modeled, and practiced in each session to ensure that parents will experience success in their special play sessions at home. For the novice filial therapist, there are significant benefits to employing a coleader to help share the responsibility of covering the required weekly curriculum, while attending to group dynamics and individual parent needs.

Another important attribute for the successful CPRT facilitator is spontaneity and creativity. Parents are more motivated to learn these new skills when the information and skills are presented in the context of their own lives. When the facilitator can seize the opportunity to teach or reinforce a skill as an issue spontaneously presented by a parent, the potential for learning is enhanced. The potential for learning can be further heightened if the facilitator uses the opportunity to explore feelings and emotional reactions in the group. Encouragement of even the smallest success must be offered throughout the process. Generalizing a specific comment made by a parent to include the other parents' experiences is another important strategy the facilitator should utilize to maximize learning. Chapter 5 provides the reader with an in-depth description of the group process component and provides case examples to illustrate the process.

Group Format

The basic format is six to eight parents and the therapist sitting in a circle (avoid tables, which create a barrier) engaged in a discussion, with lively interaction among parents. Ten parents in a group is too large for the necessary supervision of each parent's weekly play sessions and places too many restrictions on group interaction, a prerequisite to effective group process. The group feeling that develops and group cohesiveness are important dimensions of the CPRT process. Therefore, groups are typically closed, with no new participants added after the second session. It is difficult for parents to catch up on the material missed in the first few sessions. CPRT training is also possible with an individual parent or a couple, and many times may be the training mode of necessity for professionals in private practice when getting a group together for training is not possible. One caution is that when couples are included in a training group, relationship problems may emerge in the sharing that goes on and the leader may need to work extra hard to keep the discussion focused on the training objectives.

Our preference is the group setting because of the group dynamics feature and the vicarious learning that is always available to parents; however, variations of the 10-session weekly group format are provided in Chapter 25, including the application of the principles and procedures of CPRT with individuals and couples. Other variations of the model consist of collapsing the 10 sessions into 5 weeks, with twice-per-week group training sessions, and an intensive application of the model in which sessions are held daily (specifically for use in shelters and other "in-patient" settings where parents and children are living for short periods of time). Also described is an intense 1-weekend model, as well as a researched modification of the 10-session model in which the curriculum is taught during 4-hour blocks over 4 weekends.

Training Format

Lengthy lectures are avoided and, as often as possible, the focus is kept on the parents. In addition to the set training curriculum, teaching points and training information are carefully introduced in connection with spontaneously expressed parent concerns about their children. This interspersing of information in the context of parents' current struggles results in the information being received and incorporated by parents in a more meaningful manner. Solutions to concerns and new ways to respond to children often originate within the group. Homework assignments are given at each session to help maintain involvement between sessions. Therapists are cautioned against overwhelming parents with homework or the amount of content presented during a session. Homework assignments are faithfully reviewed at the beginning of the following session to communicate to parents the importance of these assignments. Experiential activities, including demonstrations, role-play, and supervision of video-recording home play sessions are crucial to parents' success in learning the skills and are utilized liberally throughout each training session.

Supervision Format

An essential component of this model is the structure and provision of supervision, particularly the requirement for parents to video their play sessions for supervision purposes. One to two parents are scheduled each week to bring their video for viewing in the group. Preferably, the therapist arranges for the assigned parents to come to the clinic or office playroom for video; however, most parents have video cameras and can record their play sessions at home (although the chance of equipment problems or parents "forgetting" to video are greater with home sessions). There is no substitute for parents being able to view themselves and each other; the opportunity for vicarious learning is unparalleled. The ability to view parents' skills firsthand is invaluable to the therapist, and most importantly, provides the opportunity for accurate and supportive feedback.

Essential Training Elements

Our approach emphasizes the vital importance of parents experiencing success in order to gain confidence in their new role. **We carefully structure training experiences to ensure that parents feel successful and prepared to implement the new skills they are learning.** Although Chapter 5 describes the following training features in detail, we consider these six elements so important to the overall success of training that they are briefly summarized here.

1. CPRT is a strength-based parent training model, rather than a problem-focused approach. Parents are encouraged to focus on their children's strengths, as well as their own, and to build on those strengths. The focus is on the future and developing potential rather than trying to correct the past.
2. The importance of parents learning and practicing the required CCPT skills during the weekly parent training sessions cannot be overemphasized. In order for parents to feel prepared to begin their weekly playtimes with their children, we follow the **3 Ds: Describe, Demonstrate, and Do.** We first *describe* the skill, then *demonstrate* the skill through video and live example, followed by having parents *do* what they saw in the demonstration through role-play.
3. Parents are asked to practice the skills they are learning only during a weekly 30-minute special playtime. They are not asked or expected to completely change the way in which

they interact with their children; in fact, they are initially told specifically not to practice these skills outside of the playtime. This avoids the sense of failure that would inevitably ensue if parents were expected to utilize these new skills in all their interactions with their children. Typically, as parents gain confidence in their skills, they will gradually begin to spontaneously and successfully utilize their new skills outside of the play sessions.

4. Considerable focus is placed on helping parents select the time and place they will conduct the play sessions each week, focusing on helping them commit to a set time when they are not likely to be stressed or hurried and can be emotionally available to the child.
5. The combination of didactic instruction within a supportive group atmosphere provides parents an experience of safety, support, and encouragement. This type of environment is critical in order for parents to express their vulnerabilities, share their failures as parents, and begin to take risks that promote growth and change.
6. Supervision of parents' video and/or live play sessions holds parents accountable for learning and allows them to receive accurate and supportive feedback from the CPRT/filial therapist and the other group members within a meaningful context.

Selection of Parents

The research on this model (see Chapter 26) supports its use with diverse populations and a broad range of presenting issues, including incarcerated mothers, incarcerated fathers, mothers residing in a domestic violence shelter, immigrant Chinese parents, Native American parents, nonoffending parents of sexually abused children, parents of chronically ill children, and parents of children with learning difficulties, to name a few. The child-centered relationship established in the special play sessions makes filial therapy an ideal therapeutic medium for parents from different cultures.

The reasons parents are referred for CPRT training have been varied and have included many of the more typical child adjustment problems and parent-child relationship difficulties, as well as children who were experiencing behavioral and emotional difficulties. Even in well-adjusted, stable families, experiences occur that may result in temporary disruptions in parent-child interactions or emotional reactions on the part of the child that make it essential that the parents be especially sensitive to the child's emotional reactions and needs (i.e., birth of an infant; stressful academic difficulty; difficult to manage child; night fears; moving from one home to another; death of a parent, sibling, or close friend; a parent who is too involved in work and absent from home; loss of a job or major change in parent income; involvement in an auto accident). These experiences can result in children being fearful, anxious, or clingy, or they may withdraw or act out. Many parents do not know how to respond adequately in appropriate emotionally nurturing ways to such reactions or behaviors. Their natural tendency is to try to stop the behavior rather than to try to understand the child.

Many parents attend CPRT training groups simply because they want to be better parents. A recent trend in filial attendees is grandparents (and other relatives) who have recently received custody of their grandchildren. Several affluent families have sent their live-in nannies to learn how to conduct the special play sessions. Recently, a young nanny in her early 20s was enrolled by the parents of a 14-month-old who were concerned that the nanny be sensitive to the emotional development and needs of their child. She did a superb job of responding empathically to the 14-month-old in their scheduled play sessions, which were video-recorded for critique in the weekly parent group sessions. One 6-month-pregnant mother-to-be signed up for the training because she wanted "to get an early start on practicing the special play techniques." She borrowed a friend's child to practice on during the training period and was one of the most excited parents in the group. A couple expecting for the first time enrolled in another group, and both parents-to-be had weekly play sessions in their own home with the children of a relative. The parents of a 5-year-old girl sought out the training because they felt it was important for the father to build a relationship bond with his child before he began serving a prison sentence. CPRT can be a preventative approach that can be helpful for all families, not just those experiencing severe problems.

The overwhelmingly positive findings on the research for this model suggest that CPRT is a more effective intervention than traditional play therapy, and in a shorter amount of time. However, clinical rationale would prohibit the use of CPRT with all parents and children. A thorough background history and initial intake screening is essential. Parents who are experiencing severe depression or other severe emotional issues, abusing drugs and alcohol, out of touch with reality, or have a history of abusive behavior would not be appropriate candidates for a CPRT group. Parents who are experiencing a significant amount of personal distress including marital/partner conflict often have difficulty focusing on the needs of their children. In this case, parents often need to undertake their own therapy before they are capable of learning and facilitating the skills of therapeutic play with their children. Also, as most child therapists have experienced, many parents are unwilling or unmotivated to participate in their child's therapy. Issues of guilt, resentment, time, money, and effort are just a few of the reasons for nonparticipation by parents.

In addition to parental issues that prohibit participation in filial play therapy training, a child may not be best suited for this approach. On occasion, a child's emotional issues might extend beyond the capability of the parent. In a case where a child is significantly emotionally disturbed, a parent may not be able to provide a child with an effective therapeutic experience. Yet, research supports that if a child and a parent are both firm candidates, filial therapy would be the treatment of choice (Bratton, Ray, Rhine, & Jones, 2005).

Practical/Logistical Issues

Marketing CPRT

Over the years, we have used several terms interchangeably to market the 10-session model to parents, because the term filial therapy was not familiar. Marketing this program as C-P-R Training met with the most success, hence that title stuck. We also liked the play on the term "CPR," as parents readily identified that term as a method of saving a life. Similarly, we believe that the application of filial therapy training can save the child emotionally. Examples of marketing strategies, including a flyer, article, and brochure, are included in Bratton and Landreth's (2019) *Child-Parent Relationship Therapy (CPRT) Treatment Manual: An Evidence-Based 10-Session Filial Therapy Model for Training Parents, 2nd Edition,* published by Routledge.

Initial Parent Intake

We recommend meeting with individual parents prior to the first group session for several reasons—most notably, screening for group membership. Other goals of the parent intake are (a) developing rapport, (b) addressing parent questions about CPRT training and how it can benefit both parent and child, (c) establishing fees, (d) administering assessments, (e) gathering background information, and (f) obtaining informed consent. A major objective is to help the parent select the "child of focus." We believe that conducting parent intakes prior to training contributes significantly to the success of the first session. The filial therapist is freed from the majority of administrative responsibilities and can focus full attention on group process and training elements.

Training Setting

The optimal setting for conducting the training is a play therapy room in a clinic with a two-way mirror and a space for providing child care for the children of the parents in the group. This type of setting allows for live demonstrations, observations, and role-play. Critiquing trainee videos of their parent training sessions is an excellent methodology for developing trainee skills and insight. A TV monitor may be needed if the training group is larger.

Child Care

Providing child care is important, particularly for single parents who often lack financial resources and/or the necessary support systems to assist in caring for their child while they attend training. Children seem to enjoy coming to the clinic and seeing where their parents are coming to learn "special ways of playing with them." Providing child care on-site also allows the therapist to conduct live demonstrations for parents to observe play session skills first-hand. Because of the length of the training groups, snacks should be provided for the children. In some cases, with disadvantaged families, we have provided a light meal for children and parents.

Goals and Objectives

The overall goal of CPRT is to enhance and strengthen the parent-child relationship. Consistent with the principles of Child-Centered

Play Therapy, **the relationship is viewed as the vehicle for the process of change.** Therefore, the objective is to help the parent relate to the child in ways that will release the child's inner directional, constructive, forward-moving, creative, self-healing power. Overall, therapeutic goals for children include a reduction of symptoms, development of coping strategies, an increase in positive feelings of self-worth and confidence, and a more positive perception of parents. Broad therapeutic goals for parents include a greater sensitivity to their children's emotional worlds, more positive perceptions of their children, and the development of more effective parenting skills. Specific goals for parents and children, as well as the family, are as follows.

Goals for Parents

- Increase their understanding, acceptance, and sensitivity to their children, particularly their emotional worlds.
- Learn Child-Centered Play Therapy principles and skills.
- Learn how to encourage their children's self-direction, self-responsibility, and self-reliance.
- Develop more realistic and tolerant perceptions and attitudes toward self and child.
- Gain insight into self in relation to the child.
- Increase parental self-acceptance and confidence in their ability to parent.
- Develop more effective parenting skills based on developmentally appropriate strategies.
- Rediscover the "joy" of parenting their children.

Goals for Children

- Communicate thoughts, needs, and feelings to his parent through a medium of play.
- Experience more positive feelings of self-respect, self-worth, confidence, and competence through feeling accepted, understood, and valued.
- Change any negative perceptions of the parent's feelings, attitudes, and behavior through increased trust and sense of security.
- Reduce or eliminate problematic (self-defeating) behavior.

- Develop an internal locus of control (self-control), become more self-directing, take responsibility for actions, and ultimately choose more appropriate ways to express needs and get needs met.
- Develop effective problem-solving skills.

Goals for Parent-Child Relationship

- Strengthen the parent-child relationship and foster a sense of trust, security, and closeness for both parent and child.
- Improve family interactions and expression of affection.
- Increase level of playfulness and enjoyment between parent and child.
- Improve coping and problem solving.

Follow-Up Training Session

Parents briefly share their experiences in their play sessions since the last meeting, focusing on changes they have observed in themselves and in their children. The therapist utilizes this sharing time to briefly review the basic filial principles, but the primary aim is to encourage and support each parent's growth since the beginning of training. Generalizing play session skills to typical parenting struggles is also emphasized. Parents are asked for examples of when they have used their new skills successfully. If there is enough interest, another follow-up training session can be scheduled to be held in 2–3 months. Parents who are interested again address a postcard to be mailed as a reminder.

Case Study

Chapters 8 through 17 provide detailed descriptions of content and material for each of the 10 training sessions. To provide the reader with an opportunity to examine the 10-session therapy process as it was lived out by an experienced filial therapist and a group of parents, a partial transcript is provided at the end of each chapter. This is a rare opportunity in filial therapy literature to "get inside" the personal perceptual world of individual parents and follow them in their experiential journey through CPRT training. The therapist was Dr. Garry L. Landreth and the training sessions were held in a play therapy room in the Center for Play Therapy at the University of North Texas for video-recording purposes and to provide ready access to toys for role-playing practice and demonstration experiences. The CPRT training group featured in the transcripts was composed of seven mothers, all of whom completed the 10 weeks of weekly, 2-hour training sessions following CPRT methodology. The dynamics of providing CPRT training, dealing with unexpected happenings, responding to parents' emotional expressions, answering questions, the importance of being flexible in responding to parental needs, and the role of the therapist in providing therapeutic dimensions as well as training dimensions cannot be communicated in a description of the content to be covered in each training session. These dimensions can only be known by going inside a functioning CPRT group.

Excerpts selected from each training session focus primarily on only a few of the parents in the group to provide insight into the dynamics of the experience for individual parents and the CPRT process across the 10 sessions of training. For clarity, the following are the names and presenting issues for the "child of focus" for each of the seven parents (all names are pseudonyms): Debbie and 4-year-old Rachel, described as demanding and bossy (also mentions her infant, Josh, throughout the training); Sonya and 2½-year-old Jenny, described as fearful; Emily and 4½-year-old foster son Chris, described as abused, neglected, and angry; Nita and 3-year-old Jeff, described as acting out and having a low sensory threshold; Kathy and 4-year-old Cody, described as angry and acting out; Kim and 4-year-old Toby, described as developmentally delayed and diagnosed with attention deficit disorder; and Laura and 6-year-old Dawson, described as angry, demanding, and jealous of his 2-year-old sister. In each session, attention is focused especially on one mother, Debbie, to highlight her personal struggles, the learning process as she experienced it, her development of insight, and the dynamic changes in her attitude and behavior.

Case of Debbie and Her Daughter

Debbie was a married, stay-at-home mother with two children, 4-year-old Rachel and 3-month-old Josh. Her initial intake at the clinic revealed that she felt isolated, depressed, angry, and overwhelmed by parenting. The marriage relationship is characterized by lack of communication and inability to connect with each other on most matters of importance. Debbie felt as though she was parenting by herself with no support from her husband in efforts to parent. "I do all the parenting by myself. He undermines me. I put Rachel to bed at night, later she wakes up, he decides she is hungry and feeds her. Then she's wide awake and tearing around the house, and I'm supposed to take care of her." (Several years later, Debbie described this time as "the darkest period of my marriage.") She felt out of control and felt everything in the home was out of control. Many little factors seem to create an explosive situation. Debbie felt powerless to create the kind of home and be the kind of parent she would like to be because "I don't know what a home and family is supposed to look like. I don't know what is normal for a family. I have no role model."

She wanted a sense of peace and calm in her home but didn't know how to make that happen. "I have no building blocks to create a home. I have no routine in my life." Debbie didn't have a sense of home, didn't know how to stay home and create order and routine. "When Rachel was a tiny baby, I would put her in a car seat and be gone all day long. I would come home just before my husband came home from work. The house was always a disaster area."

Debbie didn't know how to build routine into her life, her home, and her children. Yet, she wanted this desperately. "I want to figure things out, to make my home better, to be a better parent. I need skills so I won't feel so overwhelmed and angry toward my children. I need to know what I am supposed to do. I'm hungry for information."

Chapter 23 provides a more in-depth assessment of the parent–child relationship struggles and the impact of CPRT on Debbie and her child. Included in the chapter are (a) an interview shortly after the conclusion of the 10 training sessions to assess the immediate impact of the CPRT training on Debbie and her daughter and (b) a 4-year and a 13-year follow-up interview with Debbie to provide the reader with an unusual opportunity to evaluate the continuing and long-range effects of 10 sessions of CPRT training as experienced by Debbie.

References

Bratton, S., & Landreth, G. (2019). *Child-Parent Relationship Therapy (CPRT) treatment manual: An Evidence-Based 10-session filial therapy model* (2nd ed). New York, NY: Routledge.

Bratton, S., Ray, D., Rhine, T., & Jones, L. (2005). The efficacy of play therapy with children: A meta-analytic review of treatment outcomes. *Professional Psychology: Research and Practice, 36*(4).

Guerney, B., Jr. (1964). Filial therapy: Description and rationale. *Journal of Consulting Psychology, 28*, 304–360.

Guerney, B., Jr., & Stover, L. (1971). *Final report on filial therapy for grant MH18264-01*. Pennsylvania: Pennsylvania State University.

CHAPTER 8

CPRT TRAINING SESSION 1: TRAINING OBJECTIVES AND REFLECTIVE RESPONDING

Overview

Parents are introduced to the basic premises and objectives of CPRT, emphasizing children's use of play to communicate their experiences, thoughts, and feelings. Training focuses on helping parents develop sensitivity to their children's emotional world through the skill of reflective responding. Parents are taught the essential "Be-With" Attitudes—I'm here, I hear you, I understand, and I care—as the way to nonverbally convey empathy to their children. Parents introduce themselves and their family and briefly discuss parenting concerns. The primary objective in Session 1 is to structure the group training format to create a safe and comfortable environment for parents to share, with particular emphasis on linking parents' experiences to help them see that they are not alone in their parenting struggles. This chapter concludes with the partial transcript of CPRT Session 1 for the group of parents introduced in Chapter 7 and illustrates the focus on group dynamics, with key concepts and teaching points skillfully woven throughout.

Materials

Suggested materials include: *CPRT Session 1—Treatment Outline*; name badges for parents; *C-P-R Training: Parent Notebook* (we suggest printing the complete parent notebook with 10-session training materials and homework in a three-ring binder for parents); parent information form with list of parents/child of focus/age, etc. (with room for additional notes); and Session 1 handouts and homework, including: *Session 1 Parents Notes and Homework*, *Feelings Response: In-Class Practice Worksheet*, *Feelings Response: Homework Worksheet*, and *C-P-R Training: What Is It and How Can It Help*. Additional materials include: *Life's First Feelings* video (video source and locations of segments on the video are found in the *CPRT Treatment Manual, 2nd Edition*) and video clip demonstration of play session skills of reflection of feeling and allowing the child to lead (optional).

> *Note: The* CPRT Treatment Manual, 2nd Edition*, that is available through the publisher, Routledge, provides the complete curriculum for CPRT, including detailed training session outlines for each of the 10 sessions, reproducible parent handouts, and additional supplemental handouts and materials for each training session. Included with the treatment manual is a companion website containing all parent handouts and leader's outlines for ease of reproduction of materials. References for supplemental resources to enhance training are also included in the* CPRT Treatment Manual, 2nd Edition.

Content and Procedure

Since many of the training points and skills listed in the procedure sections for each CPRT training session are described in detail in Chapter 6, "CPRT Skills, Concepts, and Attitudes to Be Taught," or in the transcripts at the end of Chapters 8 to 17 that describe the 10 training sessions, a complete description of a training point may not appear in the procedure section for each of the CPRT training sessions. The reader is reminded that the transcripts of filial therapy sessions contain only portions of the interactions in the 2-hour CPRT training sessions. Therefore, some of the material described in the training format may not show up in the partial transcript. Including a complete transcript for each session would have been too cumbersome.

Informal Greeting and Group Sharing

Session 1 begins informally with the therapist greeting parents as they arrive, distributing name tags and parent notebooks, and facilitating casual conversation between parents in order to begin to build rapport and connections. Remind parents that it is critical that they bring their notebooks with them weekly. As an option, refreshments can be served as parents arrive and fill out any necessary paperwork that is missing from their files (consent forms, background information, child behavior checklists, etc.). Prior to this first group meeting, the therapist should have talked with each parent, either by phone or in person. The goal of the initial parent interview is to screen parents for appropriateness for CPRT training, to begin to develop rapport with parents, and to briefly explain what CPRT training is and how this approach can help alleviate child and/or family difficulties (refer to Chapter 7 for more information on screening parents and the initial interview). At this time, parents can be provided with the handout, *C-P-R Training: What Is It and How Can It Help*. Ideally, all necessary paperwork will be obtained from parents prior to the first training session, either at the initial interview or, for those parents contacted by phone, by mailing packets to complete and return prior to the CPRT start date. If all else fails, schedule parents who have not completed required forms to come early to the first training. The objective is to take care of the majority, if not all, of the administrative activities prior to the beginning of class. *Allow approximately 15 minutes for this informal sharing time before introducing training content. This informal sharing is a weekly ritual aimed at helping parents feel supported and connected.* The transcript included at the end of this chapter illustrates how an experienced CPRT therapist who is also an experienced group leader facilitated group dynamics during this initial sharing. This kind of interaction would not be possible if the therapist had not met with parents individually and obtained necessary paperwork prior to the first group session.

CPRT Training Objectives and Essential Concepts

Begin by giving a brief overview of the basic premises that CPRT is based on. Refer to Session 1 handouts when appropriate, reminding parents to take notes about assignments and main points. The main points (discussed below) can be elaborated on or explained in simpler terms, depending on the needs of the particular group of parents. Refer to the handout, *C-P-R Training: What Is It and How Can It Help*, but do not overwhelm parents with lengthy explanations. It is not necessary to try to anticipate all the questions parents might have or explain the entire CPRT process. *Encourage parents to ask questions and use their questions as a springboard to emphasizing key points. Training points do not necessarily need to be introduced sequentially or all at once, and they are never delivered lecture style.* That would be boring to parents. Provide a bit of information here and there so parents don't get overwhelmed. Encouraging parents to ask questions helps maintain interest and enthusiasm. Ideally, parents' questions and comments are utilized to link parents' experiences and facilitate group dynamics, with teaching points interspersed as illustrated in the transcript at the end of this chapter. Major points are always more powerfully delivered when introduced at a relevant point in the discussion. *However, depending on previous group therapy and psychoeducational experiences, the beginning CPRT therapist may initially feel more comfortable adhering to a more structured outline; the CPRT curriculum allows for both structure and flexibility in presentation.*

The importance of facilitating a group process where parents feel supported, while presenting key concepts, cannot be overstated. **The Rule of Thumb for the day is "warm acceptance and lots of encouragement."** Recognize that a major strength for these parents is simply that they are there—their presence and willingness to take time out of their busy schedules communicates their love and care for their children. The following key concepts should be introduced during Session 1. Again, these points do not have to be delivered in order or all at once. **The ideal is to intersperse teaching points within group process.**

- **Play is the child's language.**
  Children use play to communicate their experiences, thoughts, feelings, and wishes. Although children use both

words and actions to communicate, **young children communicate more meaningfully through the concrete world of play and activity.** Play is more than just fun for children, they can also use play to make sense of a confusing or disturbing event and work through their problems. CPRT focuses on helping parents to be "keen observers" of their children's play. Learning to understand their **children's play provides parents with a window to their children's inner worlds.**

- **The goal is to prevent problems by teaching parents to understand what their children need.**
  CPRT training gives parents the tools they need to better understand their children—to better understand what their children are saying through the toys. When children feel understood, they feel better. There is a direct connection between how children feel and how they behave. **Children who feel better behave better!**
- **CPRT training strengthens parent-child relationships.**
  Parents are the most important and influential people in children's lives. A secure, loving relationship with a parent is the greatest predictor of a child's future happiness and success in life. A strong relationship is especially important in times of stress! Filial play sessions ***provide closer, happier times for parents and children—and build warm, special memories!*** Ask parents what they want their children to remember most about them 20 or 30 years from now.
- **Focus on the donut, not the hole!**
  The focus in CPRT is on the relationship (the donut—the good stuff), not the problem (the hole—what's missing, what needs to be fixed). The greatest strength a parent brings to parenting is her relationship with and love for her child; no matter how difficult the situation, the desire for a close parent-child relationship is a strength to be built on. The importance of encouraging parents by focusing on what they are doing right is critical to the success of CPRT training. Only then will parents be able to do the same for their child. The most significant growth in parents over the 10 sessions of training generally occurs in this area.

Note: Donuts can be served as a refreshment, allowing the therapist to demonstrate this concept by holding the donut up and asking parents, "What is the first thing you notice about the donut?" The majority of parents respond "the hole." The therapist uses parents' responses to emphasize that is what we do as parents—focus on the hole, what is missing—rather than the donut—all the good stuff.

Emphasize to parents that during these 10 sessions they will be focusing on their strengths and their children's strengths.

- **The goal is for parents to change what they do for only 30 minutes each week.**
  This element of CPRT training is what sets it apart from other parenting training models, with the idea that setting aside a carefully chosen 30 minutes a week to practice these skills will promote consistency and ultimately contribute to parent success. Emphasize to parents that they are not expected to change everything they do with their children. No one could do that! Therapists, who are also parents, can use personal stories to emphasize this point. Emphasize that it will be **the most important 30 minutes per week that parents will ever spend.** Parents committing to spend only 30 minutes per week of focused attention playing with their children really does make a difference! Research shows that these once-per-week special playtimes significantly improve children's behavior, significantly impact the parent-child relationship, and significantly reduce parenting stress (see Chapter 26). CPRT is based on the premise that as the parent-child relationship is strengthened, children develop more confidence and self-control, and, as a result, behavior problems improve.
- **Parents can learn play therapy skills and become therapeutic agents for their children.**
  Explain to parents that in 10 sessions they will learn the same basic play therapy skills that graduate students learn in a 15-week semester course. In this method, the parent is viewed as the therapeutic agent for the child, rather than the professional. Emphasize that parents will not be play therapists when finished with training, but that they will have learned some of the skills play therapists use to help

children experiencing problems. Research shows parents can be just as effective in learning basic play therapy skills (Elling, 2003) and just as effective (in some cases more effective) as professionals in helping children with their problems (Bratton, Ray, Rhine, & Jones, 2005). Explain that role-play and video demonstrations of play sessions will be used to teach skills. Reassure parents that they will have many opportunities to observe and practice before they start their play sessions. The filial therapist's encouragement and modeling of the courage to be imperfect is critical in this initial stage of training. If the filial therapist is a parent, using personal stories to report the therapist's own failures as a parent helps parents feel less threatened and more willing to take risks.

- **CPRT skills help parents regain control as a parent.** The idea of "control" is very appealing to parents. Our experience is that the majority of parents come to CPRT training feeling out of control as parents and feeling that their children have far too much control. They think what they want is to be in control of their children! *The therapist's job is to help parents understand that regaining control as a parent means developing control over themselves and how they respond to their child.* Let them know that the skills they will be learning will give them the tools they need to respond purposefully and effectively to their children in difficult situations. They will know what to do and what to say—that is what is meant by control. This concept is easily introduced during the group sharing time, as there will always be a parent who reports events that allow the therapist to respond, "Sounds like there are times that you don't feel in control," as a segue into discussing how CPRT training will help.

Emphasize that not only do these new skills help parents feel more in control, they also help parents teach their children self-control. To illustrate this point, introduce the **Rule of Thumb: Be a thermostat, not a thermometer, in your child's life.** *Respond (reflect) rather than react. Your child's feelings are not your feelings. When your child's feelings and behavior escalate, you can respond in a helpful way, rather than simply reacting and allowing your feelings and behavior to escalate, too.* In-control parents are like thermostats in their child's life. Out-of-control parents are like thermometers. They only react to what is there.

> *Note: You can introduce this concept by asking parents, "What is the difference between a thermometer and a thermostat?" Thermometers simply react to the temperature: the temperature goes up, the thermometer goes up—it doesn't do anything to regulate or help the situation (room temperature). On the other hand, thermostats respond to the slightest change in temperature, taking immediate action to respond in a way to help the situation (room temperature). Thermostats create an environment that is more comfortable and pleasant.*

Emphasize to parents: **In 10 weeks you will be different and your relationship with your child will be different!** (Modify the statement, if needed, to reflect the actual length of training.) Using metaphors, Rules of Thumb, visuals, stories, or demonstrations to illustrate points often helps parents understand more readily and, most certainly, helps them retain the learning.

Getting Acquainted: Parent Introductions and Selecting Child of Focus

Parents introduce themselves and describe their family. Avoid going around the circle asking each person in turn to share. In describing their families, parents are asked to select one child they will focus on during the 10 sessions of training. This is the child that the parent will have special play sessions with, one per week for 10 weeks. Usually the child of focus is the child most in need of help or the child to whom the parent is having the most difficulty relating. Some parents who have more than one child in the desired age range for filial play sessions, 2 to 10 years of age, may need help in deciding which child needs them most right now. To facilitate consistency for the child, **parents are instructed to work with only one child during training**. This strategy is also designed to insure parent success in applying CPRT skills, by focusing all their efforts on one child in their play session each week.

Initially, most parents are eager to have play sessions with all of their children, but the therapist must hold firm. Allowing parents to commit to conducting play sessions with more than one child per week is setting them up for failure. Most parents have difficulty in consistently conducting a 30-minute play session each week with one child, much less two or more. However, some parents can be very resistant to the notion that their other children will be left out. Suggesting that parents plan special activities of another nature (e.g., baking cookies) for children not receiving special play sessions minimizes resistance. Parents are instructed that they may start play sessions with other children at the end of the 10 weeks. Parents often need help in understanding that it is OK for one child to need them more right now and that the other children are learning a valuable lesson in delayed gratification. They, too, will get to have special playtimes with "daddy," but they will have to wait seven more weeks (for younger children, marking on a calendar is helpful).

When both parents attend a CPRT training group and have only one age-appropriate child, each parent has a weekly special playtime with the child. When both parents attend and there are two age-appropriate children, each parent chooses a child of focus. All play sessions are conducted by the same parent. Alternating sessions between parents interferes with the building of trust and the development of themes across sessions. Helping parents select their child of focus during the initial parent interview avoids lengthy discussions that detract from time allotted for parents to share what has brought them to CPRT training.

In their descriptions of their children, parents generally focus on the problems they are having. These descriptions usually result in strong emotions being shared. "I am so angry at my son! I can't stand him!" Such feelings should be quickly generalized in the group by the therapist. "Anyone else ever get really angry at your child?" This protects the parent and helps to prevent overwhelming guilt by **normalizing the parent's experience**. In this way, parents quickly begin to perceive that **they are not alone in their struggles**. As parents share, the therapist clarifies and reflects content and feelings related to parent disclosure, listening carefully for underlying messages that reveal what the child really needs, rather than the problem presented. The therapist must skillfully limit the amount of time each parent shares by acknowledging the parent's concern or feelings and refocusing back to the group. For example, "*Debbie, sounds like you really have your hands full, and we're going to be helping you work on that in your special play sessions with Rachel.*"

Use what parents disclose as an opportunity to explain more about the training and special play sessions and work in a few teaching points. At an appropriate point, introduce the **Rule of Thumb: The most important thing may not be what you do, but what you do after what you have done.** We are certain to make mistakes, but we can recover. It is how we handle our mistakes that makes the difference. (This Rule of Thumb and the accompanying story are described in the transcript of CPRT training Session 1 at the end of this chapter.) The therapist can use personal stories to effectively illustrate "Rules of Thumb" and other teaching points and hold parents' attention.

Beware of falling into the trap of trying to solve parents' problems. If parents could hear a quick solution and go home and apply it successfully, they wouldn't need to attend CPRT training. They can find lots of advice on TV, in magazines, and in books—advice that focuses on the problem. The problem isn't the problem! It's the relationship and the parents' view of their child that needs work, and that takes time—**there is no quick fix!** An effective strategy for addressing parents' concerns is to briefly let them know you heard their concerns and that you're going to make a note of that to come back to in a few weeks. (*Always write parent concerns down and do come back to them in Sessions 9 and 10, when the focus is on helping parents generalize their play session skills to specific parenting issues.*)

The therapist records details of parents' descriptions of their child of focus for reference during training sessions. These notes are also read to the CPRT group in Session 10 to provide a benchmark for parents to evaluate their children's progress and to provide a base for discussing each parent's contribution to her child's growth and behavior change.

Reflective Responding

Reflective responding is the primary skill taught in CPRT training, a skill that teaches parents to **listen with their eyes as well as their ears** and to respond empathically to their children, **without asking questions**. Parents use reflective responding in play sessions to communicate to their child what they see their child doing, what they hear their child saying, and what they experience their child feeling. Reflective responses provide a mirror for the child to see herself more clearly. Most importantly, this way of responding **helps children feel understood, valued, accepted, empowered, and capable**.

Parents are taught the essential **"Be-With" Attitudes—I'm here, I hear you, I understand, and I care**—as the way to nonverbally convey empathy and understanding to their children. These attitudes are the foundation that reflective responding is built on. The most skillful parent response will not be effective in communicating empathy unless the child perceives these underlying attitudes. The concept of parents "being with" their child, fully and without distraction, during play sessions cannot be overstated.

Reflecting Feelings

The most difficult aspect of reflective responding is helping parents identify and reflect their children's feelings, wants, and wishes. The majority of skill development in Session 1 is spent on the skill of identifying and reflecting feelings. Chapter 6 contains more information and examples for teaching the skill of reflection of feelings.

Most parents' life experiences have not taught them to value and express emotions. When parents first begin to identify their children's feeling, instead of reflecting the feeling, "*You look sad*," their tendency is to ask a question, "*Are you sad?*" Help parents understand that questions imply "I don't understand," while reflections are much more powerful and convey, "I'm listening and I understand." Reflecting a child's feelings communicates acceptance of feelings and needs, which in turn helps the child feel understood and helps the child better understand and label his own feelings. We have found that using the analogy of a mirror helps parents understand how this works. The parent is like a mirror for her child; the parent accurately "reflects" back to the child what she heard and saw in the child's face (labels the feeling); then the child can "see" or understand her feelings more accurately from the "reflection." The more often and accurate the reflections, the more understood the child feels. The mirror can be a powerful analogy to help parents understand that a child's view of self is essentially what is mirrored back by the significant adults in his life. Children whose mirror reflects acceptance, encouragement, and affirmations will feel accepted, valued, and worthwhile.

Children whose parents accurately reflect their feelings also learn by example to verbally communicate their feelings. Conversely, children whose feelings are unrecognized by parents can learn that the expression of feelings is not acceptable. Some parents will likely express concern that if they accept their children's feelings, they will be condoning unacceptable behavior. Even if this issue is not raised, it will likely be a concern for some parents; therefore, some discussion of the difference is warranted.

Life's First Feelings Video

This video is a dramatic illustration of the importance of reflective responding and helps parents understand and identify feelings. Have the video cued to the segment in the early part of the video showing the infant's emotional reaction when the mother shows no facial affect in response to child. (Video source and locations of segments on the video are found in the *CPRT Treatment Manual, 2nd Edition.*) Ask for parent reactions to the video segment and use their reactions to emphasize teaching points. Parents generally comment on the dramatic impact of the mother's non-responsiveness to her baby. These kinds of comments provide an opportunity to discuss the importance of parents' nonverbal responses, as well as the critical importance of children being responded to in a way that matches how they are feeling. Children perceive as much or more from what they see in their parents face as they do from what their parents say.

It is helpful to ask parents if they can think back to when their child was an infant (like the one in the video) and ask, "How many of you think it was easier to understand what your child needed at that age?" "How many of you enjoyed your child more?" Parents generally respond that it was much easier to understand their children's needs as infants and that they enjoyed their children more. Explore with them what has changed (they began walking, getting into things, saying "no," etc.). Point out that with an infant you spend more time looking into their face for a clue to what they need, because they cannot tell you.

Hand out *Feelings Response: In-Class Practice Worksheet* (depicts emotions of anger, happiness, sadness, and fear). Next, show the second segment of the *Life's First Feelings* video to illustrate a variety of emotions (the location of this segment on the video is described in the *CPRT Treatment Manual, 2nd Edition*).

The segment shows black-and-white drawings of different facial expressions and identifies the emotion that accompanies the facial expression. Ask parents to specifically notice the four feelings on the worksheet and how the expression of those feelings develops in the child's facial expression. Parents have the most difficulty distinguishing between sad and angry; therefore, more time focused on these two emotions is warranted. **Stop the video periodically and make observations and teaching points**.

Feelings Response: In-Class Practice Worksheet

The facilitator should read scenarios provided on the worksheet with obvious emotion expressed in voice and non-verbals, and then ask parents, as a group, to identify how the child is feeling. After parents have agreed on the feeling—for example, "excited"—have them write it in the blank. Next, ask the group to use the feeling word and begin with "you" or "you're" and make a short reflection of feeling response, "*You're excited*," or "*You're excited that Grandma and Grandpa are coming*." Follow the same procedure to complete the other three examples. Parents are then given the handout, *Feelings Response: Homework Worksheet* (see Figure 8.1), and instructed to use the format on the practice sheet to identify those same four emotions in their child of focus this week and make a reflective response for each emotion (being a mirror for the child's emotions). Remind each parent to (a) look into her child's face for a clue to what the child is feeling, (b) identify a feeling word, and (c) matching the child's intensity of feeling, make a short reflection of feeling beginning with "you" or "you're" and using the feeling word they identified. Parents are then to use the homework sheet to write down what the child did or said, what the child felt, and the parent's response. The importance of going through this step by step cannot be overemphasized—parents have great difficulty with this seemingly easy assignment. Remind parents of the importance of bringing the completed sheet to the next training session. If time permits, more practice on identifying and reflecting feelings is beneficial—parents have the most difficulty with this skill. A very effective training strategy is to find three or four video clips, each depicting a situation where a child is obviously showing a feeling. Stop the video after the "happening" and ask parents how the child was feeling and then help them turn the feeling word into a "you" statement.

C-P-R TRAINING FOR PARENTS

Feelings Response: Homework Worksheet - Session 1

Directions: 1) Look into child's eyes for clue to feeling. 2) After you've decided what child is feeling, put the feeling word into a short response, generally beginning with "you", "you seem sad", "you're really mad at me right now". 3) Remember the importance of your facial expression & tone of your voice matching child's (empathy is conveyed more through non-verbals than verbals).

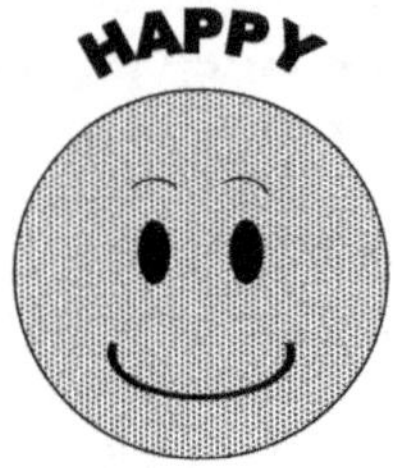

Child: *(what happened/ what child did or said)* ______________________

____

____

Child Felt: ______________________

Parent Response: ______________________

____

____

Corrected Response: ______________________

____

____

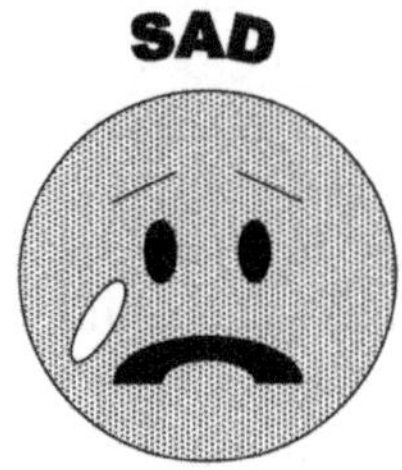

Child: *(what happened/ what child did or said)* ______________________

____

____

Child Felt: ______________________

Parent Response: ______________________

____

____

Corrected Response: ______________________

____

____

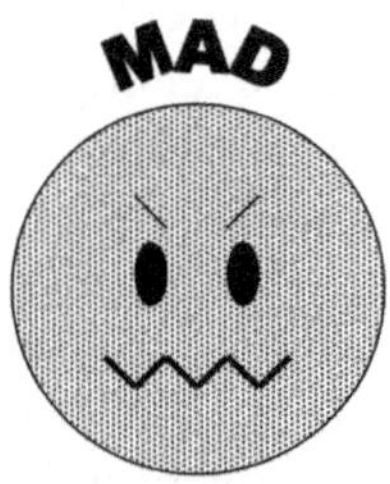

Child: *(what happened/ what child did or said)* ______________________

____

____

Child Felt: ______________________

Parent Response: ______________________

____

____

Corrected Response: ______________________

____

____

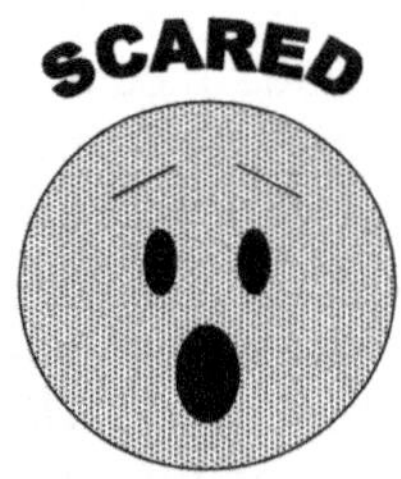

Child: *(what happened/ what child did or said)* ______________________

____

____

Child Felt: ______________________

Parent Response: ______________________

____

____

Corrected Response: ______________________

____

____

Figure 8.1 C-P-R Training—Feelings Response: Homework Worksheet #1.

Role-Playing Experiences

Role-play and demonstrations are critical experiences for parents. When working with individual parents or couples, parents can practice with their children, but the group format does not generally allow for the space or time to accommodate this activity. Instead, parents need many opportunities to role-play with each other, after first seeing the therapist demonstrate what they are expected to do. Coleaders are invaluable for this activity.

In Session 1, parents are asked to practice reflective listening and responding by first role-playing an adult listening to an adult. That assignment is generally less threatening than starting out asking parents to role-play their children. Allow time for parents to role-play reflective responding, and introduce the activity by saying, "Let's practice reflective listening and responding." Group parents in pairs. The therapist first role-plays with a parent volunteer to demonstrate reflective responding (or with a coleader, if available). Ask the parent to talk about something that happened at home this week with a child. *Ask parents to watch and listen closely to what you do, as this is your way of teaching them what you want them to do in practicing reflective listening with their parent partner.* Role-play and then ask parents to identify what they saw and heard you do. Parents then role-play. Ask parents to talk about something that happened with their child that week, and the parent partner is to reflect content and feelings. Listeners are instructed that they may not offer any solutions, suggestions, or stories of their own. After 3 minutes, parents switch roles. Then the group reacts to the role-playing. If time permits, a video clip demonstration of reflecting feelings and/or allowing the child to lead can be shown.

Homework Assignments

1. *30-second burst of attention.* Tell parents that you have a special homework assignment for them to do with their children—and that it will only take 30 seconds! Ask parents how many have had difficulty with their child wanting their attention at the least opportune moment; for example, when the phone rings. Generally, all hands go up! Explain to parents, "The next time your child wants your attention while you're on the phone, ask the person on the phone, 'Can you hold for thirty

seconds? I'll be right back.' Then bend down to your child and for 30 seconds focus your undivided attention on your child, prizing what your child is saying or showing you, as if that is most important in all the world to you at that moment. When the 30 seconds are up, let the child know that you need to finish talking on the phone and go back to your conversation." (See transcript of CPRT session at end of this chapter for a transcribed example of how to present this to parents.) Let parents know that this may not work all the time, but it does work for many parents. This assignment is offered in the first session because it is easy for parents to grasp and it really does work most of the time. This assignment also gives parents a brief experience of the power in providing for their children's need for focused attention. **Giving parents a useful skill to try after 1 week of training that has a high probability of success also encourages and motivates them to want to learn more.** Ask parents to report back next week.

2. Notice a new physical characteristic about your child of focus—could be freckle, shape of ears, etc. Explain that the reason for this assignment is to have parents practice becoming keen observers of their children during the special play sessions. The value in parents' simply noticing their children is not to be underestimated. Most parents will initially protest that there couldn't be anything physical about their children that they hadn't seen before. We have never had a parent who came back without finding something!
3. Bring a favorite picture of your child of focus. Instruct parents to bring in a picture that makes them want to smile, the one that most tugs at their heart when they look at it. Explain that they will share their pictures of their children the following week.

   Note: Most parents bring pictures of their children as infants or toddlers, which provides for additional teaching points for the following week!

4. *Feelings Response: Homework Worksheet.* Remind parents to complete and bring the following week. End by reminding parents to bring their C-P-R Training: Parent Notebook the following week and ask them for any paperwork (given at initial parent intake) that they did not return prior to class. Suggest

that if they haven't already told their children about why they are coming to CPRT training, they should tell their children, "*I'm taking a class to learn how to play with you.*" Optional: Close session with a motivational story or poem, which can be used to motivate parents to do something different *now* to make a difference in their relationship with their children, instead of looking back and wishing they would have done things differently. Parents need to leave Session 1 motivated to commit to the 10 weeks. You are asking them to make a huge commitment.

5. Remind parents of the Rule of Thumb for this week.

Introduction to the CPRT Transcripts

The partial transcripts at the end of the chapters that describe the process and content of the CPRT training sessions are from a single filial therapy training group with seven parents, no spouses. The therapist was Dr. Garry L. Landreth and the training sessions were held in a play therapy room in the Center for Play Therapy at the University of North Texas for video-recording purposes and to provide a comfortable and safe atmosphere for the parents. A secondary benefit of this setting was that role-playing practice and demonstration experiences could be easily entered into.

Excerpts selected from each training session focus primarily on only a few of the parents in the group to provide insight into the dynamics of the experience for individual parents and the CPRT process across the 10 sessions of training. In each session, attention is focused especially on one mother, Debbie, to highlight her personal struggles, the learning process as she experienced it, her development of insight, and the dynamic changes in her attitude and behavior. Chapter 7 provides an overview of Debbie's struggles and a revealing look into the dynamics of some of her child's behaviors. An interview shortly after the conclusion of the 10 training sessions affords an opportunity to assess the impact of the CPRT training on Debbie and her daughter. A 4-year and 13-year follow-up interview with Debbie in Chapter 23 provides an unusual opportunity to evaluate the continuing and long-range effects of 10 sessions of CPRT training as experienced by Debbie. This is a rare opportunity to "get inside" the personal perceptual world of individual parents and follow them in their experiential journey through filial therapy training.

The dynamics of providing CPRT training, dealing with unexpected happenings, responding to parents' emotional expressions, answering questions, the importance of being flexible in responding to parental needs, and the role of the therapist in providing therapeutic dimensions as well as training dimensions cannot be communicated in a description of the content to be covered in each training session. These dimensions can only be known by going inside a functioning CPRT group. These transcripts provide an opportunity to examine the CPRT process as it was lived out by the therapist and parents.

Partial Transcript of CPRT Session 1

(Group met in a play therapy room.)

Dr. L.: Let me tell you a little about this training and then I would like to answer any questions you have. My objective is not to change your life or change everything you do with your child, but to teach you in 10 weeks as much as I possibly can about how to structure a special playtime with your child. Play is important because toys are like words for your child and play is their language. I'll teach you skills that I teach my beginning play therapists on this campus, because I believe that what we do as a professional in this room, and what I do in this room with children like yours and other children, is helpful. So I am going to teach you what I know about play therapy. Not that you will be play therapists, but you'll have some of those skills so that when you have these special playtimes you will know how to reflect your child's feelings and communicate what you see your child doing.

The purpose behind that is so that your child will feel that you understand, that you are interested in what they do, that you are interested in them, and that you care. So, we'll be working on your relationship with your child. We have found that these special playtimes help improve children's behaviors. And then as we go along, we will work on some of the things that you are concerned about. Your special playtimes will begin in another couple of weeks.

I'll teach you what to do in the special playtimes before I ask you to have the special playtimes with your child. I'll do some role-playing here with you to practice new skills, we'll watch a video or two of my playtimes, and I'll let you see me demonstrate the skills with children like yours. Then you will begin your special playtimes at home.

I guess most of all I want you to know right off I'm not trying to change your life or that the things we do here you must go home and do every hour. I couldn't do that, I don't do these things all the time with my children either. But I will expect you to do them for 30 minutes once a week. Does that sound like something you could try, for 30 minutes?

I talked with each one of you a little on the phone, but you may still be thinking, "Well, I still don't know exactly what he meant or what I'm supposed to do." And I'd like to answer any of those questions if you have any.

Kathy: Will this help us learn how to set limits and improve our children's behavior when they're out with us?

Dr. L.: I gather by the way you are asking that question that's something that happens quite a bit for you.

Kathy: Yes, it does. Like last night, we went to get ice cream, and he ran behind the counter to choose his toppings. I had to run back there to get him. And sometimes some of the things he does like that I feel kind of silly. You know, having to go behind the counter and get him.

Dr. L.: Any of the rest of you ever have your child do something out in public that was awkward for you or that you felt a little embarrassed about?

Group: Yes.

Dr. L.: It happens to all of us, doesn't it? Children don't always do things just the way we would like for them to. I've noticed that and I'm sure you've experienced that, too. Kathy, the answer to your question is yes. One of the things we will work really hard on is called therapeutic limit setting. We won't get to that today. But we will in a few weeks, and I will teach you how to help your child learn self-control. I think that's what you're after.

Kathy: That's right. Like when I say it's time to come in off the bicycle, he doesn't think I mean it. His reward for being good is going to do something special, and then if his behavior hasn't been what it's supposed to be, then we don't go. How do we live with each other after that? He knows that will push my buttons. He just pushes my buttons until we fall apart.

Dr. L.: Until you feel like exploding.

Kathy: Right, and he does, too. He just gets angry and angrier the longer and longer we don't get to do it. But he knows he's not going to because his behavior hasn't been appropriate.

Dr. L.: Sounds like there are some times when you don't feel in control.

Kathy: There's a lot of times, a lot of times, yes.

Dr. L.: One of the things we will work on is returning control to you. Not necessarily always controlling your child. Because control means . . .

Sonya: (nods her head and smiles)

Dr. L.: Sonya, go ahead and finish that.

Sonya: Controlling yourself, or your reactions and feelings with a child.

Dr. L.: Because you will know what to do. When you know what to do and how to apply a new skill, then that gives you control. One of the things we will work on, Kathy, is how to help your child follow through without bribing.

Nita: (nods her head)

Dr. L.: You struggle with that some, Nita?

Nita: We go on spells. We have to use a lot of bribery.

Sonya: I have a question. So we will never actually have the children in here?

Dr. L.: Yes, once or twice during this training, I will ask you to bring your child to this room and be video-recorded in a playtime. The purpose will be for us to see each other. I'm going to let you watch me, and then after you have practiced your skills here and you're more comfortable, you will bring your child in here, and we'll make a video and then bring the video to one of our sessions for feedback. After the first three training sessions, we'll watch a parent play session every time we meet.

Debbie: What is the purpose of the play therapy? What's the objective?

Dr. L.: I don't expect you all to be play therapists, but I will teach you some of the skills I know so you will be a therapeutic agent to your child, you'll be helpful to them. The purpose of the special playtimes is to build a better relationship with your child and to work on things like teaching your child self-discipline. Your child might start throwing sand on the floor and sand is not for throwing on the floor; so I'll teach you how to set limits so your child will stop themselves rather than you having to jump up and stop them. It'll help you teach your child self-control. Are there some other questions?

Nita: I don't like to say I'm bossy, or controlling, but I am an over-functioning type of personality, and I see that a lot in my relationship with my son Roger. I'm really intent on becoming more self-aware and changing more things with me than I am with him.

Dr. L.: That's what we'll be working on. When I talk about returning control to you that means first you must become aware of what you do before you can be in control.

Nita: So we will address our behaviors and reactions, too? All mothers know children can just do things that can send you way off into outer space. If you weren't so busy and pressured, and could take some time to think about it, you might be able to think it through and understand the behavior. But in day-to-day life, it's not so easy. And really, I think my son's biggest problem sometimes is me. He's a lot like me, too.

Dr. L.: I hear what you're saying there about pressure, and one of the things I want you all to know is I believe parents are doing the best they can under the circumstances. Sometimes the circumstances are not very good, you have a lot to do. I heard you say, Emily, you have five foster children?

Emily: I have three foster, two biological.

Dr. L.: You have your hands full. My experience is that children don't always wait until we're at our best to ask for something they need. How many of you have children that are 4 years old or younger? When do 4- and 3- and 2-year-olds seem to want your attention the most? When you're doing what?

All: Cooking, on the phone, in the bathroom.

Dr. L.: It seems automatic, doesn't it? When the phone rings, that's when they discover something they must show you at that moment and no later. There is a little technique that you can use when your child must have your attention, like when you're on the phone. It's called a 30-second burst of attention. It works this way: You're on the phone, here comes your child and must show you their startling discovery right now, and so you say to your friend on the phone, "Excuse me, I'll be back to you in 30 seconds." You put the phone down, and you give your child 30 seconds of undivided attention. You prize what your child is saying or showing you, and then you say, "Thank you so much for showing me that, thank you for telling me that, now I'm going to talk on the phone," and you pick the phone up.

This will not work all of the time with all children, but it will work most of the time with most children. If you don't put the phone down and give your child a 30-second burst of attention, what will you do? (Parent demonstrates hand pushing away.) We keep pushing our child away for 10 minutes while we try to carry on a conversation and in the process we are rejecting our child, which is not what you really want to do. You don't want your child to feel rejected by you. So, better that your friend waits for 30 seconds than for your child to feel rejected. One of your assignments this week is to give your child a 30-second burst of attention and tell us next week how it worked out. You will need to bring a notebook each week to write down your assignments and points to practice in your special playtimes. Some of you don't have a notebook with you, so here's some paper to write on today.

Dr. L.: To get better acquainted, let's go around the circle and you tell us about your family, how many children you have, and what their names are. While you do that, begin to think about the child, age 2 to 10, that you would like to have these special playtimes with. I know you don't have time in your busy week to have special playtimes with five children. I ask that you choose one child to start with. Later we'll talk about adding a second child to have a special playtime with. Think of the child who needs you most or the child you seem to be having the most difficulty with, and that's the child we will call the child of focus that you will have your special playtime with every week, without fail. Once you start having your special playtimes, I'll ask you not to let anything interfere.

Debbie: I'm Debbie and I have a 3½-month-old son and my daughter Rachel, who is 4. She is going to be the child that I do my special playtime with.

Dr. L.: Tell us about your daughter.

Debbie: I think she is a sensitive child, but she is extremely strong willed, and I've gotten to the point where I am rejecting her as a person because I am having so many problems with not knowing how to deal with her. I have always thought if you just spank a child, they'll do what they are supposed to do and everything will be fine, but it just does not work. I have to learn what she needs. She would throw sand and go past her 30 seconds and onto the next minute, and she would tell me to clean it up.

Dr. L.: So she's demanding and bossy.

Debbie: Very.

Dr. L.: How do you react when she is bossy?

Debbie: Extremely loud. I become a 3-year-old, too. We're like these two kids that are having a fight, and it doesn't matter what I say, she doesn't do it.

Dr. L.: Sounds like you get angry sometimes. Do any of the rest of you get angry at your children?

All: Yes.

Dr. L.: Sonya, what is it like when you get angry at your child?

Sonya: Sometimes I yell at her, and I know I shouldn't.

Debbie: I don't know what to do. When we're picking up pizza at the store and she wants a toy, when I tell her "No" she just sprawls herself out on the floor and just lays there in a screaming fit, and I have a choice. I can publicly beat her, or I can ignore her. I'm feeling very frustrated and very angry. She's making a demonstration and there's something that has to be done. But I'm wishy-washy, and sometimes I'll ignore her or sometimes I'll have to leave. And I don't think that's right.

Dr. L.: So you're left feeling angry, frustrated, and defeated.

Debbie: Isn't she winning?

Dr. L.: Not the way we will work it out.

Emily: Have you tried to validate her feelings by saying, "I understand that you want this toy"? Then explain why she can't have it and then set up an odd job she can do to earn the money. Maybe that will increase her self-respect.

Debbie: I haven't got into the earning money because she just turned 4.

Dr. L.: So money may not be that important to her.

Debbie: Yeah, for the last 2 years, she has slept in our bed, and it is my husband's problem. I'm working with my own inabilities and also against my husband who thinks our daughter is a friend.

Dr. L.: So he has trouble following through with discipline sometimes.

Debbie: It just doesn't exist.

Dr. L.: Debbie, I hear several people reacting and the reaction is, "You have your hands full."

Debbie: That's why I'm here.

Dr. L.: And we're going to work on that. Let's go on. Nita, tell us about your family.

Nita: My name is Nita, my husband and I have a son who turned 3 a few weeks ago. My son was one of those babies who didn't get over colic until he was 4½ months old. He would cry an average of 8 to 9 hours a day, every day. He did not sleep more than 4 hours a day until he was 26 months old. So it is just his temperament. He is very active; he walked very early, and crawled by 5 months. He's very intense; everything is life or death with him. Always has been, always will be, I guess. He has a very low sensory threshold. I was so sure it was me and the experts say no, he is a more difficult child.

Sonya: When you say "low sensory threshold," do you mean he takes in everything easily, like sense of touch and sense of sight?

Nita: In order to get him to sleep, his room has to be pitch black, and he has to have a sound machine on. He will be half asleep, the sun will go behind a cloud, and he will sit up and say, "Where'd the light go, Mom?" He is real light sensitive, also about clothing and bright colors. He gets worked up so easily that he can't enjoy a lot of things. I have to protect him in a way, and he is kept on a very rigid schedule. If he gets off his schedule, he just disintegrates, and he gets a sensory overload.

Dr. L.: He feels out of control.

Nita: I'm a little concerned about his self-esteem. He used to be good about working on things and trying. But since we've been remodeling the house, and I've been in the hospital with this pregnancy, I've been getting more tired and cranky. He just seems to be giving up faster and saying, "I just can't do it, Mommy. I just can't do it!" I used to think that would not be a problem for him, self-esteem, but I'm beginning to think that's not as strong as I thought it was.

Dr. L.: So you're exhausted, the house is in turmoil, and he seems to be reacting to all of that. Kathy, tell us about your family.

Kathy: My son is 6, and right now I feel that sometimes he's more in control of me than I am of him. We're going through him saying "No" and "Shut up." There are a lot of things I don't like that he's telling me, like "I don't have to." I feel like he is stronger physically than I am. He's built a lot like his dad. We're in the process of a separation right now. And that's hard on him. I've got him for 2 weeks at a time all to myself. If I have my back turned for a minute, he knows what he can sneak into that will fire me up, and he will do it. He wears me out physically. He gets angry, kicks me, pinches, and scratches when he can't get what he wants. I am having a hard time setting limits.

Dr. L.: Sounds like you feel he is out of control.

Kathy: At school he has been mean and hateful, so they put him in time out.

Dr. L.: So whatever he's reacting to, he's reacting to it everywhere.

Kathy: Sometimes I lose my patience and I just yell at him.

Dr. L.: Let's work on that. Along the way I am going to share with you some **Rules of Thumb,** and there is one that really fits right here: **The most important thing may not be what you do, but what you do after what you have done.** I, like you, am an emotional person. You are not to go away thinking, "Oh, Garry Landreth does all of those wonderful things with his children all the time." I don't.

I do some of these good things some of the time when I can remember to. But there are times that I yell at my kids just like you yell at your children, and I don't mind you knowing that.

Let me show you how this Rule of Thumb works. I came home one afternoon and my wife had had it up to here with our 5-year-old daughter, and in about 30 minutes, I had had it up to here with our 5-year-old daughter. The next thing I know, I'm yelling at her. I have never taught parents, "Go home and yell at your children. It's good for them." I don't believe that. But, here I was doing something I don't believe in. And the next thing I knew, I was threatening her: "If you don't stop that I will. . . ." Does that sound familiar? Here I was doing two things that I don't believe in and I don't teach.

I blew the relationship right there; we had this big break in our relationship that afternoon. But I don't believe that was the most important thing that I did that day with my daughter. Two hours later, I was sitting on the side of her bed, and I said, "Karla, this afternoon when I yelled at you, I shouldn't have done that. I know better. But Karla, this afternoon, I was so angry at you, I couldn't think of anything else to do." She was lying there taking all this in. When I finished, she said, "Daddy, you could have said, 'I'm mad at you,'" which is exactly what I teach. And I had to be reminded of that by a 5-year-old. What did my 5-year-old daughter learn that day?

Emily: That even Dad makes mistakes.

Dr. L.: That Dad makes mistakes, and . . .?

Debbie: That you can say, "I'm mad at you."

Dr. L.: That you can say, "I'm mad at you," and . . .?

Sonya: To apologize?

Dr. L.: That it's OK to admit you made a mistake. Don't you wish all children and adults could do that? That's hard to do. And there's only one way our children will learn to do that. Someone must teach them by doing it. I believe that you are your child's best teacher. I want you to free yourself to use yourself more effectively. My daughter also learned that you can recover a relationship. The most important part of that day was the recovery of our relationship when I sat on the bed. I just described something important there. If you have something important to say to your child, sit down. If you stand in the room, the message to the child is, "She's not going to be here very long." If you sit down on the bed, the message to your child is, "She's going to be here for a while. I may have to compromise." If you stand up, they think, "She will leave quickly." If you sit down, they think, "This is going to take a while."

(Parents continue to discuss the Rule of Thumb and the implications for themselves.)

Kim: I'm Kim and I have three children, 4 years, 3 years, and 2 months. The reason I am here is my oldest son was born premature. He is in the early childhood intervention program. He has been diagnosed with attention deficit disorder, and he had real bad ear infections for 2 years. His speech has been diagnosed at 24 months. He's in physical therapy and speech therapy, and I'm going to help him at home, so he's going to be the child I'll be working with. My 3-year-old is extremely precocious and very smart. And she adds to the problem because she's way ahead, and he's behind.

Dr. L.: Tell us some more about what your son is like as a person.

Kim: When he had his ear infections, we thought he could hear us, but he couldn't. So he's completely in his own little world. Some of his symptoms are like autistic symptoms.

Dr. L.: Just thinking about him as a person, what is he like?

Kim: He doesn't have very good self-esteem. He's behind; so you have to look at him like he is at a 2-year-old level.

But he's large for his age, and he's adorable. You have to keep telling yourself, "He's 2, not 4."

Dr. L.: What else is he like?

Kim: He's real affectionate, real well meaning, and real sweet.

We have a new baby, and he's aggressive with her. But it's not to be mean; the doctors say his sensory skills are low, and he has to touch and feel his world.

Dr. L.: So he likes contact, and he likes to feel. What bothers you most about him?

Kim: His low self-esteem. I'm real worried about him, and my husband is real worried about him, too.

Dr. L.: How do you know he has low self-esteem?

Kim: He's very frustrated; he wants to do what his sister is doing. His motor skills are at about 24 months. I think he knows he is behind.

Dr. L.: So he's impatient with himself?

Kim: Very. You would think he was autistic, if you didn't know everything.

Dr. L.: The special playtimes will be a wonderful opportunity for him to learn to be patient with himself as you are patient with him. And as you are patient with your child, he will become more patient with himself. You will get a chance to work on that in the playtimes.

Kim: We were never taught to be parents.

Dr. L.: Sometimes that is frustrating, because nothing has taught us to be parents. It's just expected we will know it. In here, we are going to work on some things that are helpful for parents to do. Emily?

Emily: I have two biological children. They are 4 and 10. I don't have any problems with them. They are pretty good, well-rounded kids. I have three foster children, ages 4½, 6½, and 7½. I think the 4½-year-old is the one I'm going to concentrate on. He came into foster care after being abandoned by his mother eight times. Because of that, he has very poor respect for anything of authority, starting with the mother figure, which is me. He has been diagnosed with posttraumatic stress and pervasive developmental disorder. He is about a year behind chronologically where he should be functioning. He is an extremely intelligent child. He has been with us for 1 year and we will be adopting him in 1 month.

Dr. L.: You love him a lot.

Emily: I do. He is a special kid, and he can be a brat and a half. I think what I want to focus on is his anger toward his mother because of the physical abuse and the abandonment that has happened to him.

Dr. L.: What is he like on a daily basis?

Emily: He is a charmer, but . . . he's as big as our 6-year-old girl. He's a gorgeous kid, and he knows it.

Dr. L.: You said he's a charmer, but . . .

Emily: He goes through severe bursts of anger. I feel it's not the issue of he can't have a cookie after supper that night. It's more of an issue of at some point in his life, his mother didn't let him have a cookie, and therefore he pitched a fit and got beat up for it. And he tests me on a day-to-day basis. "How bad do I have to be?" About 6 months ago, he was peeling the wallpaper, peeling the carpet up. This kid has a lot of problems. I set the limits, I had followed the limits, and I had not lost my cool with him. When it was all over that evening and I said, "No matter how angry I get, no matter how mad you get, and no matter how destructive you are, I will always love you." And he said, "No, you won't."

Dr. L.: So it's almost as if at times he's trying to find out if you really love him. What I'm hearing most, Emily, is that you are understanding of this little boy. Even when he's angry and difficult to deal with, you understand that it's not necessarily you that he's angry at. OK, Laura.

Laura: I'm a single parent and I still like to say I have five children and one's in heaven. I have a daughter that's 15 and a son that was 9 that died January 1st, and a son that is 6, another son that is 4, and a daughter that is 22 months. Dawson, the 4-year-old, will be my focus child. The problems that he and I have are that I hung onto him like he was my last child and the 22-month-old came. She was my bonus. Dawson has a lot of anger and is very resentful of the time I spend with the 22-month-old. He is very demanding of my time. He is difficult to control. Sometimes he will just disappear out of the house at all hours and go hide under other trailer homes in our area. I put deadbolt locks on the doors of our house, but he can still get out the windows. One time he was gone for 2½ hours before we found him.

Dr. L.: That must have been a really frightening situation.

Laura: Yeah. When I found him, I just held him and cried. He has been a real challenging and trying child.

Dr. L.: What makes him challenging, Laura?

Laura: He tests me a lot, and I feel physically and emotionally drained after I have had to deal with him.

Dr. L.: Sounds like several of you have children who test you and push the limits a lot.

Laura: I know that if I stay with the limits and keep insisting that he abide by the limits, they will work. But it's really hard to do. I think that if a child knows you will give out or give up in 3 hours, the child will test you for 3 hours until you fall apart.

Dr. L.: That sounds like a frustrating and exhausting situation with Dawson. Is there anything he does that particularly bugs you?

Laura: He is very demanding of my time.

Dr. L.: I'm not sure you're saying this, but it sounds to me like you are saying, "I can never escape from him."

Laura: Sometimes he will even get into my bed or grab my hair to keep my attention focused on him.

Dr. L.: He wants all of you, and that's really draining on you. That's something we will work on. Sonya, tell us about your family and your child of focus.

Sonya: My name is Sonya, I have two girls; they're cute and sweet. One is 2½ and the other is 1 year old. I've been a single parent for almost a year now. The divorce is pending, but there will be no reconciliation. It's harder than I thought it would be. Being a single parent wasn't planned. Right now I'm concerned with the 2-year-old because I think she's trying to tell me something.

Dr. L.: And you're not quite sure what it is.

Sonya: Right. Sometimes she'll talk about being scared. Every once in a while she will get very clingy, and she's usually not like that. She is very articulate, and she does a lot of things that 4-year-olds do. We use time out a lot. We don't use physical discipline. Ever since we've been separated, there's no consistency in visitation. She loves her daddy, he's just not there, and he never really was very available physically or emotionally. It's hard for me to separate emotionally what's her pain and what's mine. I try to open up the arena for her to talk, but I think she senses that some topics aren't OK, like if she's missing her daddy or if she's scared or angry. She has started doing some things I am a little confused about.

Dr. L.: Seems as though you are trying to be all things to her, and that's not quite possible.

Sonya: Yeah, it makes me tired.

Dr. L.: It also seems to me that you are saying that you would like so much to understand what your daughter is trying to say to you, but she can't just sit down and say it. And that's one of the things I'm going to work on, to help you all understand your child's play behavior. For the 30 minutes of your special playtime, you will be a keen observer of your child's play. You will learn as much about your child as you possibly can through their play because play is the way that children talk.

They will act out the message with these toys. I will ask you to make notes about your special playtimes, and you will bring your notes here and say, "This is what my child did with these toys," and I will try to help you understand what your child is trying to say to you so that you become a reader of your child's play behavior. Let me shift gears with you. (Emily leaves the session.) It is so important that we notice our children. (Debbie leaves her chair beside Dr. L. and moves across the room into Emily's chair.)

Debbie: No offense. (group laughs)

Dr. L.: No offense taken. You can see better over there.

Debbie: You do look like Mr. Rogers.

Dr. L.: Well I take that as a compliment. I admire Mr. Rogers. Your assignment is to notice something physical this week about your child that you have not noticed before. You may notice a dimple or a freckle you hadn't noticed before. Study your child and try to find something physical you hadn't noticed before. My reason for this assignment is to have you practice becoming a keen observer of your children. When you start your special playtimes, I will say, "Now I want you to become keen observers of your child's play. I want you to listen to your child with your eyes." What your child sees in your face is also important. Let me show you how important this is. (Turns on VCR and shows segment of *Life's First Feelings* video showing an infant's emotional reaction when no emotion is shown in the mother's face.)

Nita: That almost makes me sad, because part of the reason I'm here is because when my son was younger than 2, I was tuned into him and able to pick up on his cues even though he screamed night and day, and now I can't do that. I thought somehow that when he got over all these difficulties that I would be more tuned in, but I don't feel as connected. Maybe you just don't connect when they're not nursing anymore.

Dr. L.: One of the things you will learn here is how to be more in tune with your child, and that begins by watching what shows on your face, because our children react to what they see or don't see on our faces.

Debbie: My daughter will say "Mommy!" and move my face to look at her.

Dr. L.: And that's the message I wanted you to get, that children react to what they see on our faces. The second assignment is to identify these four emotions in your children this week. (Dr. L. hands out the *Feelings Response: Homework Worksheet.*) Before we work on this sheet, let's watch more of the video to identify your children's emotions. (Shows more of the video depicting facial expressions that accompany emotions and stops.) If you saw that emotion in your child, you would let your child know what you saw in her face by saying, "*You're interested in that.*" As you see each one of these emotions, begin to practice responding in your mind: "*You're angry, you're interested, you're sad.*" Whatever the emotion is, start with "You" and then say it in your mind.

Let's watch some more of the video and you can practice responding in your mind to what you see. (Plays more of the video and stops.) Many parents mistake anger for unhappiness. The child in the video has been left, Mom walks away, and the child reacts with anger. The mom comes back and tries to make the child happy, but it doesn't work because the child is angry, not unhappy.

Debbie: I don't know how to differentiate between unhappy and angry.

Dr. L.: And I don't expect you to, yet. I'm just trying to introduce you to the whole range of emotions. (Plays more of the video and stops.) What I would like for you all to do this week is identify in your child the four emotions on this sheet. Let's make sure we are all on the same track. The first emotion on the sheet is . . .

Group: Happy.

Dr. L.: If you see your child being happy, how could you respond?

Kim: You look happy.

Dr. L.: You look happy. You're happy. You're happy about that. Have you noticed the word I start with almost every time?

Group: You.

Dr. L.: "You" points to the child and says, "I understand you're happy. You really like that." And the second feeling on the sheet?

Group: Sad.

Dr. L.: If your child is sad about something, you will say . . .

Sonya: You look sad.

Dr. L.: You look sad. You're sad about that, or you're really sad. I noticed, Sonya, as you said, "You look sad," your eyebrows squinted and feeling showed in your face. Remember, as was shown on the video, your child responds to what shows in your face. And, Sonya, you looked like you understood the sadness. (*The remaining feelings depicted on the worksheet are identified and discussed.*)

Nita: I just realized I do that, except, I make it a question and say, "Are you sad?"

Dr. L.: And that says you don't understand.

Nita: Why do I do that? Why do I have to put everything into a question?

Dr. L.: It's typical. It says, "I don't understand," and yet, you already know the answer. When you ask, "Are you sad about that?" you already see sadness. It is a lot more powerful to say "You're sad" than to say "Are you sad?" because the question says "I don't understand." There are four healing messages I will remind you of each time we meet, because we are going to work really hard on conveying them to your child. The first message is "**I'm here**. I am fully here. I won't be distracted." The second message is "**I hear you**. I hear your emotions. I hear your play"—and you hear that with your eyes—"I'm here. I hear you." The third message is "**I understand**." When you say, "*You look sad about that*," or "*You're angry*," you are saying, "*I understand*," rather than asking, "Does that make you angry?" Have you ever had an adult do that to you? You were so angry and they said, "Are you mad?" as though they had no idea you were mad. We want to communicate I'm here, I hear you, I understand. And the fourth message is "**I care**." If you communicate the first three messages, then the fourth one falls into place.

This week when you see one of these emotions, respond and reflect back to your child their emotion, sort of like looking in that mirror and reflecting back to your child their emotion. You're going to hold their emotion up to them and show it back to them by putting a label on it. After you have done that, write down what your child did and what you said. It might be "My kindergartener was really happy about the paper she brought home and I said, '*You're really happy about the happy face on your paper.*'"

Bring the faces sheet with you next time, and we will go over this assignment. Let's practice reflective listening. (Puts parents into groups of two.) The person closest to me in each pair, you talk about something that happened with your child this week. The other person is the listener, and you reflect what you hear. Here's the way it will work. Kim, tell me something that has happened in your home this week. You all watch me, and you will see what I want you to do.

Kim: My son took out a dozen eggs and decorated the kitchen floor with them. It was yuk.

Dr. L.: Sounds like a frustrating thing to have eggs all over the floor.

Kim: I overreacted. It was just a dollar's worth of eggs.

Dr. L.: You wish you hadn't reacted so strongly because it was only some eggs. What did you all hear me doing? I'm mirroring back what Kim is saying. Mirror back the words.

Now you try it in your groups. Listeners, for 3 minutes you may not tell anything that happened to you or offer a suggestion to fix a problem. (Parents practice in pairs.)

Dr. L.: Sometimes your child will play without saying anything. They're just playing in the sandbox. (Dr. L. scoops up sand in the sandbox and pours it into pile.) You would say, "*You're just scooping that sand and pouring it right there and making a big hill of sand.*" You just state what you see. That's called tracking. Our reflecting back is like what they see in our face. Let's change roles and reflect back.

(Parents practice in pairs.)

(Group discussion about role-playing.)

Dr. L.: I sense that you all want to learn everything there is to learn today, and I don't expect that. I just want you to try this on, see how it feels, come back next week, and we will talk about it. Next week, I will give you a list of toys to put together for your special playtime.

(Dr. L. ends the session by going over homework assignments.)

References

Bratton, S., & Landreth, G. (2019). *Child-Parent Relationship Therapy (CPRT) treatment manual: An Evidence-Based 10-session filial therapy model* (2nd ed). New York, NY: Routledge.

Bratton, S., Ray, D., Rhine, T., & Jones, L. (2005). The efficacy of play therapy with children: A meta-analytic review of treatment outcomes. *Professional Psychology: Research and Practice*, *36*(4).

Elling, E. R. P. (2003). A comparison of skill level of parents trained in the Landreth filial therapy model and graduate students trained in play therapy. (Doctoral dissertation, University of North Texas, 2003). *Dissertation Abstracts International*, *64*(06), 1983.

CHAPTER 9

CPRT TRAINING SESSION 2: BASIC PRINCIPLES FOR PLAY SESSIONS

Overview

The primary focus for Session 2 is to begin preparing parents to conduct their 30-minute home play sessions by reviewing reflective responding and familiarizing parents with the basic principles for play sessions. Next, the therapist emphasizes the importance of structuring and setting the stage for conducting a successful home play session, which includes parents gathering the special toys needed for their filial play kit and deciding on a consistent time and place to hold their weekly play sessions that will ensure privacy and freedom from distractions from other family members.

The partial transcript of CPRT training Session 2 found at the end of the chapter illustrates essential therapist skills needed to facilitate a supportive atmosphere while presenting key concepts and points to be covered. Important therapist skills and attributes demonstrated include encouragement and support of parents' initial attempts at reflective responding; the ability to balance parent support with teaching new concepts, spontaneity, and immediacy in presenting concepts in teachable moments; and a sense of humor. The importance of setting the stage for the first play session is emphasized, and the basic structuring skills of facilitating the child's freedom to decide and allowing the child to lead are demonstrated and role-played. Parents are reminded of the importance of conveying the four messages taught in Session 1: I'm here, I hear you, I understand, and I care.

Materials

Suggested materials include: *CPRT Session 2—Treatment Outline*; parent information form with pertinent notes on each parent (with room to add additional notes); homework assigned in Session 1, including extra copies of any homework worksheet; and Session 2 handouts and homework, including: *Session 2 Parent Notes and Homework, Basic Principles of Play Sessions, Toy Checklist for Play Sessions*, and an optional practice worksheet on reflective responding skills. Additional materials include: an optional display poster of the "Be-With" Attitudes, a sample filial play kit, photograph of toys set up for a play session, and an optional video clip that demonstrates structuring and setting the stage in a play session (creating an environment of permissiveness and allowing the child to lead). If a video clip is not available, arrange ahead of time to demonstrate with a child of a parent in the CPRT group.

> *Note: It is helpful for the therapist to make a demonstration video that specifically demonstrates basic CPRT skills that parents need to learn in preparation for their first play session. We do not recommend using a play therapy demonstration video, and it goes without saying that a play therapy client video would never be used for demonstration purposes. Alternatively, for therapists without a training video, therapists can purchase CPRT Parent-Child Play Session Skills Demonstration Video (Bratton & Landreth, 2019b) or show the last 5 minutes of the video* Child-Centered Play Therapy *by Dr. Garry L. Landreth (see CPRT Treatment Manual, 2nd Edition, for source information) or arrangements can be made ahead of time to demonstrate with a child of one of the parents.*

All handouts listed above, as well as a training session outline for the therapist, additional supplemental parent handouts, and resources for this training session are found in the CPRT Treatment Manual, 2nd Edition, *and accompanying Companion Website.*

Content and Procedure

This session begins, as do all sessions, with the therapist facilitating approximately 10 minutes of general discussion of how each parent's week has been, with a goal in mind of building rapport with parents, providing support, and facilitating connections between parents. This informal group discussion time also allows a few minutes for latecomers to arrive before reviewing weekly homework assignments and, in this session, provides the therapist an opportunity to model reflective listening and responding to feelings as a lead-in to reviewing parents' homework assignment to notice and respond to their children's feelings. This informal sharing time in the group provides an opportunity to check in with parents to see if anyone had a chance to use the 30-second burst of attention strategy. Since this skill is not directly related to what parents will be asked to do during their home play sessions, there is no need for the therapist to spend a lot of time on this activity. Remember, the goal in introducing this in the first session was to give parents an easy-to-use skill that they could immediately put to use outside of play sessions, generally with a measure of success.

As stated in Session 1, it is the therapist's responsibility to **find something to support and encourage in each parent's response** as they share about their week—when possible. Some parents' responses would challenge even the most experienced CPRT therapist, so those responses are best ignored! Continue to utilize the strategy of saying, "*That's something we'll work on later. I'm going to make a note, so I won't forget,*" when parents get off topic and want the therapist to give them a quick solution to a problem.

Reminder: it is very important to write down parents' concerns and come back to them in Session 9 or 10 when you are helping parents generalize their skills to responding to issues that arise outside of their play sessions. Your goal is to let parents know you heard them, their problems are important, you care, and you will address their concerns later.

Review Homework

Begin the session by asking parents to turn to the *Feelings Response: Homework Worksheet.* We have found that most parents have difficulty with this assignment; therefore, it is important to spend time reviewing the skill. The therapist must be encouraging and supportive as parents make their first attempts at sharing their reflective responses in front of group members by focusing on the part of a parent's response that was appropriate and ignoring the part that wasn't. For example, in the Session 2 transcript that follows, Kim shares her response to her child's happiness, "*You look happy there. Are you excited about that?*" The therapist offers encouragement and helps the parent feel successful by focusing only on the first part of her response, "I heard you begin with 'You.' 'You look happy . . .'" and proceeds to turn that part of her response into a teaching point. **Remember: Encouragement is the order of the day!**

A parent may share a concern that when she reflected her child's feeling, the child didn't respond. It's important to emphasize to parents that when they are using these new skills, **they should not expect something back from their children.** Explain to parents: "Your child probably won't say, 'Yeah, you're right.' But your child hears you and takes it in. Sometimes you may get a smile or a nod that lets you know your child heard you, but sometimes your child may just take it in and continue what she was doing."

A typical problem that arises as parents begin to use the skill of reflective responding is that some parents report that reflecting their child's feelings didn't seem to help. Of course, all parents would like to see quick and dramatic results for their efforts, but for some parents this is more of a need than for others. The therapist must caution parents to be patient, that **these new ways of responding therapeutically to their children are working, even when they seem not to be working.**

In essence, the therapist is asking parents to **trust the process**, when most parents have had no similar experience on which to base their trust. The therapist may find it helpful to use an analogy that parents can relate to, such as asking parents what they do when they cut their finger badly. Parents know from experience that although you respond immediately by putting some medicine and a bandage on the wound, it doesn't work (heal) immediately. But they would not remove the bandage and wash off the medicine after a few hours, just because the wound had not healed yet; they would trust that over time, by continuing to apply the medicine, the wound would heal. Their experience has taught them that they have to be patient and trust the process of healing; and the deeper the wound, the longer the process of healing. This analogy is used in the partial transcript of Session 2 at the end of this chapter.

For parents who are having difficulty identifying and responding to feelings, remind them, again, to first stop and think of the feeling word that best describes what they see in their children's faces and/or hear in their children's voices, and then take that word and make a short statement, beginning with "you." (Parents often get confused and depersonalize their attempt at reflection by saying: "David is really angry" or "My, *we* really are angry today!") *Remind them that beginning with "you" personalizes the response: "You are really angry."* The therapist can also demonstrate reflective responding with a parent volunteer role-playing as her own child or use a demonstration video clip to reinforce this skill (refer to Chapter 6 for more examples and strategies for teaching reflective responding). Typically, a few parents will not have completed this assignment or will have forgotten to bring their worksheet, but encourage them to participate by giving an example of a time during the week when they remember their child feeling ____ and help them formulate a response. **The message is that homework and practice are important—and you will hold them accountable!**

Share Favorite Picture and Physical Characteristic of Child

Next, ask parents to report on their second homework assignment, to notice something new about their child, a physical characteristic that they hadn't noticed before. Introduce the purpose of this activity by discussing the power of simply noticing and really *seeing* their child. Just by using their eyes, they can begin to know and understand their child better. This discussion can be coupled with having parents show their favorite picture of their child as they report on something new they noticed in their child. Our experience is that parents typically bring pictures of their children as babies or toddlers, which can lead to a brief but lively discussion of why that stage in their children's development holds more special memories than their children's current developmental phase. (Hint: fewer discipline problems and power struggles!) Sharing pictures is another way of enhancing parent connectedness in the group and developing rapport among group members. In addition, this activity focuses parents on children's strengths—what they love most or enjoy most about their children.

Filial Play Sessions—Basic Principles and Structuring of Play Sessions

The major portion of Session 2 is spent on helping parents begin to prepare for their home play sessions. The therapist begins this process by introducing the *Basic Principles of Play Sessions* handout. (See this complete handout in Session 2 of the Therapist Notebook in the CPRT Treatment Manual, 2nd Edition.) This handout introduces four basic principles that are critical to parents' successes in conducting play sessions with their children. Focus primarily on the four principles (*parents can read over play session goals later at home, if group time is limited*).

1. **Parent sets the stage.**
2. **Parent's major task is to empathize with the child.**
3. **Parent communicates understanding to the child.**
4. **Parent is clear and firm about limits.**

Goals of Filial Play Sessions

1. To allow the child—through the medium of play—to communicate thoughts, needs, and feelings to his parent; and then, for the parent to communicate that understanding back to the child.
2. For the child to experience more positive feelings of self-respect, self-worth, confidence, and competence through

feeling accepted, understood, and valued, and ultimately develop self-control, responsibility for actions, and learn to get needs met in appropriate ways.
3. To strengthen the parent-child relationship and foster a sense of trust, security, and closeness for both parent and child.
4. To increase the level of playfulness and enjoyment between parent and child.

Selection of Toys for Filial Play Kit

Next, the therapist introduces the importance of setting the stage for a successful play session by careful planning and preparation, which begins by collecting the required toys. The therapist provides parents with the *Toy Checklist for Play Sessions* and gives a brief discussion of the overall rationale and importance for inclusion of specific toys and materials within three broad categories:

1. real-life/nurturing toys;
2. acting-out/aggressive release toys; and
3. creative/expressive toys.

The Toy Checklist for Play Sessions in Session 2 of the Therapist Notebook in the CPRT Treatment Manual, 2nd Edition, provides a more detailed description and complete list of toys in each category.

Explain briefly that the toys included in the filial play kit were carefully selected because they provide opportunities for a wide range of expression, mastery, imagination, fantasy play, creativity, and activity. Caution against including mechanical toys that limit children's creativity. Remind parents that the toys collected for the filial play kit should be selected with safety in mind to keep limit setting to a minimum. Emphasize that toys need not be new; in fact, old is better! Lastly, inform parents that the filial play kit toys are to be used only during play sessions to convey the specialness of this time. Landreth (2012) provides additional information on rationale for toy selection criteria, but avoids lengthy explanations. Additional rationales can be provided as toys are demonstrated.

Parents need to see the actual toys they are being asked to collect. Be sure the demonstration kit reflects the instructions given to parents by including old toys, broken crayons, and inexpensive toys found in dollar stores. If the training sessions are being held in a play therapy room in a clinic, the therapist can point out the difference in quality of toys for the playroom (which are purchased for durability) and the quality of toys for the filial play kit. Under no circumstances should you use the playroom toys to show parents what toys they need to collect—parents tend to be literal and will think they must find the same quality toys. Playroom toys are generally far too expensive and many would be hard to find. Parents find it helpful for the therapist to briefly show each toy and explain the rationale for including specific toys, particularly the nursing bottle and the dart gun. These are the toys parents generally express the most concerns about including in the play sessions. As each toy is shown, this is a good time to briefly demonstrate how to respond to a child's verbalization or play activity involving the toy.

We find it helpful to be very specific in all matters related to toys by demonstrating such things as how to store the toys, how to arrange the toys, etc. A small, sturdy cardboard box with a lid, such as the type that reams of copy paper are delivered in, is free and can double as a dollhouse and container for toys. The deep box lid can be used as the dollhouse by drawing lines on the inside to designate rooms and drawing or cutting out windows and doors on the sides *(again, it is helpful to show parents exactly what you are describing)*. Toys need to be kept in a container that can be easily stored out of sight to avoid the child's wanting to play with the toys at other times during the week. The therapist can suggest a location such as the parent's closet or the trunk of a car to avoid conflicts over the use of toys outside of play sessions. In either this session or the next it is helpful for parents to see the filial play kit arranged for a play session. A photo example of a filial play kit arrangement is included in the *CPRT Treatment Manual, 2nd Edition*, for ease of copying for parents. Parents are instructed to find an old quilt or blanket to arrange the toys on, to serve as a boundary for the play area, and to protect the carpet. The therapist can also suggest that parents provide a cookie sheet or similar flat, easy-to-clean surface for children to use for playdough (to contain the mess) and to be used as a hard surface for drawing on.

The therapist will need to provide suggestions on places to obtain toys, emphasizing that they do not need to be new. Focus on sources where toys can be obtained at little or no cost to the parent, such as from attic storage, neighbors, relatives, garage sales, "dollar" stores, and toy aisles at grocery stores and drugstores. The filial toy checklist also includes inexpensive ideas for making toys or using common household items to substitute. Some toys on the list can be obtained from toys the child already has; however, parents are to make sure the child understands that **toys and materials put in the special playtime box can only be played with during the special playtime**. For an older child, parents can add more craft items. Adaptations for younger children are primarily related to safety and messiness due to lack of experience or coordination with art materials.

Unless emphasized, most parents will not understand the rationale for the toys being used only during play sessions and may be tempted to haphazardly pull some toys from the child's room for weekly play sessions. Remind parents that the requirement for a special kit of toys is very important to maintaining the specialness of the parent-child play sessions and for providing children with a variety of toys specially selected to facilitate their children's expression. Because **children use play to express their thoughts, feelings, and needs to parents**, the selection of toys is important. **Toys are the child's words!** This is also a good time to discuss children's need for opportunities to learn to delay gratification. The therapist can use this opportunity to briefly role-play what limit setting would look like in the case of the child wanting to play with toys outside of a play session: "*I know that you really want to play with the special toys now, but these toys are for our special playtime; you will get to play with them tomorrow right after school.*" The therapist ends the discussion of toy selection by asking parents to commit to gathering the majority of all of the toys listed by the next week's class.

Choosing a Place and Time for Filial Play Sessions

The therapist then introduces the second critical element in setting the stage for a successful play session: planning ahead for where and when parents will have their play sessions. Suggestions are made for suitable locations to hold play sessions—locations that insure privacy, freedom from distractions, and minimal worry about mess and breakage of treasured or expensive items. The location chosen is also dependent on whether other family members are home at the time the play session will be held. Ideally, play sessions can be held when no one else is at home, particularly siblings. In this case, the kitchen area is ideal, because it meets the criteria stated above and has the added bonus of having easy access to water for cleanup. If play sessions must be held when other children are in the home, the location must be in a room with a door that can be closed during the sessions. Locations to avoid are the child's room, because of the distractions of other toys, and the living room, where there are too many concerns about mess and breakage of family possessions.

The therapist emphasizes **the importance of consistency in holding play sessions on the same day and at the same time each week**, a time that the child looks forward to and can count on. This time should be a time the parent can commit to without fail and ideally will be a time free of interruptions from other family members. Consistency builds a sense of predictability and routine for the child; these are necessary conditions for children to feel secure. Play sessions should not be scheduled during the first 30 minutes after the child arrives home from school. Children, like adults, need time to unwind. Most importantly, the therapist asks parents to choose a time when they are generally feeling the most rested and patient and the least stressed and rushed, a time when they can be most emotionally available and free to focus fully on their children, without distractions. Introduce the **Rule of Thumb: You can't give away that which you don't possess.** *As your child's most significant caregiver, you are asked to give so much of yourself, often when you simply don't have the resources within you to meet the demands of parenting. As parents, you may be deeply aware of your own failures, yet you can't extend patience and acceptance to your child while being impatient and unaccepting of yourself.*

Introduce this analogy by asking parents what the flight attendant says when demonstrating the use of oxygen masks in the case of emergency (having one as a prop adds interest). Most parents answer that the flight attendant informs passengers to first put the mask on themselves and then put the mask on the child. Use this analogy to reinforce the concept that parents cannot help their children unless they first take care of themselves. With this in mind, the therapist asks each parent to give *careful* thought to deciding on a time and place to hold his play session and to report back the following week on what he has decided.

Role-Play and Demonstration of Basic Filial Play Session Skills

The therapist needs to make sure to allow time in the training session for demonstration and role-play of the skills covered in *Basic Principles of Play Sessions*, most importantly, the structuring skill of "allowing the child to lead" without giving suggestions or asking questions. This is a difficult role for parents to assume, because their experience as a parent is that it is their job to be in charge, have all the answers, make the decisions, and tell the child what to do. *Asking the parent to follow the child's lead requires a huge role shift for parents; therefore, much practice and patience is needed.* Remember that parents must first stifle their natural urge to direct and initiate before they can begin to apply these new skills successfully. Remind parents that the attitude of fully being with their children goes along with the attitude of allowing children the freedom to lead the play. Both are necessary elements for setting the stage for successful filial play sessions. Review the "Be-With" Attitudes: I'm here, I hear you, I understand, and I care.

The therapist helps parents generate possible responses to anticipated scenarios involving their children asking them for help, or wanting parents to solve a problem for them, or even the inevitable "Why is . . .?" These kinds of situations are pitfalls for parents to slip back into the comfortable role of problem-solver (refer to Chapter 5 for strategies and examples of how to teach parents to follow their children's leads and various responses to challenging situations). The therapist can either conduct a live demonstration with one of the parents' children (if on-site child care is provided) or show a demonstration video clip focusing on these skills. If time permits, it is helpful for the therapist to briefly role-play with a parent, with the parent assuming the role of the child. Parents are then paired up for role-play, taking turns being the parent and the child, practicing play session skills learned thus far. **(Role-playing should occur in each training session.)**

Homework Assignments

1. Ask parents to collect toys and materials on filial play kit checklist—brainstorm ideas and sources and suggest parents share resources.

2. Ask parents to select a consistent time and an uninterrupted place in the home suitable for the play sessions and to report back the following week.
3. Remind parents to complete a worksheet on reflective responding (parents are given several scenarios of what children have said or done in play sessions; they are to write their responses, practicing their reflection skills).

   Note: the *CPRT Treatment Manual, 2nd Edition*, contains sample worksheets.

4. Remind parents of the Rule of Thumb for this week.
5. Close with motivational book, story, or poem, such as *Love You Forever* by Robert Munsch (1986). This children's book provides a lighthearted, yet touching, example about the importance of the parent-child relationship. Parents need to leave this session motivated to begin preparing for their home play sessions. **In order for parents to be successful in their first home play session after training Session 3, it is critical that parents leave Session 2 prepared and motivated to gather the required toys and begin to plan for when and where they will have their play sessions, including making plans for other family members that will insure privacy and a minimum of distraction.**

Partial Transcript of CPRT Session 2

Dr. L.: Well, how has the week been?

Debbie: Pretty good.

Dr. L.: What made it a pretty good week?

Debbie: When I got home Monday, Rachel came in from day care, and I just did 30-second bursts of attention when she'd want my attention. I didn't go follow her around when she wanted my attention. In the past, she has acted like a little witch in public, and this time she acted like a little lady. We went to the awards banquet, and she sat and ate her cookies. She sat in her chair through the awards ceremony, and she was just an angel. It was unbelievable.

Dr. L.: Really different.

Debbie: It was really different.

Dr. L.: It sounds like she was controlling herself. She sat in the chair.

Debbie: Uh-huh, she did, and she had her little dress on, and usually that's just another explosion point.

Dr. L.: Disaster time.

Debbie: Yeah, yeah—embarrassing. And when she said "Mommy, this," "Mommy, that," I just gave her the 30 seconds of attention, and she would go on. That was the interesting thing; she didn't want anything more than just that little speck of attention. She just wanted to say something, and we enjoyed the awards banquet.

Dr. L.: Sounds like a really delightful time for you, and, I gather, for a change.

Debbie: Yes, for a big change.

(Nita enters late. She is 8 months pregnant and is carrying two pillows.)

Dr. L.: Come in, come in.

Nita: I'm gonna have to just get comfortable because I've been hemorrhaging again.

Dr. L.: Oh, bless your heart.

Nita: So, I just brought my pillows, and I'll just kind of recline. (She sits on the floor and leans back against a table.)

Dr. L.: That's fine. You just make yourself comfortable. I'm glad you're here.

Nita: Well, I wasn't gonna come, but I thought, oh, I hate not to come because we've had a really rough week, and

I thought you all wouldn't mind because I'm sure you've been in similar circumstances.

Emily: With the exception of Dr. Landreth, maybe.

Dr. L.: No, I can't say I've been there. (Group laughs.) Are you OK?

Nita: I'm OK, yes. It's gonna be rough getting to 36 or 40 weeks, so I almost feel like I need this more than ever. Because Jeff's starting to—

Dr. L.: He's starting to react.

Nita: To feel the tension. Never knowing if I'm gonna have to go to the hospital and not knowing whether or not there will be a nursery or a bathroom; we have our whole house torn up right now, because we assume that I will go the 40 weeks.

Dr. L.: So everything's disrupted right now.

Debbie: How many weeks are you?

Nita: I'm 32, so I have a good chance of the baby surviving, like 90% chance, if he were to come now.

Kim: I had one at 32 weeks, and he's fine.

Nita: How long did he stay in the hospital?

Kim: Twelve to thirteen days, and he went back after three months, but he's fine. He's huge.

Nita: Good, that makes me feel better. When they said he'd be about 5 pounds, I thought, "Oh!"

Emily: Still, 5 pounds is a good size for a preemie. It really is. A lot of full-term babies barely weigh 5 pounds.

Nita: It seems tiny.

Dr. L.: I hear what you're saying, though, it's a scary time.

Nita: Yes, not knowing is, I think, almost worse for us than if we knew exactly what we were having to deal with; it's just not knowing.

Dr. L.: Um-hum, I guess that's true in a lot of our experiences, isn't it? If we could just know what's around the corner.

Nita: Right.

Dr. L.: In this case, what's around the corner in the pregnancy, but also what's around the corner with what's your child going to do next, or, will it get any better after this? Well, let's check on what it was like for you to identify emotions this week. Did everybody bring their sheet with you? OK, what I'd like to do is go around and each one of you share with us what happened, and what you said in reflecting the feeling to your child in the first episode, the happy situation. Sonya, you want to start? We'll just go around.

Sonya: My daughter is Jenny. She's 2½, and for Valentine's Day I got her this big huge balloon. It's almost as big as she is, and it was a surprise when she got home from preschool. She looked real surprised and then, when she said, "Is that for me?" I said, "Oh, I see a happy face," and she said, "I am! I am!" and she was hopping up and down.

Dr. L.: So, she knew that you understood she was happy.

Sonya: Um-hum.

Dr. L.: And I gather, from what you said there, that seemed to increase her happiness.

Sonya: Yeah.

Dr. L.: Generally, when you're happy and someone understands that you're happy and verbally reflects your happiness to you and shares it with you, what happens to your happiness?

Sonya: It feels better.

Dr. L.: Yes, it increases. What happens when you share your sadness with someone, or if you've been hurt and you share your hurt with someone, and they understand?

Laura: For me, I am able to get rid of more of it.

Dr. L.: It decreases—that's very interesting the way we're made. You share your hurt and it decreases. It's less hurtful because somebody understands. You share your happiness and it increases your happiness because somebody understands. Debbie, did you get a chance to reflect happiness?

Debbie: I didn't write it down, but I told Rachel we would take her to McDonald's when we picked her up from school, and she was real happy, so I said, "I see you're happy," and she said, "Oh, yes, I'm happy."

Dr. L.: So she knew you understood.

Kim: My experience is the same. I usually don't stop and just talk to him. I could tell he was thinking, "Why are you talking to me?" I noticed he was happy, he smiled bigger. He was happier.

Dr. L.: What did you say to him when he was happy?

Kim: Well, we were taking cupcakes to school. We made cupcakes for Valentine's, and he was just bouncing. I told him, "You look happy there. Are you excited about that?" And he just got more happy.

Dr. L.: I heard each one of you begin with "You." "You look happy," which helps your child identify "this is for me."

Sonya: Jenny has just recently potty-trained herself, and I would tell her, "I am so proud of you," and so now, when I go to the potty, she tells me, she says, "I am so proud of you, Mommy. Thank you."

Dr. L.: What we want to do is give our children credit. They need to feel good about what they've done because of the effort they've put into it, not because of whether or not it makes us proud.

Kathy: We went skating, and Cody learned how to do an airplane with one foot. I was real proud of him for learning a new trick, and I told him, "I'm really proud of you."

Dr. L.: I'm not a skater, but having tried it once or twice, I can tell you that took great effort. He had to work hard to do that.

Kathy: Oh, he did.

Dr. L.: So, instead of saying, "I'm proud of you," you could say, "You really worked hard to do that just right."

Debbie: So that's like what you told us last week about telling our children what we see them doing. "Oh, I see you're coloring that picture," and "I see you're doing this," sort of adds to what they're doing. Is that like giving them credit?

Dr. L.: Yes, you noticed your child. Since we've touched on that, let's go back to that first assignment. Your first assignment was to notice something new about your child. This all fits together. Your words say, "This is what I notice with my eyes, what I see," or "This is what I hear with my ears." You notice things about your child with your eyes. What did you notice about your child? Kim, did you notice anything new or different about your child?

Kim: Yes, I noticed that Toby pulls his ears forward when he's playing, if he's thinking about his cars or whatever. So, I took him to get his ears checked Friday morning, and the doctor said they're clear; so, it's just a character trait. He pulls his ears forward and she said, well, a lot of little boys do that, pull their ears forward. I never noticed that before.

Dr. L.: I hear a very sensitive mom in what you described. You noticed something you needed to check out. Sonya, what did you notice?

Sonya: While I was trimming Jenny's toenails, I noticed how really pretty her feet are. Her younger sister has Fred Flintstone feet. They're square, but Jenny's are really pretty. I had never really noticed her feet.

Dr. L.: But, this time, you did. You took them in. You appreciated her feet.

Sonya: Yeah, they were pretty.

Dr. L.: And, the important thing is that we see what we're looking at. Lots of times we look, but we don't see. We just know our children are there. I hear you saying, "I really saw her feet."

(All parent reports of what they noticed about their child are not transcribed here.)

Dr. L.: Well, I hear some moms who have really studied their children. The important thing is that you study your child, because in the special 30-minute playtimes once a week, beginning in one more week, I'll ask you to study your child with your eyes and notice everything about your child and everything they do for 30 minutes. Well, let's go back to the sheet, and do the second one. How about sadness? Did anybody see that this week?

Emily: Oh, yes.

Dr. L.: Emily, what did you see?

Emily: It's real important for me to prepare Chris for events that are going to happen, and I was trying to prepare him for the event that he's no longer going to have a caseworker. That lady will leave. It will be another loss and separation for him to experience, and when I told him that Cindy would no longer be his caseworker, he just immediately began to cry, and I said, "Chris, that makes you very, very sad," and he just cried, and he shook his head, yes.

Dr. L.: I was listening to you and thinking, my, you really handled that well. You recognized his feeling.

Sonya: I noticed from the film we watched of the kids, a lot of times when I think my kids are sad, they're angry. That squared-off mouth look. We were getting ready for preschool, and she didn't want to go. She had started crying, and I said, "Oh, Jenny, you look so sad," and she said, "I'm not sad, I'm angry." I thought, oh, she's sad because we're going, and she was very clear that she was not sad, she was angry. I have been noticing since then with my little one, I think she's sad and I try to comfort her, and she's mad as hell. She pushes away from me, like, "Let me be angry," and when she really is sad, she'll allow me to comfort her.

Debbie: Well, our big dilemma is really bedtime. We're talking 2 and 3 hours of this debating and talking. You can talk about this until the cows come home, about her feelings and how she feels about going to bed, but the fact is, Rachel still has to go to bed.

Dr. L.: Exactly.

Debbie: But, that didn't change this week. That is one of the hard-core problems. Saying "I know you're not happy about going to bed" didn't change anything.

Dr. L.: And it's not expected to in one or two times. These responses work even when they seem not to be working. Let me explain. Have you ever cut your finger? You put medicine on it, a bandage, and 30 minutes later you take the bandage off. The cut is still almost exactly like it was; so you wipe the medicine off, throw the bandage away. You ever do that?

Emily and Sonya: No.

Dr. L.: You leave the medicine on. Why?

Sonya: Because it will slowly heal the cut.

Dr. L.: You assume it will eventually begin to be helpful. Have you ever gone to the doctor because you have a really sore throat or head stuff and he says, "Take this twice a day for 7 days." You take it for 1 day, you wake up the next morning and your throat's still sore, so you throw the pills away. No, you don't do that. Why?

Kim: You know you have to give it time.

Dr. L.: You assume that it's going to work, and it is working. You just don't see an immediate result. And with these responses, you won't always see immediate results. Some of you will see quick results, like with your daughter, Sonya. She even corrected you because you were trying to understand. It doesn't change the circumstances that it is bedtime, but, over time, Rachel will come to realize you understand, and she won't have to push so hard to get her message over to you, Debbie. We will work on the bedtime routine later. I'm going to make a note, and we will come back to that.

Sonya: Good, because I have problems with that, too.

Kathy: Good, good.

(All parent reports of their responses to emotions are not transcribed here.)

Dr. L.: Let's move on to something else. One of the things that we need to work on today is getting ready for your play sessions, which will happen not this coming week, but the next week. So I have several assignments for you. The first assignment is to put together a play kit similar to what I have here. This is a list of toys for the play sessions. (Hands out *Toy Checklist for Play Sessions.*) I want you to go home and tell your child, "I'm taking a special class to learn how to play with you, and I go to class every Monday afternoon. My teacher is teaching us how to play with our children, and he gave us this special list of toys for our special playtime. We're going to have a special playtime once a week."

Then, you get a box, it can be about this size (points to box), and ask your child to help you collect these toys. Some of them, your child already has in his or her room. If you select toys your child has, you will need to explain the toys will be placed in a special box and can only be played with during the special playtime. Other toys, you can borrow from a neighbor or a friend whose children have outgrown them. A few of these, you may need to buy, and I suggest you take your child shopping with you. You might find some of these toys in a garage sale. Let's go over the items. I want you to get playdough, and you'll probably find it in little containers of four, but you only need to put one of these out at a time. Put the other three somewhere else. Your child doesn't need to play with all four of them at the same time.

Sonya: You can't make your own?

Dr. L.: Oh, yes, that would be great. Make your own. How do you feel about your child playing with playdough in your house? Does that bother any of you?

(Brief reactions)

Dr. L.: If the place you choose in your home for the special playtime is carpeted, you'll need a towel, or a cookie sheet, and when your child pulls the playdough out, you say, "The playdough is for playing on top of the towel." You just set a limit. It can only be played with in the place you designate. Put some crayons together, and your child probably already has some.

Debbie: Like, how many?

Dr. L.: Just a few, six or eight, that's all you need. Sixty-eight crayons are too many choices. If your child has a bunch of crayons, choose some colors and break the crayons in two pieces, peel the paper off so the sides show, and break the points off the crayons. This will give your child a message that says, "You don't have to be careful." Points say, "Be very careful, be neat," and in this special time, your child can color with the side of the crayon. He can be messy. He doesn't have to color between the lines. You need some paper, and it can be like paper in your notebook there, or the backs of computer sheets, or some newsprint. Find a pair of blunt scissors. I want you to get a nursing bottle. If you have some tucked away somewhere, just pull one out of the closet. Laura, you're reacting.

Laura: Yeah, because Dawson was never a bottle baby, but last fall, I guess just because of different stressors, he wanted to suck on a bottle.

Dr. L.: And that will be OK for your child to do for this special 30 minutes.

Debbie: Really? Are you serious?

Laura: Yeah, he's serious.

Dr. L.: Some children, even 8 or 10 years of age, wonder what that used to feel like, and so they'll suck on the bottle. It is a quick way for them to find out how patient you will be with sucking on the bottle and how accepting you are during these 30 minutes. So, I really do want you to get a nursing bottle with a regular nipple on it. Your child may look at the nursing bottle and say, "There's nothing in there." What's your child really saying? "I want . . ."

Emily: A drink?

Dr. L.: Yes, "I want something in here to suck on," and you could say, "Well, we can go to the kitchen and get juice or water. Which would you like to have?"

If your child wants to suck on the bottle for the whole 30 minutes, he can. This is the child's time to choose. But, no other time.

Kim: That's what I was gonna ask.

Dr. L.: Whatever goes in this box stays in the box, and after the session, the box is put in the closet, or if you really have trouble, and you can't keep your child from getting into the box, lock the box in the trunk of your car. They can play with these toys only during the special 30-minute playtime. The reason for this rule is that it makes the playtime really special. The second reason is, and this may be more important, you're going to help your child learn how to delay their need for gratification.

Sonya: Jenny still takes a bottle when we're reading a story. We worked on her giving the bottle up about 6 months ago, and it was 2 weeks of hell. I decided I didn't have the energy, and I know I'm not going to wean her at this point. My question is, should I have a special bottle?

Dr. L.: Yes, a special bottle for the playtime.

Sonya: OK, I'll do that.

Dr. L.: I also want you to get a dart gun, something like this. It doesn't have to look exactly like this one, but these are probably easiest to find.

Emily: They've got those at the dollar store for a dollar.

Dr. L.: You all have small children, so your child may have trouble pulling this plunger on the gun back, that is hard to pull back, and it would be OK for you to help your child. In fact, you may even have to show your child how to pull that back. Kim, how do you feel about having a dart gun?

Kim: I just know Toby's gonna go for my 2-month-old with that.

Dr. L.: It can only be used in this 30-minute playtime, and the other children won't be around. Just you and your child, so you won't have to worry about another child getting shot with it.

Dr. L.: With this toy gun, you get a chance to teach your child that people are not for shooting. Your child may start to shoot you with it, and you get a chance to say, "I'm not for shooting," and then your child learns something really important.

This toy gun also gives you the opportunity to work on setting limits: "I'm not for shooting. The lamp is not for shooting." If you will practice that response ahead of time, you will be ready. "I'm not for shooting. You can pretend the Bobo is me and shoot the Bobo, or the plastic thing is for shooting," and you point to that. And they can shoot that.

Emily: Can you set the limit that, "I'm not for shooting," and if the child persists, say, "If you insist on shooting me, then I will have to remove the gun from the playroom." Can you set that kind of limit?

Dr. L.: Sounds great. We'll work more on limit setting later. You will need some toy soldiers, about 20 will be enough. Even 10 is enough. Fifty toy soldiers is too many, and the reason is, that's too many for you to pick up.

Laura: For us to pick up?

Dr. L.: I see you got the message, Laura. At the end of the session, you will pick up, because this is a special time, and your child uses the toys to express himself. The toys are like your child's words. Children use toys like words, and their play is like their language. And so, during this special 30-minute playtime, they play out messages or express themselves through play. If you say, "Now you have to clean up," then next time your child will play carefully so he doesn't have to clean up as much.

Your child may want to help you clean up, and that will be OK. If they don't want to help you clean up, that's OK, too. Helping clean up does not mean more playtime. A small cardboard box like this will serve as a place to store all the toys. Cut a door in one side and a window in another side. Draw some marks across the bottom like this and that becomes your dollhouse.

(All the other toys were shown and discussed but are not transcribed here.)

Dr. L.: Those are the toys for your special playtime. Now, let's talk about two other things. One, when you come next Monday, I want you to tell me the place in your house where you're going to have your special 30-minute playtime. It should be a place that's private, that will not be interrupted by other people in the house. If there are other people at home when you have your session, it will need to be a place where you can close the door. If everybody else is gone, it could be your kitchen. I do not recommend your living room. Use the kitchen or a den. Do not select your child's room, because all their other possessions are in there, and they will play with all that other stuff. The third assignment is to pick a time and a day for your special playtime and tell me next Monday.

Sonya: That will be kind of fun, buying all that stuff.

Dr. L.: I hope you'll be able to get most of the toys without buying new stuff. Used toys are better. So, if you can get toys in garage sales or borrow some from the neighbors, or pull some out of your attic that you've stored away, great—use that. Now, can we shift focus?

Sonya: Sure.

Dr. L.: All right, I want to show you a video of one of my play sessions. You will see me doing what I would like for you all to do. Let's watch the video, and then we'll talk about it. The child is 4 years old, and this is our first time together.

(Dr. L. plays a segment of a video that clearly illustrates the concept of allowing the child to lead, while he follows the child's lead.)

Dr. L.: (Stops video.) Now, let's talk about what you saw me do.

Debbie: You gave him space when he came in the room. You weren't crowding him, which gave him his freedom, or space.

Dr. L.: Yes, I let the child move away and settle in, and then I went over to be close to him. What else did you see me do?

Kim: You let him pick what he wanted to do.

Dr. L.: I let him choose. He's in the lead. This is his time to play with any of the toys that he chooses to play with.

Sonya: You got down to his level.

Dr. L.: Yes, I got down to his level. Don't stand. You will say to your child, "It's time for our special playtime," walk your child back to your bedroom, close the door, and say, "This is our special playtime, and this is a time when you can play with these toys in a lot of the ways you would like to." Sit down, sit on the floor. If you'd rather sit in a chair, sit in a chair. But then when your child settles in, show interest in what they're doing by moving to be close to your child. Lie on the floor and prop your chin on your hand, and fiddle with the things that your child is fiddling with, but don't take over. Your child is to be in the lead. Now, I'd like for you to listen to who leads the conversation.

(Dr. L. plays more of the video.)

Dr. L.: (Stops video.) For 30 minutes, you are not your child's answer source.

Nita: Oh, my child will just start saying "Why?" to everything.

Dr. L.: For 30 minutes, you are dumb.

Kathy: Just for 30 minutes? (Group laughs.)

Sonya: You use a lot of paraphrasing. When he asked you a question, you just said, "Gee, I don't know why." I've used that a lot with Jenny, and I'm real surprised at her answers and the joy of the answers.

Dr. L.: They'll figure it out. He's asking, "Why don't these rocks go through here?" I'm not sure I have a good answer for that.

Debbie: You wondered it yourself. You said, "Hmm, wonder why those rocks won't go through that."

Dr. L.: You caught it.

Emily: That was interesting.

Dr. L.: When your child wonders about something, you just wonder about it, too. You're studying your child so intently, and you're so caught up in what your child is doing, it's almost as if you are doing it, too. And when your child is puzzling about something, you're puzzling about that, too. He says, "Wonder why these rocks won't go through there." "Hmm, wonder why those won't go through there." As if, I'm trying to figure that out, too, and I am.

(Plays more of video.)

Dr. L.: (Stops video.) Who is leading this conversation?

(Everyone): He is.

Dr. L.: For 30 minutes, your child is in the lead. For 30 minutes, you follow.

Nita: When you describe what he's doing, is that to serve some purpose?

Dr. L.: Yes. Laura, you're reacting. Go ahead.

Laura: Well, when you acknowledge what he is doing, you're being a part of what he's doing.

Dr. L.: Yes, the message is to say, "I'm here. I understand what you're doing." Describing what your child does validates your child and the importance of what your child is doing.

Sonya: Isn't part of it, also, to say that "You're important to me." The things in my life that get my attention are obviously something I value that is important to me. And I would start showing my child that I value her and she's important to me.

Dr. L.: Sure, this is like the 30-second burst of attention. For that 30 seconds, you looked at your child and listened to your child. Now, I'm going to ask you to do that for

30 minutes. Describing or tracking what your child does says everything your child does is important to you, so that your child then feels important. You can't feel important, folks, until you're important to somebody. You must be important to somebody first. Nita?

Nita: I am a little confused. What if my son says, "You build such and such," or, "You draw a picture of baby."

Dr. L.: You stop, and you say, "Show me what you want done."

Nita: Mmm.

Dr. L.: Or, "Tell me what I am to do next." If you just start building, then you've taken over. The child may say, "You play with the toy soldiers." And I would say, "Show me what you want done with them." "Well, you take these, and I'll take these, and you line them up." "OK, show me where you want them lined up, and I'll line mine up." "Well, you line yours up right there. I'll line mine up right here." Now you know exactly what he wants done. So you start lining the soldiers up, and he starts lining his up. But you keep getting your direction from the child.

Debbie: Um-hum. It's almost like role reversal, isn't it? From what we're accustomed to.

Dr. L.: Yes, we're usually in control, we're in charge, and we tell children what to do.

Nita: I'm so used to taking over his play.

Dr. L.: Usually, we tell our children what to do and how to do it, but for 30 minutes, they get to find out what it is like to lead. That's called self-responsibility. Do you see what you're teaching your child? Something important.

Laura: So we expect them to do it.

Dr. L.: Yes, you expect them to be able to take the lead and be responsible. And I believe they can figure it out, to be the way they want it to be.

(Plays more of video.)

Dr. L.: (Stops video.) Let's suppose that you're the parent, and I'm the child (picks up handcuffs), and I say, "What is this?" Now, we haven't worked on this, so let me give you a standard response. The standard response in these 30-minute play sessions is, "That can be whatever you want it to be." You are to free your child. If your child says, "What is this?" don't say back, "What do you think that is?" because your child will say, "I don't know. What do you think it is?" If your child says, "What is this?" and you say, "That can be whatever you want it to be," your child is free to say, "Oh, it's a space ship, and this is where you drop the bombs through." And you think, "Well, I would never have thought of that." You are to free your children's creativity. "That can be whatever you want it to be." "Can I play with this stuff?" (Dr. L. picks up a can of playdough.)

Debbie: "On the towel."

Emily: "If that's what you choose, if that's what you choose to play with right now."

Dr. L.: Yes, "If you want to, that's for you to decide, on the towel." Your child will begin to realize for 30 minutes, I get to make decisions. "That's for you to decide." "I'm gonna take this guy and this guy falls right in the bucket." (Drops toy soldier into sand pail.)

Emily: "Did you hear how loud it hit the bucket?"

Dr. L.: Or, if it made no sound at all, you'd still say what?

Sonya: "I see you dropped that in the bucket."

Dr. L.: You just state what you see. That's called tracking. You could drop the words "I see."

Kathy: "He fell in the bucket."

Sonya: "He's in the bucket."

Dr. L.: Let's practice tracking and responding. Pair up with someone. One of you is the parent and the other is the child. What I'd like for you to do, children, is try to get your parent involved. Ask them some questions and give them a chance to practice giving the leadership back to you. And, other times, just play with the toys and let them practice reflecting what they see.

(Group role-plays.)

Dr. L.: OK, folks, you can stop, and children, tell your parents something you heard from them that you thought, "That sounds like a neat response. That's what we've been talking about here." Don't just say, "That was great," or, "You did a good job." That's generic praise, and it doesn't help. State something you heard, be specific. "When you said _____, that felt good," or, "That's the kind of response we've been working on." OK, kids, give your parents some feedback.

(Discussion)

Dr. L.: All right, everybody stop, and children, you're now the parents. We're gonna reverse roles now, and parents, you're now the children.

(Role-playing)

Dr. L.: OK, children, give your parents some feedback. Tell them something specific you heard that you thought, "That's a neat response."

(Discussion)

You have a lot to do this week. Next week, I'll show you some more of this play session, and we'll talk about where you're going to have your session, when you're going to have it, and do you have the kit ready. I have a list of Dos and Don'ts for your special playtime, and we'll go over that next week. Then, the next week, you'll have your first play session with your child.

Nita: It's just too hard.

Sonya: I know you can do it.

Dr. L.: It's different.

Nita: I'm just so used to directing his play, and he's just so used to, "Well, Mom, you show me."

Dr. L.: What you're saying is, it's hard to change, and that's OK. It's hard for all of us to change. Well, I'll see you next Monday.

References

Bratton, S., & Landreth, G. (2019a). *Child-Parent Relationship Therapy (CPRT) treatment manual: An Evidence-Based 10-session filial therapy model* (2nd ed). New York, NY: Routledge.

Bratton, S., & Landreth, G. (2019b). *CPRT parent-child play session skills demonstration video*. Denton, TX: Center for Play Therapy, University of North Texas. Retrieved from: www.cpt.unt.edu

Landreth, G. (2012). *Play therapy: The art of the relationship*. New York, NY: Routledge.

Munsch, R. (1986). *Love you forever*. Willowdale, Ontario, Canada: Firefly Books.

CHAPTER 10

CPRT TRAINING SESSION 3: PARENT-CHILD PLAY SESSION SKILLS AND PROCEDURES

Overview

The major focus for this session is preparing parents to be successful in their first 30-minute home play session, including specifics on what to tell their child and procedures for setting up and conducting play sessions. Basic "skill" guidelines for the play sessions, which includes eight "Dos" and "Don'ts" for parents to focus on during play sessions, are introduced and illustrated through demonstration and role-play. Play therapy skills of structuring/setting the stage, allowing the child to lead, and reflective responding are reviewed and practiced. Limit setting is briefly introduced and demonstrated. The partial transcript included at the end of this chapter illustrates many of the same therapist skills focused on in Session 2, including immediacy in presenting teaching points and the use of humor. Session 3 is unique in the amount of content that must be covered; therefore, of primary note is the therapist's careful balance between encouraging and supporting parents and covering the didactic content that is essential in order for parents to be prepared to conduct their first home play sessions.

Materials

Suggested materials include: *CPRT Session 3—Treatment Outline*; parent information form with pertinent notes on each parent; homework assigned in Session 2, including extra copies of any homework worksheets; and Session 3 handouts and homework including: *Session 3 Parent Notes and Homework, Play Session Dos and Don'ts* (print on yellow), and *Play Session Procedures Checklist* (print on blue). Additional suggested resources are included in the *CPRT Treatment Manual, 2nd Edition.*

> Note: Because these two handouts are the most used and referred to, it is helpful to run them on colored paper for easy reference.

Additional materials include: *Special Playtime Appointment Cards*, demonstration video of play session skills (helpful, but optional), one fully equipped filial play kit (and additional toys as needed to facilitate role-play and demonstration of skills), and a photograph of filial play kit set up for a play session.

> Note: It is helpful for the therapist to make a demonstration video that specifically demonstrates basic CPRT skills that parents need to learn in preparation for their first play session. We do not recommend using a play therapy demonstration video, and it goes without saying that a play therapy client video would never be used for demonstration purposes. Alternatively, for therapists without a training video, therapists can purchase *CPRT Parent-Child Play Session Skills Demonstration Video* (Bratton & Landreth, 2019b) or show the last 5 minutes of the video *Child-Centered Play Therapy* by Dr. Garry L. Landreth (*see CPRT Treatment Manual, 2nd Edition, for source information*) or arrangements can be made ahead of time to demonstrate with a child of one of the parents.
>
> *All handouts listed above, as well as a training session outline for the therapist, additional supplemental parent*

handouts, and resources for this training session are found in the CPRT Treatment Manual, 2nd Edition, *and accompanying Companion Website.*

Content and Procedure

This session begins, as do all sessions, with the therapist facilitating approximately 10 minutes of general discussion of how each parent's week has been, with a continued goal of building rapport with parents, providing support, and facilitating connections between parents. This informal group discussion time also allows a few minutes for latecomers to arrive before reviewing weekly homework assignments. This informal sharing time in the group provides an opportunity to check in with each parent's progress on collecting toys for their filial play kits and facilitate sharing of ideas for toys that parents had difficulty finding.

Continue to utilize the strategy of saying, "*That's something we'll work on later. I'm going to make a note, so I won't forget,*" when parents get off topic and want the therapist to give them a quick solution to a problem. Avoid suggesting that parents try any of the play session skills in response to reported child behavior problems. **Remember that the problem is not the problem—keep the focus on the relationship!**

Review Homework and Skill Training from Session 2

The therapist begins the session with a discussion of homework assignments and review of CPRT skills, focusing on reflective responding. Most parents have difficulty making appropriate empathic, understanding, reflective responses; providing parents with examples that list multiple-choice responses is a strategy we have found helpful.

> Reminder: Asking parents to first identify the feeling, and then to make an empathic or reflective response using that feeling word, is a highly effective strategy. *Again, a primary aim in CPRT training is structuring activities that facilitate parents feeling encouraged and successful in their efforts.*

Next, parents are asked to report on arrangements for their special play sessions—when and where they will be held—and report on their progress in collecting the toys provided on the checklist. The success of the first home play session depends on the parents obtaining a majority of the toys on the checklist and carefully selecting a day, time, and place that is free of distractions for both the parent and child. In our experience, some parents will not have given serious thought to when and where they will hold their play sessions. We cannot overstate the importance of spending time ensuring that parents have carefully thought out a time and a place to hold their weekly play sessions! Parents are reminded of the importance of consistency in children's lives and asked to choose a day and time that they can commit to without fail, a time when they are rested and have the emotional energy to fully focus on their children—and a time when their children are rested and not missing out on activities that are especially important to them.

Generally, we recommend that special playtimes not be scheduled until at least 30 minutes after the child comes home from school, so that the child has time to unwind and have a snack. As parents share the locations they have chosen for their play sessions, listen carefully for potential problem areas, such as rooms where making a mess or breaking fragile items might be a concern for the parent or a place where interruptions by others in the household is likely. If necessary, review the guidelines for selecting a play session location covered in training Session 2. The therapist must anticipate any other potential problems that would interfere in the parents' successes and address these before reviewing basic procedures and practicing skills to be utilized in the play sessions.

Play Session Dos and Don'ts

Parents are given the handout, *Play Session Dos and Don'ts*, for conducting special play sessions. This handout includes the overall goal of the play session for parents, basic "Dos" and "Don'ts," and reminders about the four messages that parents should convey to their children during special play sessions. This handout is the most used of all training materials; therefore, we suggest reproducing it on bright yellow paper that parents can easily locate and refer to. As suggested in the Materials section, making a poster of the *Play Session Dos and Don'ts* is a helpful visual aid in teaching these essential skills.

Goal of Filial Play Session for Parent

Parents' major tasks are to keenly observe their children's play and to communicate their understanding of their children's thoughts, feelings, and behavior, through their words, actions, and presence. The following "Dos" and "Don'ts" are considered essential to parents learning to successfully conduct home play sessions. Briefly cover each, but focus most on the following: do set the stage, do let the child lead, and do join in the child's play as a follower. It is imperative that the therapist briefly cover how to state a simple limit.

- **Dos:**
  - **Do set the stage.**
  - **Do let the child lead.**
  - **Do join in the child's play actively, as a follower.**
  - **Do verbally track the child's play** (describe what you see).
  - **Do reflect the child's feelings.**
  - **Do set firm and consistent limits.**
  - **Do salute the child's power and encourage effort.**
  - **Do be verbally active.**

Examples and descriptions of each "Do" can be found in Session 3 of the Therapist Notebook in the CPRT Treatment Manual, 2nd Edition.

- **Don'ts:**
  - Don't criticize any behavior.
  - Don't praise the child.
  - Don't ask leading questions.
  - Don't allow interruptions of the session.
  - Don't give information or teach.
  - Don't preach.
  - Don't initiate new activities.[1]
  - Don't be passive, quiet.

Remind parents that it is their attitude and intent in their responses that is most important. The therapist emphasizes that these play sessions (and the new skills they are learning to apply) are relatively meaningless if applied mechanically and not as an attempt to be genuinely empathic and to truly understand their child. Review the "Be-With" Attitudes by asking parents to list them:

- I am here.
- I hear/see you.
- I understand.
- I care.

Video/Demonstration of Filial Play Session Skills and Role-Play

After reviewing the basic guidelines for the play session, parents view a video-recorded demonstration play session or a live play session conducted by the therapist in order to observe play session skills in action. If a video is used, stop the video frequently to point out the "Dos" by pointing to the poster and asking which "Do" have they seen you demonstrate. If a coleader is utilized and you have access to a two-way mirror, learning is enhanced by the coleader pointing out the "Dos" while parents observe a live demonstration play session. A child of one of the parents in the group can be used for the demonstration if on-site child care is provided during the CPRT training. In either case, parents are encouraged to verbally note when they hear the therapist using any of the "Dos" listed on the handout (or optional poster). Parents are encouraged to share their observations and ask questions and then to immediately put their knowledge into action by role-playing, taking turns being parent and child. In cases where space permits and the parents' children are in child care at the site of the CPRT training, parents can role-play with their children.

Filial Play Session Procedures Checklist

Parents are given the handout, *Play Session Procedures Checklist*, with additional tips for ensuring a successful play session. This is a handout that parents will refer to often; therefore, we have found it helpful to reproduce it on colored paper. The following information is presented by the therapist (most of which is included in the parent handout, but with less detail):

- Plan ahead to avoid interruptions: encourage the child to use the bathroom prior to the play session, put pets outside or in another room, arrange for other children to spend special time with other parent or relative, **turn the phone off**, and **don't answer the door** during the special playtime. These actions convey the importance of the playtime to the child and communicate that the child is special.
- Tell the child 1 to 2 days ahead about the upcoming play session and explain that you will be having these "special" play sessions because "Mom (or Dad) is going to class to learn some special ways to play with you." Reinforce the "specialness" of this time together by assisting your child in making a **"Special Playtime—Do Not Disturb"** sign to be put on the front door during the playtimes. Marking the day and time on the family calendar and giving the child a *Special Playtime Appointment Card* are other activities that communicate the importance of this time with your child. Explain to parents about filling out the appointment card and giving it to the child the same day they make the "Do Not Disturb" sign with their child, suggesting the child tape the appointment card in a place the child will see it, such as the bathroom mirror or refrigerator door.

  Note: Reproducible appointment cards are included in the Companion Website that accompanies the CPRT Treatment Manual, 2nd Edition, and depicted in Figure 10.1.

- Allow sufficient time to set up for your first play session so that you are not rushed and can begin on time. Follow the suggestions in "Do set the stage" and check video equipment to insure that the entire play area is in view and that the camera is operating. Parents are encouraged to video-record every week to become comfortable with the process.
- Begin the session by telling the child, "*This is our special playtime for 30 minutes. You can play with the toys in a lot of the ways you would like to*," and let the child lead from this point.

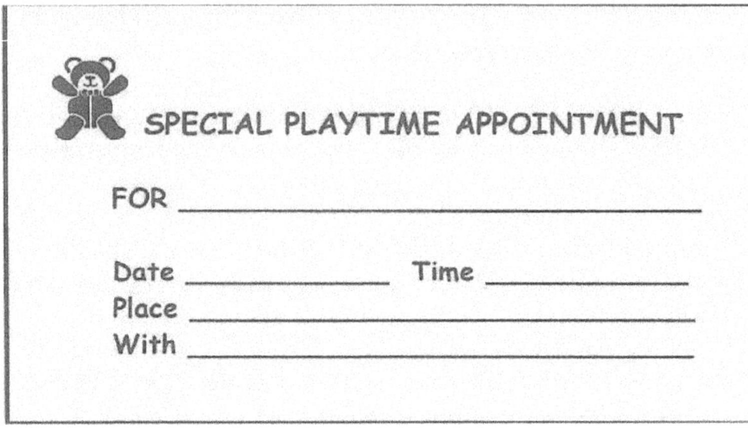
SPECIAL PLAYTIME APPOINTMENT

FOR ______________________

Date ____________ Time ____________
Place ______________________
With ______________________

Figure 10.1 Special Playtime Appointment Card.

Reminder: **For 30 minutes, your child is your teacher and you are the student;** your child is the director, and you are the actor who hasn't seen the script and must look to the director for what your "role" is. For 30 minutes, you don't know the answers to any questions. **For 30 minutes, you are dumb!**

- Set limits on behaviors that make you feel uncomfortable. If you don't set limits, your child will sense your discomfort and think you are upset with him.
- Avoid identifying toys by name because this can limit your child's expression and creativity—instead, *refer to the toys as "it," "that," "them," "her," "him."*
- Give the child a **5-minute advance notice** before ending the session to allow the child to have time to finish or complete an activity, but never exceed the time limit by more than 2 to 3 minutes. When time is up, verbally state, "*Our special playtime is over for today*," while standing up and helping the child transition to another activity. Remind parents that stating that time is up while continuing to sit in the play area with the child may encourage the child to continue playing. Standing up nonverbally communicates to your child that the playtime is over and it is time to leave the play area. If the child has difficulty leaving, reflect your understanding, but **remain firm in your responsibility to end the play session on time**:

"Billy, I know that you wish you could play longer, but our special playtime is over for today." In some cases where the child has had previous experiences (pre-CPRT training) of the parent giving in with repeated pleas or whining, the child may be persistent in pleading to play longer. However, stand firm—and never give in! The child learns that the parent will follow through on stated limits, and that no amount of pleading and whining will work.

Note: Parent is responsible for keeping track of time, so no timers allowed!

- Cleanup after the sessions is the task of the parent. Children may assist if they choose but may not continue to play after the time has ended. Generally, parents should have an activity or snack for the child to transition to immediately after the play session to provide an alternative to the child wanting to continue to play: "*Billy, I know that you wish you could play longer, but our special playtime is over for today; we can play outside together after you have your snack.*" Or parents can provide a choice after stating that time is up: "*You can choose to go outside and play with Sam or you can choose to have a snack. Which do you choose?*"

Homework Assignments

- Play sessions begin at home this week—remind parents to arrange to video-record their sessions.
- Parents are reminded of the importance of conducting their first home play session at the same time and same place. Confirm that the time and place they chose will work and that they have made arrangements for their other children, etc.
- Ask parents to take a few minutes to review *Play Session Dos and Don'ts* (yellow handout) and *Play Session Procedures Checklist* (blue handout) prior to their play sessions.
- Parents are reminded to complete their filial play kit—get old blanket/quilt, etc.
- Parents are reminded to make **"Special Playtime—Do Not Disturb"** signs with their children 1–3 days ahead (depending

on children's ages) and give children the *Special Playtime Appointment Card* 1–3 days ahead.

- Remind parents of the Rule of Thumb for this week.
- Parents are instructed to make notes immediately following the play sessions about specific happenings in the play sessions, noting what their children did or said, their responses, and their emotional reactions. Parents are reminded that **the new skills they are learning are to be practiced only during the once-per-week special playtimes**. In addition, the first parent—or two (depends on the size of your group)—is scheduled to come to the clinic/office to be video-recorded or to video-record his/her play session at home. Our preference is to have the first volunteer parent(s) come to the office/clinic playroom to be video-recorded after having one home play session. For the parent's convenience, the parent can conduct the first play session at home during the prearranged time and then video a play session to be shown during group immediately prior to training Session 4. This practice allows the first parent(s) to be video-recorded to have extra practice and support from the therapist.
- **Remember, structure all aspects of CPRT training to ensure maximum parent success!** In very rare cases where video-recording is not available, parents can conduct play sessions during CPRT training with the rest of the group watching from behind a chair or table, something to form a barrier of separation. *Note: The filial therapist should select the first parent to be video-recorded, rather than asking for volunteers.* Select a parent in the group who seems to readily pick up on the skills being taught and seems open to feedback. Most parents are apprehensive about being video-recorded, knowing that their video will be viewed by the entire group of parents at the next week's session; therefore, much encouragement and support is needed throughout the process. Again, having the parent come to your office/clinic to be video-recorded allows you to provide extra support and encouragement for the novice parent. In rare cases, there may not be a parent ready to demonstrate his/her new skills on video this early in the training process; therefore, video-recording can be delayed one week. *Some flexibility in the structure of training is necessary to ensure that parents experience success.*

- End the session by emphasizing the importance of this first home play session and asking parents to make a commitment to keep this appointment with their children, as if it were a very important business meeting or doctor appointment. The therapist emphasizes that play sessions must never be used as a reward or punishment for the child's behavior. Close with the reminder about the Rule of Thumb for the week. Although this Rule of Thumb was covered in Session 1 as a teaching point, it is useful in helping parents focus on their goal for the first play session—to establish a different kind of environment for their children; that for 30 minutes this week, they are going to be like a thermostat, responding to their children's thoughts, feelings, and needs.

Partial Transcript of CPRT Session 3

(Parents began by discussing toys and reporting on times and places they had chosen for their playtimes.)

Dr. L.: This week I want you to make a sign with your child's help that says "Special Playtime—Do Not Disturb." You can use a piece of paper like you are writing on and tape a string to it to hang on the door knob when you go into the room for your playtime. If you are home alone, hang the sign on the front door. Tell your child, "*Our special playtime is really important. If the phone rings, I'm not going to answer the phone.*" You could even disconnect the phone. If someone rings the doorbell during your playtime, say to your child, "*They will come back.*" You can only answer the doorbell if you hear someone yell, "Fire!" The message you are communicating is your child and the special playtime are so important you won't allow anything to interrupt.

Debbie: How large does the area for the playtime need to be?

Dr. L.: The space does not have to be a big area. If you did not have any other place, the playtime could be in your bathroom.

Laura: The bathroom is the smallest place in the house.

Dr. L.: Yes, it does not have to be a big area. What were you thinking about, Debbie?

Debbie: I was thinking about having my playtime in my bedroom, because I can close the door and have more privacy.

Dr. L.: What's going to happen if you have to miss one of your playtimes?

Emily: We'll have to pay for it. (group laughter)

Dr. L.: What are you going to do?

Sonya: Reschedule as soon as possible.

Dr. L.: Yes, reschedule. The playtime is just as important as an appointment with your doctor. If he cancels, you reschedule as soon as possible. If you miss a playtime, you say to your child, "Oops, I forgot or I had a meeting. Let's pick another time for our special playtime."

(Parents fill out *Special Playtime Appointment Card* to be given to their child.)

Dr. L.: Prior to your special playtime, display the toys, and then go get your child and the sign and say, "Let's hang this on the door." Then you walk into the room where your session is going to be and you say to your child, "This is our special playtime. This is a time when you can play with these toys in a lot of the ways you would like to." Please do not say to your child, "You can play with these toys any way you want to." They can't, right?

Kathy: Right. (laughs)

Dr. L.: They can't do anything with these toys they want to do. They can't throw the toys into the lamp. They can't try to break something. They can't mark on the walls with the crayons. So, you will avoid saying to your child, "You can play with these toys anyway you want to." What will you say to your child?

Sonya: "Many of the ways you would like to."

Dr. L.: Or "a lot." The child's word is "a lot." "You can play with these toys in a lot of the ways you would like to." And then you sit down (gestures toward the floor) on the floor, or if that's not comfortable, you can sit in a chair, but do not remain standing. You sit down. And then once you have done that, there are rules for your sessions. (Hands out *Play Session Dos and Don'ts* for play sessions to parents.)

Kathy: What if he's not ready to come in and start playing at 7:15? What if he's doing something else or says, "I don't want to right now?"

Dr. L.: Then you negotiate.

Debbie: Don't you think that after the first session this would be something they would be excited about?

Dr. L.: Yes, they will look forward to it. But if your child resists, and they may have something special that is just developing, then you say to your child, "Let's do this: Let's have 10 minutes of our 30-minute special playtime. At the end of that 10 minutes, you can decide whether you want to have the rest of the special playtime or stop." So you let the child continue to choose and make a decision. But you compromise, "We'll have 10 minutes and then you can decide." Your child may resist at first, but begin playing and have a good time. When you say, "Well, our 10 minutes are up. You can decide if you want to have the rest of our special playtime or stop," your child will probably choose to continue the special playtime. Look over the list of "Don'ts" and pick the one you think you're going to have the most trouble with.

(Group discusses principles they will have difficulty implementing and Dr. L. gives suggestions.)

Sonya: I'm going to have trouble with the "Don't praise your child."

Dr. L.: Give your child credit for what he does rather than praise him. Praise causes your child to want to please you and doesn't teach your child to be creative. You want your child to grow up feeling good about what she has done. Let's work on this for just a minute. (Walks over to sandbox and bends down.) If I pick up the sand scoop, and

I scoop a bunch of sand over into one place, how can you give me credit for doing that?

Debbie: Say, "You're piling up the sand."

Dr. L.: You just track what you see me do.

Debbie: "I see you're making a pile in the sand."

Dr. L.: Or maybe the first thing you said, "You're piling the sand up just as high as you want it to be." That gives me credit, "as high as you want it to be." If I stack this up (stacks cans on edge of sandbox), and it's kind of hard to make it stack, and it falls off, and I stack it again, you can now say what to me? "There, you . . ."

Sonya: "You did it. There, you did it."

Dr. L.: "There, you did it." Or there might be three or four blocks. "There you stacked those blocks way up high."

Sonya: It feels good just hearing you say that. I mean, if I was a little kid doing that, I would feel brave enough to do something else. I'd want to do something else.

Dr. L.: It builds up your child's self-esteem. And you don't have to say, "What a wonderful job you did." (returns to chair)

Sonya: I always say that. Now I feel terrible. "That was a good job, Katie, that was such a good job." But I can see now where there's more.

Dr. L.: Yes, there's more to it, and you're going to learn a different way to respond. This new way of responding is not going to feel very comfortable at first, but that's OK. What else are you going to have trouble with?

Debbie: Don't give information.

Dr. L.: Most parents want to teach their children.

Kathy: That will be a hard one.

Dr. L.: For 30 minutes, you may not tell the child how to work the Tinkertoys, or how it's supposed to be done, or "That doesn't look like this picture so you need to put this one here and make it look better." That's giving information.

Debbie: OK.

Dr. L.: For 30 minutes, you're kind of dumb. For 30 minutes, you're not an information source. You don't have any answers. Ever get tired of giving information?

Sonya: Yeah.

Dr. L.: For 30 minutes, I give you permission not to give information.

Sonya: That'll work.

Dr. L.: It can be the way your child wants it to be. That's a phrase I'd like for you all to use a lot. Your child picks up an object you have in your toy box (picks up a dragon puppet) and says, "What is this?" And you can say, "That can be . . ."

Parents: "Whatever you want it to be."

Dr. L.: (puts puppet on hand) And then I can say, "Oh goody! It's a frog!" Well, if you had identified the puppet, you probably would have said it's a dragon. Or I might say, "Oh goody! It's a space man!" It can be whatever I want it to be for this 30 minutes. That way you help me to be creative.

Dr. L.: (picks up plastic Coke bottle) (to Kathy) What's this?

Kathy: I don't know.

Dr. L.: Begin with "that." Kathy: That . . .

Dr. L.: Can be . . .

Sonya: Anything you want it to be.

Dr. L.: And it doesn't have to be a Coke bottle. It can be scrambled eggs if I want it to be. I may throw it in the pot here and say, "I'm scrambling this; I'm going to make eggs out of this." Or it could be a bowling pin. It could be a rocket ship. It can be whatever I want it to be. (Puts Coke bottle down and picks up plastic elephant.) What is this?

Parents: It can be anything you want it to be.

Dr. L.: I want you all to say that enough times that if you were sleeping and I suddenly whispered in your ear, "What is this?" you would say, "That can be whatever you want it to be." (laughter) The idea of what we're trying to do is free your child, to free their creativity so they can learn what it's like to make their own decisions. When you tell me it can be whatever I want it to be, you give the decision making back to me, and you put me in the lead.

(Parents continue to discuss items on "Don't" list that they believe will be hardest for them to avoid, and Dr. Landreth responds by providing a rationale for the "Don't" and demonstrating what to do instead.)

Dr. L.: If you say the wrong thing, you can recover. **Rule of Thumb: The most important thing may not be what you do, but what you do after what you have done.**
Any of you ever do something and realize, "That wasn't the way I really wanted to do that?"

Parents: (agreement)

Laura: You feel stuck.

Dr. L.: You can recover. It's OK if you make mistakes. I have really worked hard at trying to live by that **Rule of Thumb: The most important thing may not be what I do, but what I do after what I have done.** Let's see, what else is on the list? Number 7; nobody mentioned that one, "Don't initiate new behavior."

Sonya: What do you mean by number 7, "Don't initiate any new behavior?"

Dr. L.: Initiating new behavior would be like saying, "Well, you haven't played with the Tinkertoys yet. Maybe you'd like to play with them." That would be to initiate new behavior. You are a follower for 30 minutes. You don't suggest, "We've had four special playtimes, and you still haven't colored anything. Maybe you'd like to draw a picture." You don't do that. For 30 minutes, you can't suggest anything for your child to do. They have to figure it out. In the process, what will your child learn?

Sonya: Problem solving.

Dr. L.: Yes, problem-solving skills. How to figure things out for themselves. What it feels like to make decisions. Let's take a look at the "Dos." Would you pick the one that you think you're going to have the most trouble with?

Several parents: Tracking behavior, be a follower.

Dr. L.: For 30 minutes, you are the follower, and they are the leader. So that means if the child picks up this can, hands it to me, and says, "Go put that stuff over there," I'll say, "Show me where you want it put." And he may say, "In the sandbox." If the child says, "Go to the store and buy some groceries," I'll say, "What do you want me to get?" "Well, you get some eggs, some bacon, and some potatoes." You might have thought "hamburgers, bananas, and oranges." You always ask the child, "What do you want me to do?"

(Parents discuss "Dos" on list.)

Dr. L.: When your child is doing something, you track what they do. In this 30 minutes, you are to reflect what you hear with your eyes. If the child were to (picks up the can and drops it in the sandbox): "Oh, you just dropped that right there in the sandbox." (Dr. L. scoops up sand.) "Looks like you scooped some sand in it." Those would be your tracking responses. So that your child then knows you saw, took in, and recorded what they did. So what are the four messages we're working on? **I hear you with my ears, I hear you with my eyes—in this example it was hearing with eyes. I'm here with you, I understand, and I care.** And how does the child know we understand? Because of what you give back to them. (walks over to the sandbox) "You just dropped that in the sandbox there, and you scooped up some sand in it." Then the child knows you understood what they did. If your child is banging on the Bobo and saying not one word and you see anger, you would say, "You look angry," then the child knows you understand.

Kathy: What if my child wants to go get another toy to bring into the playtime?

Dr. L.: You can say, "I know you would like to play with the army truck in your room, but the army truck is for staying in your room. You can choose to play with it after our special playtime."

Kim: How do you handle the time? Do you have a timer?

Dr. L.: I am so glad you asked that. I almost forgot that. You will need a watch or clock, no timers. Why not set a timer for 30 minutes?

Laura: Because it makes a ticking sound and would be distracting.

Dr. L.: Yes, and the tendency is to attribute the cause for stopping to the timer. "Oh, shucks, the timer went off. We have to stop." Ending is your responsibility. Your child has been in the lead during the playtime, and now you're in charge. You will help your child get ready to end the playtime by giving a 5-minute alert 25 minutes into every playtime. "We have 5 more minutes in the playtime and then it will be time to stop." And then your child can get ready to bring the playtime to a close. The ending of the session returns control and responsibility to you all.

Kim: What if the child is not ready to end the session?

Dr. L.: We're going to make that a bit easier by doing three things: When time is up, you say, "Our special playtime is up for today," and you stand up, giving a second message that time is up. If you stay seated, the message to your child is time really isn't up. So you stand up, move towards the door and say, "It's time to go to the kitchen for cookies and milk." Then your child has something desirable to move toward. You may not have to do that every time, but it might be helpful the first couple of times. As you walk out of the room, you say to your child, "I'll come back and clean up." If your child says, "I want to help," that's OK, but no more playing. The rule of thumb at ending time is patience. If it takes several minutes for your child to walk away from the special playtime, that's OK. You walk towards the door, stop, and say, "I know you would like to play longer, but our time is up for today." Any more questions about your playtimes? Well, I have given you a lot to do today. I feel as though I have given you the whole course in one session.

(Group views a video segment of one of Dr. L.'s play sessions, and he explains what he does in the playtime.)

Dr. L.: Now, let's practice. You two are partners, you two are partners, and you two are partners. One of you is the child and one is the parent. (Group role-plays a play session, and Dr. L. moves from pair to pair listening and giving suggestions.) Next week when you come back, I will ask you, "How did your special playtime go? What happened in your special playtime? Did you have any problems?" So you will need to make notes after each one of your playtimes. I'd like to know what your child plays with or stories they play out. I need two volunteers to come here to the Center this week and be video-recorded in your play session before we meet next time. (Dr. L. briefly scans the group and makes eye contact with Emily.) Emily, would you be willing to come to the Center with Chris this week? Then the group will watch part of your playtime next week.

Emily: I can do that.

Dr. L.: Thanks, Emily, I'll meet with you briefly after group to set up a time for you. Each week I will ask for volunteers, and the playtime here will be your session for that week. I'll see you next week. I think your special playtimes are going to be fun for you.

(Dr. L. selects a second "volunteer.")

Note

1 "Don'ts" 1–7 are taken from Guerney, 1972.

References

Bratton, S., & Landreth, G. (2019a). *Child-Parent Relationship Therapy (CPRT) treatment manual: An Evidence-Based 10-session filial therapy model* (2nd ed). New York, NY: Routledge.

Bratton, S., & Landreth, G. (2019b). *CPRT parent-child play session skills demonstration video*. Denton, TX: Center for Play Therapy, University of North Texas. Retrieved from: www.cpt.unt.edu

Guerney, L. (1972). *Filial therapy: A training manual for parents*. Unpublished manuscript.

CHAPTER 11

CPRT TRAINING SESSION 4: SUPERVISION FORMAT AND LIMIT SETTING

Overview

The major focus in this session is for parents to report on their first special playtime with their children, with the most time spent reviewing the video of the parent who volunteered to be video-recorded. All skills introduced in training Session 3, as well as underlying principles of CPRT therapy, are continually reinforced by the therapist as parents report on their play sessions, but the major strategy is to encourage parents as they share their play session experiences, finding something positive to comment on in each parent's report. The partial transcript of CPRT training Session 4 found at the end of this chapter provides the reader with a glimpse into this process of balancing didactic instruction and dynamic support and encouragement of parents as they struggle to learn these new skills. Limit-setting skills are taught and demonstrated, and play session skills are reviewed and practiced, based on the needs of the group.

Materials

Suggested materials include: *CPRT Session 4—Treatment Outline*; parent information form with pertinent notes; homework assigned in Session 3, including extra copies of any homework worksheets; Session 4 handouts and homework, including: *Session 4 Parent Notes and Homework*, *Limit Setting: A-C-T Before It's Too Late!*, *Limit Setting: A-C-T Practice Worksheet*, and *Play Session Notes*. Additional materials include: display posters for both *Play Session Dos and Don'ts* and *Play Session Procedure Checklist* (or laminated color copies of each can be used in lieu of poster), video clip of limit setting (optional), and video clip or live demo of play session skills.

> *Note: All handouts listed above, as well as a training session outline for the filial therapist, additional supplemental parent handouts, and resources for this training session are found in the CPRT Treatment Manual, 2nd Edition, and accompanying Companion Website.*

Content and Procedure

This session begins, as do all sessions, with 10 minutes of parents sharing how their week went as they arrive. By this fourth session, parents generally feel more comfortable openly and honestly sharing their parenting struggles, and the therapist utilizes this time to support and encourage parents. Resistant parents often share behavioral problems they are having with their children, often citing examples of how they tried to use a skill and it didn't work—"Nothing works with my child." Remind parents of the Band-Aid—that it's working even when they don't see it working. Ask them to trust the process, and not to take the Band-Aid off yet! The therapist can also use a resistant parent's reports of frustration with her child's behavior as an opportunity to reflect that what she is doing doesn't seem to be getting the desired results. Ask the parent to consider that her child may have special needs that require a different response, and that the 30-minute special playtime will teach her a new way to respond to her child's needs. This is a good time to introduce the **Rule of Thumb: When a**

child is drowning, don't try to teach her to swim. Ask parents what they would do if their child *were* drowning. Do you look into the pool and try to tell them what to do and try to give them a crash course in how to swim? Of course not! You would jump in and save your child. Liken the 30-minute special playtime to the parent jumping in to save the child (hence the name of the course: CPR). The special playtime is a time for parents to respond to their children's needs, without trying to teach a lesson, change behavior, etc. Reflective responding is the tool that parents use to respond to their children's needs. When a child is feeling upset or out of control, that is not the moment to teach, preach, or impart a rule.

The facilitator must be sensitive to the difficulty parents have with the concept of focusing only on the special playtimes, when they are having significant behavior problems that they want solved, and NOW! Continue to affirm their frustrations and struggles, writing down their concerns, and assuring them that you will come back to those issues in a few weeks. An exception to the rule regarding the use of skills outside of play sessions is the introduction of the concept of choice giving to address a relevant problem expressed by a parent. Choice giving is a skill that is relatively easy to learn and often produces immediate results. Although we typically teach the skill of choice giving in depth in Session 6, this skill can be covered briefly as early as Session 4, depending on the needs of the group. Choice giving is one skill that parents are encouraged to use outside of their play sessions and, as with many teaching points, this skill is more powerfully learned when introduced or reinforced in response to a parent's expressed concern, as illustrated in the partial transcript at the end of this chapter. **Some flexibility in presentation of content is often necessary in order to most effectively respond to parents' needs.**

Filial Play Session Reports

The majority of this session is focused on parents' reporting on their first special playtimes with their children. Parents are asked to report on such things as making their "Do Not Disturb" sign with their children, and their children's responses to parents' explanation of the specialness of the playtimes, etc. Each parent is asked to briefly describe the first play session with her child, with the "parent of focus" (parent who video-recorded a play session) going last. The therapist carefully listens for parent strengths, finding something positive to comment on in each parent's report. Remember that the **donut analogy** applies to parents, too. They will have lots of "holes" at this point in the training, but the therapist's job in this session is to focus completely on "the good stuff."

Look for every opportunity to use parents' comments to forge connections and help them see that they are not alone in their struggles to try out these new skills. Find a part of a parent's report to respond to and build on in order to reinforce the filial play session "Dos." For example, Debbie reported that during her first play session, her daughter climbed up on the bed close to her with the doctor kit, and that she (Debbie) responded, "I don't know what to do." Her daughter then responded, "Well, you lie down here, and I'll tell you." Although Debbie's response was not a perfect example of "*Do* let the child lead," the leader used this opportunity to encourage Debbie and reinforce a teaching point by responding, "So, you let Rachel know that it was up to her to decide what to do, and she let you know that she knew just what she wanted you to do!" Then, the therapist turned to the group and pointed to the poster of "Dos" and said, "That was an example of . . .," and two of the parents responded in unison, "*Do* let the child lead."

During the reporting of happenings in their first play session, parents typically ask for help with how to respond to specific situations. **The emphasis of CPRT training is on learning by experience and observation.** Therefore, role-play is utilized to address specific questions, with the therapist playing the role of the parent who presented the question and the parent playing the role of the child. The filial therapist may also introduce new teaching material that is relevant to parents' questions. For example, in the Session 4 transcription given at the end of this chapter, choice giving was introduced in response to Debbie's power struggle with her daughter about her clothes. Debbie was so frustrated with Rachel's behavior throughout the week that she could not keep her focus on her play session report. In response, the therapist reflected how frustrated Debbie seemed and suggested that Debbie try giving Rachel two choices of clothes to wear. After much discussion from Debbie about why choice giving will not work with Rachel, the therapist asked Debbie to work on choice giving, adding that he will check in with her next week (*and made a note to himself to do so*).

Following through on promises made to parents, such as this one, is important and models the value of parents following through on their promises to their children. This strategy also serves the purpose of ending the discussion and brings the topic back to Debbie's special playtime. Writing down parents' unsuccessfully resolved problems and other concerns helps them feel heard, conveys that their concerns are important, but most importantly, allows the therapist to refocus on the task at hand. *Our experience is that successfully conducting a CPRT group is a continual and delicate balance between providing didactic instruction and supervision that helps parents learn the skills necessary for success and facilitating a dynamic process so that parents feel supported and understood.*

Filial Play Session Video Critique

The next and most important training element in this session is viewing the video-recorded parent play session. An advantage of video-recording is that parents get to observe themselves, an experience that can produce tremendous insight. Other benefits of video-recorded supervision are enhanced opportunities for vicarious learning for all group members and the opportunity for parents to give, as well as receive, help from each other. The experience of watching themselves on video usually produces considerable anxiety for parents, but the other parents in the group are always extremely supportive and the anxiety quickly dissipates. A major objective of therapist feedback is to provide support and encouragement and to be sensitive to the feelings parents experience. Correction is kept to a minimum. **Encouragement is the order of the day**. As mentioned earlier, while viewing the parent video the therapist carefully listens and watches for parent strengths and opportunities to offer encouragement and to reinforce the Dos and Don'ts listed on the poster.

In the viewing of the first video-recorded play session, the therapist often has to work hard to find strengths to reflect. For example, Emily was the first parent to show her video, and after watching her video for several minutes, commented that she was much quieter than usual, because she wasn't sure what to say.

The therapist stopped the video and encouraged Emily's periods of silence between her brief responses by commenting, "Emily, that shows me you were thinking about how you should respond, instead of responding how you typically would—that's the first step! Just now, as you watched your child playing with the playdough, what were you aware of?" Emily quickly responds, "He's having fun rolling it and squishing it! [pause] Probably because I never let him have playdough at home." The therapist uses that opportunity to encourage Emily's understanding of her child's play and suggests that as Emily begins to trust her instincts, she will be able to respond more quickly, with understanding, to her child's play.

Group Dynamics and Support

The therapist also uses every opportunity to link parents' shared experiences, by noting and commenting on verbal and nonverbal messages that convey "Me, too." For example, in the segment described above, Laura smiled, and Kathy nodded, when Emily revealed that she wasn't sure how to respond, prompting the therapist to reflect, "Laura, seems like you understand what Emily's struggling with . . . and, Kathy, I noticed you nodding your head, too." This led to a discussion about how all the parents felt awkward with practicing this new way of responding to their children's play and, more importantly, helped them feel that they were not alone in their struggles.

An issue that is usually brought up following the parents' first play session is that a child is enjoying the play session and doesn't want to stop when the time is up. Parents are reminded that it is their responsibility to end the sessions even though children may want to continue playing, and that this happening provides a perfect opportunity to demonstrate an example of limit setting. "*Rachel, I know you would like to play with the doctor kit longer, but our special playtime is over for today. You can choose to play with the doctor kit next week.*" For the younger child, who may need a more immediate alternative, "*Rachel, I know you want to play longer, but our special playtime is over for today. We can go to the kitchen and have a snack.*" This example demonstrates how ending a play session with a reluctant child leads into instruction of the skill of limit setting.

Limit Setting

The importance of parents establishing consistent limits with their children is briefly discussed: **consistent limits provide a predictable, safe environment and a sense of security**. The A-C-T model of limit setting is taught and demonstrated in this session. The handout Limit Setting: A-C-T Before It's Too Late! in Session 4 of the Therapist Notebook in the CPRT Treatment Manual, 2nd Edition, includes detailed information about the A-C-T method of limit setting and strategies for teaching this important skill. Parents are given the handout, *Limit Setting: A-C-T Before It's Too Late!*, to refer to as the therapist teaches the three-step process of the A-C-T method of limit setting. (What follows is only an outline of the A-C-T model.)

Three-Step A-C-T Method

Begin by providing parents with a limit-setting scenario that might occur *during* a play session. Do not give a scenario that would take place outside of a play session; parents have enough difficulty resisting the urge to try this new skill to deal with problematic child behaviors. Example scenario: *Billy has been pretending that the bop bag is a bad guy and shooting him with the dart gun; he looks over at you and aims the dart gun at you, then laughs and says, "Now, you're one of the bad guys, too!"*

1. ***A***cknowledge your child's feeling or desire (*your voice must convey empathy and understanding*). **"Billy, I know that you think that it would be fun to shoot me, too."** *The child learns that his feelings, desires, and wishes are valid and accepted by his parent (but not all behavior)*; simply empathically reflecting your child's feeling often defuses the intensity of the feeling or need.
2. ***C***ommunicate the limit (be specific and clear—and brief). **"But, I'm not for shooting."**
3. ***T***arget acceptable alternatives; provide one or more choices (depending on age of child). **"You can pretend that the doll is me [pointing at the doll] and shoot at it."**

The goal is to provide your child with an acceptable outlet for expressing the feeling or the original action, while giving him an opportunity to exercise self-control.

Why Establish Consistent Limits

Providing children with consistent limits helps them feel safe and secure. This method of limiting children's behavior teaches them self-control and responsibility for their own behavior by allowing them to experience the consequences for their choices and decisions. Limits set in play sessions help children practice self-control and begin to learn to stop themselves in the real world.

When to Set Limits

During play sessions, limits are set only when the need arises, and for four basic reasons:

1. To protect the child from hurting himself or his parent.
2. To protect valuable property.
3. To maintain the parent's acceptance of the child.
4. To provide consistency in the play session by limiting child and toys to play area and ending on time.

Before setting a limit in a play session, ask yourself:

- "Is this limit necessary?"
- "Can I consistently enforce this limit?"
- "If I don't set a limit on this behavior, can I consistently allow this behavior and accept my child?"

Avoid conducting play sessions in areas of the house that require too many limits. Limits set during play sessions should allow for greater freedom of expression than would normally be allowed. The fewer the limits, the easier it is for you to be consistent. **Consistency is very important**. Determine a few limits ahead of time (practice A-C-T): no hitting or shooting at parent, no playdough on the carpet, no purposefully breaking toys, etc. Hint: Children really do understand that playtimes are "special" and that the rules are different—they will *not* expect the same level of permissiveness during the rest of the week.

How to Set Limits

Limits are not punitive and should be stated firmly, but calmly and matter-of-factly. After empathically acknowledging your child's feeling or desire (very important step), you state, "*The playdough is not for throwing at the table,*" just like you would state, "*The sky is blue.*" Don't try to force your child to obey the limit. Remember to provide an acceptable alternative. In this method, it really is up to the child to decide to accept or break the limit; however, **it is your job, as the parent, to consistently enforce the limit**. (See A-C-T Before It's Too Late! for details.)

Limit-Setting Demonstration, Practice, and Role-Play

Provide parents with three to four written or oral examples of limit-setting scenarios and how to respond using A-C-T. Time may not permit a thorough review of the rationale for limit setting and when and how to set limits. Limit setting generally is an area of concern for parents and will continue to be a topic of focus for several weeks. Parents are asked to reread the handout for homework and note any limit they think they might need to set with their child. The therapist demonstrates limit setting through role-play, as with every skill that is introduced, and if time permits, a short video clip of limit setting is shown. Parents are typically very interested in limit setting and generate many questions about the use of this skill in everyday struggles with their child. However, the therapist uses humor to explain to parents that under no circumstances are they to try this outside of the play session! On a more serious note, remind parents that the goal is for them to be successful in learning to apply these new skills during their 30-minute special playtimes with their children.

In some cases, the experienced CPRT therapist may introduce the limit-setting skill earlier in this session in response to a parent's concern, rather than wait until the end of the training session. Opportunities to teach and reinforce limit setting arise on a regular basis. There is no need to try to teach all limit-setting concepts all at one time in one session. Again, using relevant moments to teach skills enhances parents' learning, as illustrated in the transcription that follows. Debbie was expressing frustration with her daughter's screaming when she doesn't get her way. The therapist suggested that when that happens again, Debbie respond to Rachel by saying, "*Sounds like you need to scream, but the kitchen is not a place for screaming. It hurts my ears. You can scream in your room.*" A very brief overview of the A-C-T model of limit setting is provided at that time, but the therapist continues to focus the process on parents' reporting of play sessions, letting parents know that limit setting will be taught in more detail later. Again, some flexibility of content delivery is allowed in order to respond to the unique needs of a particular group of parents.

Allow at least 15 minutes for parent pairs to role-play, each parent taking a turn being the child playing with toys and responding as the child to limit-setting situations. Since this week has been the parents' first opportunity to practice their new skills, they usually have so much they want to share about the experience that the time for specific training is minimal. Time constraints may require that the therapist provide more detailed instructions, practice, and role-play of limit setting during Session 5.

Homework Assignments

1. Parents are reminded of the importance of conducting their play sessions at the same time and same place (no excuses!), likening the play session to a weekly staff meeting with the boss (a meeting that no one would dare miss!), and parents are reminded to video-record their sessions.
2. Parents are reminded to take a few minutes to review the following handouts prior to play session: *Play Session Dos and Don'ts* (yellow), *Play Session Procedures Checklist* (blue), and *Limit Setting: A-C-T Before It's Too Late!* (Optional assignment: Provide parents with a handout with several scenarios of children's behaviors in play sessions requiring limit setting, which they are to respond to in writing and bring the following week—this can be done in class the following week or given as homework after Session 5.)
3. Remind parents to notice one intense feeling in themselves this week; also, if they needed to set a limit during their playtimes, describe what happened and what they said or did, and think about what limits they think they might need to set for their child.
4. Parents are reminded after conducting the play session to complete the *Parent Play Session Notes* and bring to group the following week.
5. One to two parents are scheduled to video-record their play sessions to be shown in class the following week.
6. Remind parents of the Rule of Thumb for that week.
7. Close with a motivational poem or story (optional).

Partial Transcript of CPRT Session 4

(Informal group sharing and the first part of parents' reporting on home play sessions are not included.)

Debbie: How is Nita, the pregnant mom?

Dr. L.: Nita called and wanted everyone to know she's fine. She has an appointment with her doctor, but she's fine. Let's continue talking about your sessions. I'd like to hear from each one of you about how your sessions went, how you got started, what your child played with, what the playtime was like for you. We're going to see your video, Emily, so we'll skip you for now. Debbie, what was your session like?

Debbie: Rachel was bouncing off the walls. I set the playtime for 10:00 in the morning because my husband's schedule is so flexible, and I like him out of the house. But she was so excited about the playtime; she started bouncing off the walls at about 8:30. It was just horrible. I finally set the timer on the microwave and said, "Now, when it beeps, you can go in the room, and we can get started." I took the baby next door and I said, "Now, I'm going to be in the bedroom, and when it beeps, you come in there." Well, I heard it beep twice. She was at the microwave turning it off, so it would be time. (laughter)

Dr. L.: Good for her. She's eager, and I would suggest next time, don't set the timer ahead like that with a beeper to go off. You just decide when you are ready to start at a time close to the prearranged time. Display the toys, and then bring her into the room, or allow her to help you get the playtime ready.

Debbie: I don't have to start it at 10:00?

Dr. L.: You can be flexible. If she is eager to start, and you're ready to start, you may want to start 10 minutes early. We don't want to make an issue out of the time.

Debbie: I want to go back and listen to the video. I recorded it, and it was pretty good. Except, she wanted to play doctor, and she decided the thing you give shots with is for sticking in my nose. So here she is on the bed next to me close up, and I said, "I don't know what to do." She said, "Well, you lie down here, and I'll tell you." It was pretty interesting. She only played with two things. She had all these toys, but only played with two. Another real interesting thing was she took everything out of the dollhouse, but then she put everything back in the dollhouse before she went on to play.

Dr. L.: She put things away. That was unexpected by you.

Debbie: Yeah, it was. She put them all back in there and closed the door.

Dr. L.: So, what did you learn about your child?

Debbie: Nothing new, that I thought of. It was surprising that she put things away.

Dr. L.: And what does that mean?

Debbie: That she likes to be organized.

Dr. L.: That's a possibility. It also means she's capable of putting things away.

Sonya: She can put her things away before she moves on to something else.

Dr. L.: And without being told to do it. You learned that about her. That might be an important learning.

Debbie: But she doesn't put her toys away at other times.

Dr. L.: But now you know she's capable.

Sonya: Having that information, it's like oh, yeah, she can do that, but she chooses not to.

Debbie: I go through a lot of things with Rachel, like choice of dresses and stuff.

Dr. L.: It's a dressing problem in the morning.

Debbie: All the time; all throughout the day.

Dr. L.: All day?

Debbie: She goes through about five outfits a day.

Dr. L.: Because?

Debbie: She doesn't want to wear this, she wants to wear that, and when she's tired of that, then she wants to wear this, etc. It's always got to be a dress and all her pantyhose and her leotards are all ripped because that's the only thing she wants to wear.

Sonya: I have something I just want to interject: the first thing that I do, if I feel like I'm having a "struggle of wills" with Jenny, she's almost 3, the first thing I do is check on, "How important is this?" Sometimes I just have to stop and think, "Is this worth arguing over?" If it is something that is important, then I will tell her. I'm going to give this example because (to Dr. L.) you mentioned it last week. If she starts crying over the smallest little thing and says, "I want my daddy," or "You're not my friend anymore!" I stopped feeling guilty and playing the game with her like you said. I just said, "It sounds like you're very angry with me," and she just stopped in her tracks as soon as I acknowledged what her feeling was, and she didn't go on and on about "You're not my friend any more, I miss my daddy." Then I asked, "Are you going to call your daddy?" and she said, "Maybe later."

Debbie: Is it OK for her to . . .

Emily: To pitch a fit?

Debbie: Well, yeah!

Emily: Yes.

Dr. L.: Emily, you have experienced that, and Debbie, it sounds like you're really frustrated with Rachel. Perhaps you could try choice giving by giving her two choices of clothes to wear, and then how is she likely to react?

Debbie: She will scream.

Dr. L.: And you show understanding by saying, "You're really angry about your choices."

Debbie: I don't keep talking to her through the screaming, do I? Is there a point where I withdraw?

Dr. L.: You can say, "Sounds like you need to scream, and your room is the place for screaming. I'm going to the kitchen, and you can have 5 minutes to scream in your room." And if she follows you into the kitchen, you can say, "The kitchen is not a place for screaming. It hurts my ears. My kitchen is not for screaming in. Your room is for screaming in." And you take her back to her room. It's OK if she screams back there. The important thing is that you are allowing her to get rid of some of her feelings, and she learns you're not too bothered by that.

Debbie: I won't do anything to reinforce her behavior.

Dr. L.: You got it. One of the things I keep hearing from you, Debbie, is you know what needs to be done. I didn't say anything about reinforcing. You know you're reinforcing some things you shouldn't be reinforcing.

Debbie: Maybe I need reinforcement. (group laughs)

Dr. L.: You're on the right track, Debbie. You just can't change the whole world. Right now you just need to work on choice giving. I have written that down (points to notebook), and I'll check on that next week. Let's go back to your special playtime.

(Focus on an issue unrelated to the special playtimes is typically not done until the last couple of sessions unless the parent has intense feelings about the issue. If that is the case, hearing the parent and suggesting something the parent can try provides a measure of relief. The parent can then focus on the task of learning skills for the playtimes.)

Debbie: (Describes more of her child's play behavior.)

Dr. L.: Did the time seem to go slow or fast for you?

Debbie: Very fast.

Dr. L.: That's a good sign. A caution, folks, the playtimes may not always go fast. There may be some special playtimes when the 30 minutes seems like an hour, and that's OK. What that says is you may not have been very interested in what was going on, but your child probably was. The playtime can also seem long if your child is giving you a hard time. The important thing is you are together. Debbie, tell us how your playtime ended.

Debbie: I said, "We have 5 more minutes and then our playtime will be over," and she said, "Oh, I want to play some more." I didn't respond, and then when time was up, I said, "Our time is up, we can go get some cookies."

Dr. L.: Who was in charge of the ending?

Debbie: I was.

Dr. L.: Yes, as you needed to be. I would add to one thing you said. When Rachel said at the end, "Oh, I want more time," reflect her feelings. "It would be fun to have a lot more time, but you have 5 more minutes." The time is not going to change. You just show understanding, but the time is not going to change. "I know you would like to have a lot more time."

Debbie: Later she was looking at the calendar and said, "Mom, when is our next special playtime?"

Dr. L.: So the playtime is important to her already. And I can see in your face, Debbie, that you enjoyed the playtime also. Kim, tell us about your playtime.

Kim: He had a hard time settling down to one thing. He has that problem anyway, he has attention deficit, and so he has a hard time.

Dr. L.: He played with everything?

Kim: Yeah, he's never seen any of the toys before, they're all brand new. So he was just bouncing off the walls. So I put some of the toys away, and we just sat on the floor for a while with what was left.

Dr. L.: I'm not sure what you did there. What do you mean you put the toys away?

Kim: I put them back in the box. I had stuff on the table and stuff in a chair and on the floor. I left the chair stuff alone and put the table stuff away.

Dr. L.: Why did you put the table stuff way?

Kim: Because he wouldn't calm down or anything. He was overwhelmed by everything new. He couldn't concentrate on one toy.

Dr. L.: In this special playtime, it doesn't matter.

Kim: I was afraid he was going to get the hyperactivity type thing, where he won't settle down at all. But I brought them back out once he started playing on the floor.

Dr. L.: OK. I'd like to suggest that next time you leave all the toys out, and let's see what happens. Even if he gets really hyper, it will be an opportunity for him to act that out; it will also give you an opportunity to reflect a lot more. You will have more behaviors to respond to. In the rest of his world, nobody puts things away. Right?

Kim: Oh, you mean, when he's usually playing?

Dr. L.: Yeah, out there in the other parts of his world—on the playground, nobody tries to hide stuff, to put it away. He learns to cope with it. So in the special playtime, you can allow him to cope.

Kim: Yeah, I noticed he was talking about the toys. He didn't get to play with all of them, and he wanted to. For several days, he kept talking about the toys and trying to get to the top of my closet where I put the toys. I moved the box so he wouldn't know where it was, but he really wants to get to that stuff because it's all new, it's all his.

Dr. L.: The toys must be very special to him. Was there any one toy that he spent any more time with than the other toys?

Kim: The people, he likes the people a lot.

Dr. L.: What did he do with the people?

Kim: He wanted them to eat and sleep and go up the stairs. David, my husband, made stairs in our house. There's no upstairs, but there's stairs, like there was an upstairs. And Toby's very interested in stairs.

Dr. L.: So that's important to him.

Kim: For some reason. I guess it's new. I didn't try to make him go on to the next thing; I just let him play with the people for a while. They bend and so he'd try to make them lie down and sit down.

Dr. L.: One of the things I heard you say there was you let him choose.

Kim: He spent so much time on that one thing.

Dr. L.: And that kind of bothered you a little bit.

Kim: Well, there's all the other stuff there.

Dr. L.: "There's all this other stuff I got for you, show your appreciation and play with all of it!"

Kim: I didn't say it though. (laughing)

Dr. L.: (to the group) But whose time is this?

Kathy: The child's.

Dr. L.: Did the time seem to go fast?

Kim: Oh yeah, in fact we went over the time, and I didn't know it. I let him put the sign on the door with me; he was real excited about that.

Dr. L.: That makes the playtime really important.

Kim: Yeah, because everybody else was gone.

Dr. L.: How did it end?

Kim: He didn't want to stop. I had to bribe him to do something else, so I said, "You can go out and play."

Dr. L.: Well, you can just start putting things away. We haven't talked about that, but if you have some problem with your child wanting to continue to play, and your child won't walk out of the room with you, you can just start putting things away and end it. Sonya, what was your playtime like?

Sonya: It went pretty good. When I first told her we'd be having the special playtime, as soon as we got home, she taped the appointment card to the refrigerator by herself; so we have this little crooked appointment card taped on the refrigerator. The rough part about the playtime was that about 5 minutes into it, the baby started crying, but I let her cry. She cried for about 20 minutes and went back to sleep; so that was new information to me. I usually comfort her so she will go back to sleep. I started our playtime by telling Jenny to put her stuff up in her room, and while you do that, I'll fix up for our special playtime, and she did. So I quickly got everything out, and I sat on the floor in the living room. She walked in and said, "Are these all for me?"

Dr. L.: Like Christmas Day.

Sonya: Oh yes, just like it. She was real excited, and I made a comment about that and watched her get more excited as I said it. And then, strangely enough, she started moving all the toys to the middle of the floor, where I was. She grabbed the playdough first, took it out and checked it. She mostly played with the Tinkertoys, and they weren't quite what I thought they were; they're real complicated. She would say, "Ok, Mommy, let's build." I would say, "Ok, what do you want me to do?" And she would say, "Ok, these are for you, and these are for me." But every time I asked her, "What do you want me to do?" or "Show me what you want me to do," she wouldn't tell me. She moved on to something else. The message I got was, "I like you to sit here with me and watch me play, but don't get into any of that," and that was hard. I really wanted to get into it.

Dr. L.: Playing with the toys would have been more fun for you. Let's look more closely at your child's behavior. When she said, "Do this mommy," and you said, "Show me what you want done," and then she went on to something else, wonder why a child would do that? Why wouldn't she then go on with that play?

Sonya: I don't know, just trying to get the initial contact, or wondering "Are you really paying attention to me?" or "Are you really wanting to do this?"

Dr. L.: Could it be that was an old behavior of asking you to do something, and in the past you have automatically taken over and done it? Could it be that all the time your child has wanted to go on to something else?

Sonya: Yeah. And she's started saying a lot more, "I can do it myself," and I'm thinking, "Yeah, OK, well I just wanted to help you." Like with the potty thing, "I can do it myself." I've started clicking to the fact that she really wants more independence. I really thought that I had given her that, and I saw through the play session that I do too much for her. It was hard to hold back. And then she put the Tinkertoys back in the canister one at a time! *One at a time*, and I was thinking, I'm not going to say 200 times, "I see you put another one in, and another. . . ." The time went real fast, and when I told her, "We have 5 minutes left for special playtime, and then I'll need to put the toys away," she started putting the toys away.

Dr. L.: Sounds like a really active time, and there were some things that happened that were surprising to you. As with each of you, some of the things your children do are a little surprising. And you're learning some new things about your children.

(Other parents report on their play sessions and receive feedback.)

Dr. L.: Emily, let's see the video of your session.

Emily: Oh, let's not! (group laughs)

Dr. L.: Emily, tell us what it was like to come in here and be video-recorded. You're the first one to do that, and I'm sure the group would like to know what it was like for you.

Emily: I was very self-conscious for the first 5 minutes or so, and then I forgot someone was behind that two-way mirror, and that I was being video-recorded.

Dr. L.: So you forgot about being video-recorded, and then how did it go?

Emily: Very fast, because I walked in there thinking, "Gosh, this is going to be the longest 30 minutes of my life!" (Group laughs.) The next thing I knew, I was thinking it's time to give him a 5-minute warning.

Dr. L.: Emily, I really appreciate your courage. It takes courage to be first and courage to come in here and be video-recorded. I appreciate you're doing that. Let's watch your session.

(Group watches part of Emily's video. Dr. Landreth stops the video frequently to point out the skills Emily is demonstrating and to give Emily encouragement.)

Dr. L.: (Stops video.) That's the second time he has put a toy back on the shelf after he played with it. Is that typical of him at home, to put things away?

Emily: His bicycle was stolen this weekend, so he's very much into putting things back where they belong. (Group laughs.)

Dr. L.: There is a reason why children do the things they do in their play. So that's really on his mind—putting things back.

(Group watches more of Emily's video.)

Dr. L.: (Stops video.) Little comments like that may not seem to be very important, but they convey a powerful message. When you said, "You're pushing that car right on top of the sand," what did that say to the child about him?

Kim: He has the ability to do it.

Sonya: You're important to me. I noticed exactly what you did. I think my Mommy is watching me, now I know for sure. I must be important.

Dr. L.: Yes, I'm important and what I'm doing is important enough for her to pay attention to it. A child cannot feel important until he is important to someone. So, Emily, you helped your child to feel important because he is important to you. And what your child is doing becomes more important because it is important to you. There is a lot to a little statement like, "You're pushing that car right on top of the sand." Emily, you look natural in this playtime and your tracking responses are well spaced. They communicate your involvement.

Kathy: It's not natural for me. I'm an overfunctioning person. I have to take responsibility for how my child feels and what he does. I kept wanting to ask questions in our playtime.

Dr. L.: So it takes effort to track what he does.

Kathy: It's very, very difficult for me.

Dr. L.: The important thing is that you did it.

Kathy: Not very well.

Dr. L.: You think you should have done it better, but the important thing is that you followed through on your commitment, and you were with your child.

Kim: What we're doing in here kinda seeps into everything I'm doing even though I know we're only supposed to do it in the playtime. Like with my little girl, she nags, and I've noticed when I answer the first time, she doesn't go on. I used to think she was such a nag. Now if I look at her in the face and answer her, even if I tell her what she doesn't want to hear, she will leave me alone.

Dr. L.: It's enough for her.

Sonya: Just like with the telephone and the 30-second burst of attention. I've been doing that more often. I'll say, "Excuse me, let me give Jenny about 30 seconds." My friends will say, "Oh, OK," and as soon as I give Jenny attention, she leaves. My girlfriend has started doing the same thing with her son—so it's being passed on to others.

Emily: That also works when you're not on the phone. When my husband comes home from work, he helps me in the kitchen get ready for dinner. The kids are not supposed to bother us because that is our time. Chris came in one night, and my husband and I were trying to talk, and I said, "Let me try something." I turned around to Chris, and I said, "Ok, Chris, I can give you 30 seconds, what do you need?" I didn't take my eyes off him. He said what he needed to say, I responded to him, I said, "Your 30 seconds are up," I turned back to my husband, and Chris ran off.

Dr. L.: It worked. He got what he needed. You all give Emily some feedback on her play session. Tell her what you saw.

Sonya: You gave him your undivided attention. You were like radar. You tracked him with your total body.

Kim: I would have a hard time not suggesting he go on to something else. You allowed him to focus on just one thing, and you were great with the limit setting.

Kathy: Yes, you handled shooting with the gun really well.

Laura: Your tracking was right with him. I was bothered by my tracking because I sounded so repetitive.

Debbie: You allowed him to lead the whole time.

Laura: And he seemed comfortable leading.

Dr. L.: Good job practicing what we've been working on. Now, let's work on limit setting.

(Dr. Landreth explains A-C-T limit setting.)

Your child is headed toward the wall with a crayon and you say, "You would like to mark on the wall. The wall is not for marking on." This is what I call the educational approach. You just state what things are for or not for. "The wall is not for marking on." "You're angry at me. I'm not for shooting." You identify the feeling and then communicate the limit.

Then the third step is something we almost never do for children. We usually set out to stop their behavior. "Stop that. Don't do that." And we stop right there, but children still have an unexpressed feeling, want, or need. The third step is to target choices. "You'd like to mark on the wall. The wall is not for marking on." Now, what would be acceptable to mark on?

Kathy: You can mark on the chalkboard.

Dr. L.: The chalkboard is for writing on or if your child has a crayon, the paper is for marking on with the crayon. Or, "I can see you are angry at me. I'm not for shooting." And then what would be acceptable?

Kathy: The stuffed animals are for shooting.

Dr. L.: When you target an acceptable alternative, it is important to point toward the acceptable choice. "You can shoot the stuffed animals," or if there's a Bobo in the play sessions, "You can pretend the Bobo is me and shoot the Bobo," and point. Or, "I'm not for shooting. The door is for shooting." You might give a couple of choices. "The sand is not for pouring on the floor. The sand is for pouring in the sandbox or in the pail or in the funnel," and point. You can remember the steps to follow by remembering to act. The three steps are: A: acknowledge the feeling, C: communicate the limit, and T: target some choices. You just act. The light's not for shooting. Now, you give me a choice.

Kim: The bean bag is for shooting.

Dr. L.: Now suppose the child has the dart gun and suddenly points it at you. You may not have time to start with the first step and reflect the feeling. First, you state the limit. "I'm not for shooting." Then you can go back to, "I know you would like to shoot me. But I'm not for shooting." So you may not always be able to start with the first step and acknowledge the feeling. You may have to start with step two. Your assignment for the week is to write down one time you set a limit during your playtime with your child, if a limit was needed. Sometimes the only limit you will need to set is ending the session. Also, I want you to notice one intense feeling you experience during your play session and share that with us next week.

(Dr. L. summarizes feedback and teaching points, parents do brief role-playing, and Dr. L. makes arrangements for video-recording one to two parents for the following week.)

Reference

Bratton, S., & Landreth, G. (2019). *Child-Parent Relationship Therapy (CPRT) treatment manual: An Evidence-Based 10-session filial therapy model* (2nd ed). New York, NY: Routledge.

CHAPTER 12

CPRT TRAINING SESSION 5: PLAY SESSION SKILLS REVIEW

Overview

The major focus of this session is supporting and encouraging parents as they learn and practice their new play session skills. No new material is introduced to avoid overwhelming parents. As in each of the remaining training sessions, the majority of the session is spent on parents' reports of home play sessions, with the most time allocated to reviewing the video(s) of the one to two parents who volunteered to be video-recorded for this week's focused supervision. A specific focus during group supervision is on increasing parents' self-awareness of their own feelings, particularly in relation to their children. The therapist also uses supervision and feedback to review and reinforce previously taught CPRT principles and skills, with an emphasis on the filial play session "Dos." The partial transcript of CPRT Training Session 5 included at the end of this chapter provides the reader with an illustration of how the experienced filial therapist facilitates and utilizes group dynamics to spontaneously review and reinforce basic filial play session skills, including limit setting, while providing dynamic support and encouragement to parents.

Materials

Suggested materials include: *CPRT Session 5—Treatment Outline*; parent information form with pertinent notes; homework assigned in Session 4, including extra copies of any homework worksheets; and Session 5 handouts and homework, including: *Session 5 Parent Notes and Homework*, *Limit Setting: A-C-T Practice Worksheet*, *Limit Setting: Why Use the Three-Step A-C-T Method?*, *Parent Play Session Notes*, and *Play Session Skills Checklist*. Additional materials include: display posters for both Play Session Dos and Don'ts, Play Session Procedure Checklist, and optional demonstration video clips to review and reinforce basic CPRT skills.

> *Note: All handouts listed above, as well as a training session outline for the therapist, additional supplemental parent handouts, and resources for this training session are found in the CPRT Treatment Manual,* 2nd Edition, *and accompanying Companion Website.*

Content and Procedure

The therapist begins the session by asking parents to briefly share how their week has been. With so much information and activity packed into each CPRT training session, therapists may be inclined to dispense with this informal sharing time. This activity is not to be underestimated. It is an important time for establishing rapport, building trust and safety in the group, fostering connections between the parents, and, most importantly, offering support and encouragement as parents share their struggles and failures as parents. The therapist helps parents to see that they are not alone in their child rearing by referring to or linking experiences shared by several parents. **Parents who feel supported and not alone in their struggles are more likely to share openly and honestly, thus enhancing group dynamics.**

Again, the therapist is encouraged to limit advice giving and to avoid suggesting that parents use the CPRT skills outside of play sessions. Although parents are generally eager to try the skills, they simply are not ready. The crucial element in parents' readiness to generalize CPRT skills to problems they are having with their child not only requires mastery of the skill, but more importantly for most parents, requires a significant shift in attitude toward their children and how they view their children's behaviors. Most parents are not ready to begin generalizing skills until around Session 8 or 9. As suggested in earlier sessions, the need to provide parents with answers, as well as parents' sidetracking on discussions of minor child-related problems, is avoided by briefly acknowledging parents, writing down their concerns, and letting parents know their concerns will be discussed later in the training. Use parents' sharing and "stories" about the week to transition to review of homework.

Review Homework

Parents were asked to be aware of one intense feeling they experienced during their play sessions with their children. Most parents have difficulty focusing on their feelings and initially may not be able to share an intense feeling. The therapist can use parents' reports of their home play sessions to reflect and point out feelings as they describe what happened. Focusing on parents' feelings is an important part of the overall strategy in CPRT training; parents who are not aware of their own feelings will not be able to identify and acknowledge their children's feelings. **The success of filial therapy training hinges on parents' ability to embrace and apply the skill of reflection of feeling.** The development of this skill also facilitates parents' beginning to trust their own instincts—a prerequisite for effective parenting. Parents are asked to share a time they used limit setting in their play sessions (if one was needed) and how it worked out. Remind parents that because they have carefully structured the time and place so that their children can have more freedom of expression, parents may need to set few limits during their play sessions. The limit of ending the play session on time is generally the most used. Be careful in presenting limit setting so that parents don't get the idea that they should be setting many limits during play sessions. Structuring play sessions so that limit setting is kept to a minimum is what is most important!

Filial Play Session Reports and Video Critique

As is true for all remaining sessions, the majority of this session is spent on supporting and encouraging parents as they report on their play sessions, with the greatest focus on giving feedback to the one to two parents who video-recorded their play sessions. The specific goal for this session is to review and reinforce all CPRT skills taught in Sessions 1–4. **No new skills are introduced during Session 5**—parents need time to focus on the basic skills introduced in the first four sessions without being overwhelmed with new information. The therapist listens carefully for opportunities to point out parents' strengths and examples of when parents are using the basic CPRT skills taught thus far. Remember to model **"Focus on the donut, not the hole."** The focus in this session is on what parents are doing right, not what they should do differently.

Displaying the Play Session Dos and Don'ts on a poster for parents and therapist to refer to as parents report on their home play sessions aids in the review and reinforcement of CPRT skills. After each parent briefly reports on the home play session, the therapist can ask other parents to point out one "Do" they heard used. Allow plenty of time for viewing the video-recorded play sessions. This activity provides the richest learning experience for all parents and greater opportunities for vicarious learning than when parents report orally on their home play sessions. The therapist can use the supervision of video-recorded play sessions to introduce the *Play Session Skills Checklist* that parents are asked to complete at home the next week after their play sessions. Pass out extra copies, briefly explain how to use them, and ask parents to use the form to note their observations of CPRT skills demonstrated during the viewing of video-recorded play sessions. Stop the video frequently and facilitate a discussion of play session skills demonstrated, showing parents how you would use the checklist to note your observations.

Insuring that at least one parent brings a video to class is imperative; therefore, we suggest that parents scheduled for video-recording come to the therapist's playroom to do so. The therapist can keep the video to cue up for the next CPRT training session. Again, it cannot be overstated that **weekly supervision of the video-recorded sessions, along with the dynamics of group interaction, are crucial elements in the success of the CPRT training.**

Limit Setting Review, Video, and Role-Play

Although all CPRT skills are reviewed in Session 5, typically the concept and application of limit setting is an area that most parents struggle with; therefore, review and demonstration of this skill is crucial. The therapist can show another video clip demonstration of limit setting and then ask parents to role-play, following up with a homework assignment to complete a limit-setting worksheet in which parents are given limit-setting scenarios to respond to. Parents often struggle with stating limits in a concise way. This can be a good time to introduce a new **Rule of Thumb: If you can't say it in 10 words or less, don't say it** (although when the therapist teaches the skill of choice giving, this rule is broken). Parents have a tendency to over-explain to children, with the result that their message gets lost in the words. "*The doll's head is not for pulling off*" can be understood by a child, but adding a long explanation about the cost of the doll can distract a child from hearing the limit. Parents are also asked to write down one limit set during their next play sessions (again, if one was needed), noting what happened, what they said, and how their children responded. Of all skills taught, parents are most eager to try limit setting outside of play sessions before they have mastered it. Remind parents again that, at this point in their training, **they are only to practice these skills during the 30-minute special play session.** The therapist's primary training strategy throughout the 10 sessions is to structure training and experiences to maximize parents' successes. Allow 10–15 minutes for role-play to practice limit setting before reviewing homework for the next week.

Homework Assignments

1. Parents are reminded of the importance of conducting their play sessions at the same time and same place.
2. Remind parents to take a few minutes to review the *Play Session Dos & Don'ts* and *Play Session Procedures Checklist* prior to their play sessions.
3. Remind parents to practice setting a limit during their play sessions, if needed, and to write down what happened and what they said. They are also reminded to complete the limit-setting practice worksheet.
4. Parents are reminded after conducting the play session to complete the *Parent Play Session Notes* and *Play Session Skills Checklist* and bring to group the next week.
5. One to two parents are scheduled for video-recording.
6. Remind parents about the Rule of Thumb for the week.

7. Close by introducing Sandwich Hugs and Sandwich Kisses (explained in the partial transcript at the end of this chapter) and ask parents to give each of their children a Sandwich Hug and Sandwich Kiss during the week (not during the special playtime). This type of assignment is designed to meet the CPRT training goals of helping parents rediscover the joys of parenting and helping families build warm, happy memories. The authors can both attest to the effectiveness of Sandwich Hugs and Kisses, as both have grown children who still get Sandwich Hugs and Kisses on occasion and who are now passing this practice to the next generation.

Partial Transcript of CPRT Session 5

Dr. L.: What has the week been like for you?

Sonya: My kids are really good kids, but my problem is trying to do everything by myself. Taking kids to school, fixing meals, baths, running errands, putting kids to bed. My youngest is still at home, and tomorrow it starts all over again. My children are still at the age that they're still pretty needy. Beth and Jenny can feed themselves, but they can't give themselves a bath. Sometimes I get overwhelmed.

Dr. L.: So if something's going to be done, it's up to you. That sounds pretty stressful.

Sonya: I think I handle it pretty well.

Dr. L.: You're always on call even when you're overwhelmed.

Sonya: And if any emergency comes up or one of the kids is sick, I'm the one who stays up with the kid at night. I'm the one who has to make it through the next day. It's hard even when things go smoothly.

Dr. L.: Even at the best of times it's stressful and overwhelming when things go wrong.

Sonya: Yes.

(Other parents report on their week.)

Dr. L.: One of your assignments was to be aware of one intense feeling you experienced in your playtime this week. What were you aware of feeling during your playtime?

Sonya: I felt really irritated and kind of rejected because my daughter played and played and didn't once invite me to play with her.

Dr. L.: So you were a little angry with her for not including you. Anyone react to that?

Laura: I'm learning to hold myself back so I won't interfere with my son's play to make it be what I want it to be.

Sonya: Yeah, I know I have a problem needing to be included in everything so I will feel better about myself.

Dr. L.: Laura, sounds like you and Sonya are both beginning to become aware of some of your own needs. That's great progress. Sonya, for 30 minutes you are giving your daughter a very special gift: your attention, your understanding, your caring. Anyone else experience an intense feeling during your playtime?

(Other parents describe an intense feeling.)

Dr. L.: Nita, what was your special playtime like this week?

Nita: Jeff was *real* sick. And when he's real sick, he's very aggressive, very unhappy. I felt terrible, too, that day. In the evenings, I have lots of pain [she is pregnant], unless I have more control of my day, but I hadn't had any control of my day; so I was feeling lousy. He was *really* feeling lousy. He was just totally disorganized.

Dr. L.: You did the session anyway, even though you felt crummy.

Nita: Yeah, because I just knew there really wasn't another time. We had so much trouble the past 2 weeks with him coming down with this for a week, and then getting over it for a week. We ended up averaging maybe 5–6 hours of sleep out of 24 for 2 weeks.

Dr. L.: (to group) I want to tell all of you that one of the things I am reacting to is your commitment. Laura, you didn't want to have your playtime, but you did it anyway. Kathy, you had that terrible no-good happening, but you had your playtime anyway. Nita, you felt crummy, you didn't want to, but you did it anyway. That says commitment! I am really impressed with your commitment; I don't know if you would use that word to describe yourselves, but I hear commitment from each one of you. So, Nita, how'd it work out?

Nita: At the time, I didn't think it was working out at all because he kept trying to do things that he obviously knew he wasn't supposed to do.

Dr. L.: So he did some testing.

Nita: Oh yes, but he didn't just throw terrific fits or anything, like he usually does. He was too sick and too tired. He was pretty quiet and disorganized, but then he said what he's been saying for the past 2 weeks, "Mommy, I *need* you." I said, "Well what do you need me to do?" He climbed into my lap, and we just sat there. He didn't want me to say anything; he didn't want me to touch his hair; he just wanted to sit.

Dr. L.: He just wanted to be there, sitting in your lap. Sounds like a contented time in your lap.

Nita: And then finally he did get up and play.

Dr. L.: Let's talk about that just a minute. Whose time is this?

Sonya: His.

Dr. L.: He did what he wanted to do. You bought all these special toys, and your child chose to sit in your lap, that's what's important to him. It says that's more important right now than playing with a whole lot of new toys.

Sonya: Wow.

Dr. L.: What are you reacting to?

Sonya: Well, that's pretty special. To think that your kid would want to be with you a lot more than play with all these new things. He would rather just lie on you.

Dr. L.: It's also special that he got to sit in your lap and have all of you right then, even though you started out feeling crummy and would rather not have done this.

Nita: Definitely. That's really how we spent most of our time, him sitting in my lap. Well I'd been talking to him lately, in the evenings, about how I can't do a three-ring circus every evening. I haven't been able to since before Christmas. So I tell him that Mommy has pains, doesn't feel good, and that it will soon be over. So he's aware, and he plasters both of us with Band-Aids.

Dr. L.: He was sensitive to your pain and nurtured you. (addresses group) Could I suggest that in the 30-minute playtime, you all change the "Mommy" to "me," to "I"? "I don't feel good," instead of "Mommy doesn't feel good." I've heard two or three of you say, "Mommy." Change that during the playtime to "I." Let's personalize it, "I."

Debbie: I know you think I keep picking, but why can't you say, "Mommy?"

Dr. L.: It's like you're talking about someone else.

Debbie: So, it personalizes it more, makes it more real.

Dr. L.: Debbie, I continue to be struck by the fact that you have the answers. You just don't trust them.

Debbie: No, I don't.

Dr. L.: I wish I had a magic wand. I would walk over, touch you on the head and say, "Now, trust the answers you have."

Sonya: I like your questions because it always feels good when you get clarification. It confirms things for me, too.

Dr. L.: Behind your questions, you have the answers.

Debbie: I just want to know if I have the answers.

Dr. L.: And I would like to give you permission with this magic wand to trust yourself. I don't have all the answers for you all. I can help you structure your special playtimes, but you're the real key, and the most important thing is that you trust what you are doing. Nita, how did your playtime end?

Nita: I told him we had 3 minutes left, and he totally and completely fell apart, screaming.

Dr. L.: Because he wanted more?

Nita: Because he wanted me, and he thought once it was over he wouldn't have me at all. Finally, I had to pick him up and carry him into his room and start telling him a story.

Dr. L.: You handled it. Did it work out, did he calm down?

Nita: Yes, once I told him his favorite story, he settled down. Somehow, I knew it was just the issue of needing me.

Dr. L.: He's very vulnerable right now. Someone else is about to take his place and that can be scary to a child. The important thing is that you are understanding of how he feels.

Nita: It just occurred to me that Jeff's wanting to sit on my lap so much lately is because I can't get down on the floor and be close to him like I used to do. Actually, I have been concerned about him wanting to sit on my lap so much.

Laura: He wants to be close to you, especially when he is crying. He feels closer, more secure.

Dr. L.: So, Nita, you learned something about Jeff.

(Parents report on their play sessions and receive feedback.)

Dr. L.: Kim, you video-recorded your play session. Tell us what it was like for you before we see it.

Kim: It was kinda tense, but OK. I didn't know what to do. I just tried to do what we've been doing here. My son really enjoyed himself.

Dr. L.: OK. Let's see your play session.

(Group watches video.)

Dr. L.: (Stops video.) Kim, I noticed that you said a lot with your eyes. You are so in tune with your child. As your child looked up on the top of that shelf, his eyes went up, and I saw your eyes go up. You were looking at what your child was looking at. Children know when you are that involved. Just as you said earlier, Debbie, your child senses when you're sure and senses when you're not sure. Our children sense when we're with them and understanding them, and they sense when we're not paying attention. Kim, that was a very powerful message you communicated with your eyes.

(Group watches video.)

Dr. L.: (Stops video.)

Sonya: That's exactly what Jenny does in our special playtime. She will say, "Mommy, I want you to do this or that," and as soon as I say, "What do you want me to do?" she goes on to something else.

Kim: Yes, he drops it and plays with something else every time.

Dr. L.: What does that mean?

Sonya: He's saying, "I just want you to sit there and watch me."

Dr. L.: Yes, that's enough.

Sonya: It kinda hurt my feelings when she first started doing that, because I really wanted to play.

Dr. L.: You felt left out, as though your child didn't want to include or didn't care about you.

Sonya: Yes, but I know she really does.

Dr. L.: So you have to watch out for your need to be needed.

(Group watches video.)

Dr. L.: (Stops video.) Kim, before we started watching your session, you said there were some parts that didn't seem to go very well, and I'm sitting here hearing some great responses.

Kim: I'm really nervous.

Dr. L.: Even though you're nervous, I was thinking that you're doing so well. I wondered if there might be a message in that for all of us.

Kathy: You don't give yourself enough credit.

Dr. L.: You got it. You don't give yourself enough credit for what you are doing. Debbie, you said that earlier, too, that you're smarter than you give yourself credit for. And you all do a better job than you give yourselves credit for.

Sonya: I think there's something else going on there, too, Kim. You put what was going on inside you aside so you could be there for him. And you came across as being genuinely interested in him.

Kim: Yes, I knew he was having fun.

(Group watches video.)

Dr. L.: (Stops video.) Kim, you look comfortable. You might make one change there. You turned a great statement into a question, "You're taking the doll's clothes off?" The tone of voice turns it into a question and implies you don't understand. That really makes a difference. We want to let our children know that we understand, and you do that by making statements.

(Replays segment so group hears the question. Group watches video.)

Dr. L.: (Stops video.)

Kathy: Now I got it.

Dr. L.: Kim, let's see more of your session.

(Group watches video.)

Dr. L.: (Stops video.) What just happened there, Kim? (Group laughs.)

Kim: I just reached out and fixed his shirt.

Dr. L.: It's an unconscious thing. Parents reach out and do things for their children. Things should be in their place, and a shirt should be pulled down. Perhaps more than we realize, we reach out and do things for children, and the message is "You're supposed to be neat."

Sonya: Kim looked so interested in everything.

Dr. L.: What feedback do you want to give, Debbie?

Debbie: You tracked him not only physically, but verbally and with your eyes. What impressed me the most was the look on your face as you watched him. If I were your child, I would know that you cared about me, that you love me. You looked like you cared, and it was genuine.

Dr. L.: Yes, having someone focus entirely on you, for even a few minutes, can be powerful. Well, let's shift focus and do some review of last week. Last week we worked on limit setting. If those of you who were here last week will tell what you remember about limit setting, that will help the parents who were absent last week to learn it.

Sonya: ACT—he gave us an acronym, and A means acknowledging the feeling or the want of the child. Like, I know you want to hit your sister. C was communicate the limit. Your sister's not for hitting. T is target the choices. You may hit your stuffed animals.

(Parents continue to discuss what they learned last week about limit setting, but it is obvious they are struggling with understanding and believing in the concept.)

Dr. L.: Why don't we watch a parent playtime as a way to review the A-C-T method. The child in the video is 2½. Most of you are probably thinking, no way a 2½-year-old can understand and respond to this way of limit setting.

(Parents laugh, then Dr. L. starts video. A partial transcript of the video is included here because it provides such a dramatic example of a child's inner struggle and the effectiveness of the A-C-T model, even with a child this young.)

Child: (Gets a cup from the kitchen and walks to the sink.)

Mom: Kristin, we have 5 more minutes in the playtime today and then it will be time to go.

Child: (Fills the cup with water from the sink faucet.) Five?

Mom: We have 5 more minutes, and then we need to go.

Child: (Walks to sandbox and pours water from the cup into sand.)

Mom: (While child is pouring water in the sandbox) One cup of water . . .

Child: (Child walks back to sink and fills cup with water, walks to sandbox and pours water in the box.) Two . . .

Mom: Two . . . you're counting . . . you poured that slowly. I heard it make a noise.

Child: (Goes back to sink again and fills cup a third time, then walks back to sandbox and pours water into sandbox. She looks very absorbed in her play.)

Mom: Three . . . you poured three cups of water in the sand.

Child: Just one more. (Child walks back to sink and fills cup with water.)

Mom: I know you would like to pour more water in the sandbox, but you have already put three in and that is all. (Standard rule in the playroom: only three containers of water allowed to be poured in the sandbox.)

Child: (Walks to sandbox with a cup full of water and starts to pour water in the box.)

Mom: Kristin, in here the sandbox can only have three cups of water, and you have already put three. No more water can go into the sandbox. (Mother leans toward the child and shows "three" with her fingers. She gives lots of nonverbal signs to Kristin. Her voice is firmer. Child stands in front of sandbox. She is about to pour more water, but listens to her mother.) I know you really want to put more water in.

Child: OK. (She stops herself.)

Mom: But you can pretend.

Child: I just . . .

Mom: You can pour that water into the sink. That water can't go in the sandbox cause you already put three in. You can pour that water into the sink.

Child: (Seems to be struggling with the idea of pouring more water in the sandbox. She tilts the cup a little bit, trying to pour water in the sandbox.)

Mom: Kristin, I know you really want to pour that water in the sandbox, but it is not for pouring in the sandbox. You may pour that water into the sink. You already put three cups of water, and that's all the sand can have.

Child: (Is still struggling. She tilts the cup forward more and some water dribbles into the sandbox.)

Mom: I see you pouring water. (Child pours a bit more.) Kristin, that water is not for pouring into the sandbox (said in a patient, but firm tone).

Child: I just put little bit . . .

Mom: I know you just really want to put a little bit in the sandbox.

Child: (Walks back to sink and dumps rest of water into sink.)

Mom: Now, you poured it into the sink.

Child: No more. . . .

Mom: The sink is the place where you can pour that water.

Child: (Plays with water in sink.) I just pour out . . . cup . . . so I can . . . put this in it.

Mom: So you are getting more water in the cup and pouring it in the sink.

Child: Right there!!!

Mom: Right there!!!

Child: (Continues playing at the sink with water running.) Look at me. (She turns to her mother.)

Mom: I heard that! It went right down that drain. Oh . . . you're being careful . . . put it right in the drain . . .

Child: Some of it out.

Mom: Some of it out. That's where you want it to go.

Child: Two . . .

Mom: Mm-hmm.

Child: Three . . .

Mom: Three . . .

Child: Four . . . Five!

Mom: You counted to five!

(Dr. L. stops the video—end of viewing mother/child play session.)

Dr. L: You see this child struggle with wanting to pour more water into the sand. She hears her mom's calm statements indicating the rule of three containers of water in the sandbox, but she still wants to pour more water. The result is a graphic example of the age-old inner battle between doing what the child wants to do and knowing that is not appropriate. This 2½-year-old's struggle demonstrates the effectiveness of the A-C-T model of therapeutic limit setting in returning responsibility to the child to bring self under control and to say "No" to self. Yes, the child did dribble a bit of extra water into the sand, but did control her inner urge, walked to the sink and poured the remaining water into the sink. If a 2½-year-old child can bring herself under control in response to the A-C-T model of therapeutic limit setting, then surely older children will even more easily respond in like manner.

Kim: So it's really not discipline during the playtime, it's just about putting limits on your child's behavior.

Dr. L.: Well, it actually is discipline. It's a different way of disciplining. In this kind of limit setting, you're teaching your child to say "No" to self. If I say, "The wall is not for marking on, the paper is for marking on," and the child stops himself or herself, who made the child stop?

Sonya: The child did.

Debbie: And it would work later when they get angry, instead of abusing someone.

Kim: So does discipline follow if it doesn't work, or do you start all over again with acknowledging the feeling?

Dr. L.: That's a good question. There is a Step 4, but you go through the A-C-T steps several times first. Let's review those steps. What is the first step?

Sonya: Acknowledge the feeling.

Dr. L.: Yes. We always start by reflecting the child's feeling or want. "You're angry at me." And the second step?

Laura: Communicate the limit.

Dr. L.: Yes, set the limit. "You're angry at me. I'm not for shooting." And the third step?

Nita: That's the hard one; target an alternative.

Dr. L.: Yes, target an acceptable alternative, something the child can do. "You're angry at me. I'm not for shooting. You can shoot the Bobo." If you go through these three steps several times, and your child continues to try to shoot you with the dart gun, Step 4 is "If you choose to keep trying to shoot me, you choose not to play with the gun for the rest of our playtime. If you choose not to shoot me, you choose to get to play with the gun."

Kim: Then they made the decision.

Dr. L.: Yes. We'll work more on giving choices next week. Now, let's work some more on limit setting. Turn to the person next to you. One of you can be the child first. Use the toys and do something children might do to break the limit. Pretend you're going to break the toys, or pretend you're going to splash paint and let your parent practice setting limits.

(Parents role-play.)

Dr. L.: OK, folks. Everybody stop. It is really important when targeting a choice to always point toward the choice.

Sonya, role-play with me. You're the child and you start banging with that wood hammer. "I know you'd like to bang on that, but that's not for banging on. The wood over there," and you point, "is for banging on with that."

Sonya: And inside I'm feeling, "Oh, OK, I do get to do it."

Debbie: But there's a delay time, because I'm not sure what to say.

Dr. L.: That's OK. The words will come to you faster later. This is like learning a foreign language. The first few times you do this, you're going to feel tongue-tied. You may blurt out some old commands.

Sonya: Don't do that!

Dr. L.: Yes. You will sometimes go back to the old behaviors. But in this special 30-minute playtime, you try to contain that urge and go through the steps of limit setting. Now, let's switch roles.

(Parents role-play.)

Dr. L.: OK, folks, time to stop for today. I have one more really important homework assignment for all of you to do with your child and another family member. You do this sometime other than your play session—and you do this with all your children. It's called a **Sandwich Hug**. It looks like this. (Dr. L. gets up to demonstrate.) You and your husband get on either side of your child (pick your child up if she is little), and you say (playfully), "We're going to make a Sandwich Hug, you're going to be the peanut butter (or whatever sandwich child likes best) and we're going to be the bread." Then squeeze your child between you and your husband and give your child a big physical, noisy hug, "ummm—ummm!" (The noise is very important—children love that!) Be sure and give each of your children one. "One more thing, who can come to the center this week and video your play session?"

Reference

Bratton, S., & Landreth, G. (2019). *Child-Parent Relationship Therapy (CPRT) treatment manual: An Evidence-Based 10-session filial therapy model* (2nd ed). New York, NY: Routledge.

CHAPTER 13

CPRT TRAINING SESSION 6: SUPERVISION AND CHOICE GIVING

Overview

Sessions 6 through 9 follow the same general format, with the main focus on supervision of home play sessions; therefore, this section provides a comprehensive overview of the critical elements shared by these four sessions. Each session begins with 10 to 15 minutes of parents' informal sharing about their week, followed by a discussion of homework assignments and brief reporting by all parents about their play sessions. The therapist provides suggestions and points out CPRT skills demonstrated as parents describe play session happenings, attending carefully to feelings expressed by parents. Greater attention is given to common problems parents are experiencing. The partial transcript included with each training session provides the reader with a dynamic example of group process.

As parents report on their play sessions, the therapist has two primary tasks: to find something to encourage in each parent and to use parents' comments to reinforce the basic CPRT principles and guidelines covered thus far. The therapist may find it helpful to continue to display a poster with the *Play Session Dos and Don'ts* for parents to refer to during play session reporting. For example, the therapist can ask the parent to talk about one "Do" they felt they did well and pick one "Do" they want to work on in their next play session.

An essential element in Sessions 6 through 9 is the weekly viewing and critique of one to two parent videos; therefore, it is imperative that the therapist take necessary measures to ensure that at least 1 parent comes to class with a video-recorded play session. (In rare cases where a parent cannot or has not video-recorded a session, a live parent-child session can be observed by the therapist and group, with the parent receiving immediate feedback.) An objective is that each parent will be video-recorded and receive focused feedback at least once, and hopefully twice, during the 10 sessions of training. Weekly supervision of video-recorded sessions, along with the accompanying dynamics of group interaction and various learning experiences that naturally occur, is a powerful process and the cornerstone to the success of CPRT training. An invaluable part of the learning process occurs when parents begin to recognize the basic "Dos" and "Don'ts" demonstrated and/or reported during supervision and are able to give constructive feedback to each other.

Taking the time to process parents' feelings as they arise is especially important and models for parents what you are asking them to do with their children: focus on feelings. Again, the therapist's skillful balance between the teaching content and supporting parents is critical to the success of CPRT training—this skill cannot be overemphasized. The therapist helps parents to see that they are not alone in their child-rearing struggles by linking experiences shared by several parents. Reviewing and role-playing of play session principles and skills are continued each session.

As parents spontaneously begin to share happenings outside the play session that in any small way indicate generalization of CPRT skills, the therapist quickly acknowledges the newly developed coping strategy, with the aim of encouraging, empowering, and enhancing parental confidence. Enhancing feelings of parental efficacy, along with building self-esteem and self-confidence, is a primary aim for the therapist, just as a primary aim for parents in Sessions 6 through 9 is to actively respond to their children in ways that encourage and build their children's self-esteem.

As successful use of CPRT skills outside the play sessions naturally occurs (around Session 8 to 9), the therapist can begin to add homework assignments that encourage generalization of skills; for example, by giving parents an assignment to practice making a therapeutic limit-setting response to a typical happening outside the play session. As is true for all homework assignments, be specific in what you want parents to *write down* and report on the next week; and then, make sure to take a few minutes at the beginning of the next session for parents to share homework results.

Parents' growing confidence in themselves and the use of their newly acquired skills becomes evident in their interactions during the group supervision and feedback time in each session. Generally by the eighth session, parents begin to volunteer comments on changes they see in themselves, in their children, and in other parents in the group. The therapist takes this cue as an opportunity to facilitate parents' growth and learning to a higher level by asking them to give each other feedback as they watch and listen to each other's play sessions. Essentially, the therapist is moving parents into the role of peer-supervisors and helping them become more self-aware, with a goal of moving toward self-monitoring skills by Session 10.

In Sessions 6 through 8, the therapist continues to acknowledge parental concerns about long-term and crisis-related child problems not related to the special playtimes by listening and writing down concerns as they are expressed, but typically these issues aren't addressed until Sessions 9 and 10. As is true in all sessions, the inevitable sidetracking on discussions of minor child-related problems is carefully avoided by the therapist acknowledging the parent briefly with a word, but refocusing the discussion to the point at hand. In limited cases of some minor child-related problems, a brief suggestion might be offered but is not explained in a prolonged discussion.

The importance of consistency is emphasized over and over: consistency in holding play sessions, consistency in limit setting, consistency in daily routines, etc. The importance of consistency in conducting home play sessions at the same time and place each week is emphasized throughout, even if the child asks for changes and/or it would be more convenient for the parent to change the time. Parents often have great difficulty grasping the importance of consistency and predictability in children's lives.

Continually remind parents that for children, **parental consistency → predictability → security → child feeling safe and loved!** At the end of each session, the therapist gives reminders about homework for the next week and schedules one to two more parents to be video-recorded for the following week's focused supervision.

Although all essential teaching points and skills needed to conduct successful play sessions are covered in Sessions 1 through 5, new, but related, topics and homework are introduced in Sessions 6 through 9 to help solidify parents' learning and generalize their new skills to everyday happenings. The therapist can be flexible in introducing new topics and assigning homework according to the needs of the group. Specific to training Session 6, choice giving is the only new topic introduced.

> Reminder: As is true for all sessions**, avoid overwhelming parents with too much information or homework. Rule of Thumb for the successful filial therapist leader: Leave parents with no more than three or four main points or assignments to focus on between sessions.**

Materials

Suggested materials include: *CPRT Session 6—Treatment Outline*; parent information form with pertinent notes; homework assigned in Session 5, including extra copies of any homework worksheets; and Session 6 handouts and homework, including: *Session 6 Parent Notes and Homework, Choice Giving 101: Teaching Responsibility & Decision Making* and *Advanced Choice Giving: Providing Choices as Consequences, Practice Choice Giving Worksheet*; *Parent Play Session Notes*; and *Play Session Skills Checklist.* Additional materials include: a display poster of *Play Session Dos & Don'ts, Choices, Cookies, & Kids* video by Garry L. Landreth (see *CPRT Treatment Manual, 2nd Edition*) to demonstrate choice-giving method of discipline, and an optional video clip demonstrating filial play session skills focused on self-esteem-building responses and responses that return responsibility to the child. The therapist may also find it helpful to make a list of common problems often experienced by parents during play sessions to facilitate a discussion on challenging issues (refer to Chapter 24).

> *Note: All handouts listed above, as well as a training session outline for the filial therapist, additional supplemental parent handouts, and resources for this training session are found in the CPRT Treatment Manual,* 2nd Edition, *and accompanying Companion Website.*

Content and Procedure

As explained in the overview, the major focus of training in Session 6, as well as in all remaining sessions, is supporting and encouraging parents' skill development and confidence through group supervision and feedback as parents report on their play sessions; thus, the majority of the allotted time is devoted to this activity. As in all previous sessions, the initial informal sharing time is used to support parents and forge connections, while shifting the focus to a review of homework. Parents are first asked to share their experiences with giving their children Sandwich Hugs and Sandwiches Kisses, followed by a discussion and practice of limit setting using either oral or written examples (use homework practice worksheet, if assigned). As parents report on their play session experiences, they are each asked to describe any limits set during play sessions. In addition, parents are each asked to discuss one thing they thought they did well and one skill they want to focus on in their next play sessions.

The **Rule of Thumb: "Grant in fantasy what you cannot grant in reality"** is introduced to help parents understand the value of children's role-playing of behaviors during play sessions that would be unacceptable outside of the play sessions. For example, 3-year-old Margaret has a new baby sister and is naturally feeling a little jealous. During her play session, she takes the baby doll and throws her out of the play area. A helpful parent response would be, "*You just didn't want the baby to be in here,*" or "*You decided to just throw the baby over there.*" However, parents are generally disturbed by this kind of behavior, believing that if they accept this behavior during the session that their child will think it is permissible outside of session. The same is true of any aggressive or regressive play behaviors; therefore, the therapist must be careful to explain this concept in a way that parents can understand. The only new concept/skill introduced in this session is choice giving.

Choice Giving

The concept of giving children choices is introduced to build on the principles of limit setting focused on in Sessions 4 and 5 and as a strategy for empowering children to make decisions and avoid power struggles outside of play sessions. Emphasize to parents that choices given must be commensurate with a child's developmental stage.

RULE OF THUMB:

Big choices for big kids, little choices for little kids.

The skill of choice giving is most easily grasped by parents through demonstration and providing opportunities for practice. The *Choices, Cookies, & Kids* video by Garry L. Landreth is shown to clearly illustrate both the concept and the skill of choice giving. The video is approximately 30 minutes in length and should be previewed prior to use. Because of time constraints, the therapist may want to show part of the video during Session 6 and the remainder during Session 7. The Oreo® Cookie Theory of choice giving is covered approximately 6 minutes into the video and should be covered during Session 6, even if time restricts a viewing of the full video. Parents are provided with the handouts *Choice Giving 101: Teaching Responsibility & Decision Making* and *Advanced Choice Giving: Providing Choices as Consequences*. The therapist reviews the information from the handouts, clarifying the difference between choice giving to empower children and choice giving as a method of discipline.

The following topics related to choice giving and the Choices, Cookies, & Kids video are discussed and examples given for application in Choice Giving 101: Teaching Responsibility & Decision Making in Session 6 of the Therapist Notebook in the *CPRT Treatment Manual, 2nd Edition.*

- **Providing children with age-appropriate choices empowers children.**
- **Presenting children with choices provides opportunities for decision making and problem solving.**
- **Providing children with choices reduces power.**
- **Provide age-appropriate choices.**

The Oreo® Cookie Method and the following related topics are discussed and examples given for application in Advanced Choice Giving: Providing Choices as Consequences in Session 6 of the Therapist Notebook in the *CPRT Treatment Manual, 2nd Edition.*

Common Problems in Filial Play Session

We have found that there are certain common problems that parents often struggle with during special playtimes with their children or that they have questions about. Some of these are:

> My child notices that I talk differently in the play sessions and wants me to talk normally. What should I do?
>
> My child asks many questions during the play sessions and resents my not answering them. What should I do?
>
> My child just plays and has fun. What am I doing wrong?
>
> I'm bored. What's the value of this?
>
> My child doesn't respond to my comments. How do I know I'm on target?
>
> When is it OK for me to ask questions, and when is it not OK?
>
> My child hates the play sessions. Should I discontinue them?

My child wants the playtime to be longer. Should I extend the session?

My child wants to play with the toys at other times during the week. Is it OK?

My child wants me to shoot at him during the play session. What should I do?

Additional information about common problems and how to respond is in Common Problems in Play Sessions in Session 6 of the Therapist Notebook in the CPRT Treatment Manual, 2nd Edition and Chapter 24 in this text.

Limit-Setting Review

The skill of limit setting is an ongoing challenge for most parents and typically continues to be a major focus in Session 6. The therapist uses parents' spontaneous sharing of limit-setting struggles to review and practice the skill. The majority of parents struggle with following through once they have set a limit, especially when faced with their children's pleading, whining, and other behaviors that they have learned to use to manipulate and wear down their parents. Remind parents about the importance of follow-through: **When they don't follow through on limits set or promises made, they lose credibility with their child**—and ultimately, damage their relationship with their child. Trust is the foundation of a healthy relationship. When parents fail to follow through and provide consistency, the message to the child is "You really can't count on me to do what I say." Humor can be used to get this very serious point across; for example, by having parents repeat after you three times, **"When setting limits, I WILL follow through—I am tough as nails!"**

Self-Esteem-Building Responses and Video

If time permits at the end of the session, the therapist can briefly introduce self-esteem-building responses and the concept of giving the child credit as a way of enhancing the child's sense of personal power, assigning parents to practice making one self-esteem-building response in their upcoming play sessions. A brief video-recorded demonstration of the use of self-esteem-building responses in a play session provides parents with concrete examples of this skill. A brief demonstration with a parent, or, even better, with one of the parents' children, can be used in place of a video.

Homework Assignments

1. Parents are reminded of the importance of conducting their play session at the same time and same place and to video-record their session.
2. Remind parents to take a few minutes to read over *Play Session Dos & Don'ts* and *Play Session Procedures Checklist* prior to their play sessions.
3. Remind parents to practice giving one self-esteem-building response during their next play sessions (if time permitted the brief introduction of the self-esteem-building skill).
4. Parents are reminded after conducting the play session to complete the *Parent Play Session Notes* and *Play Session Skills Checklist* and bring to the group the following week.
5. Ask parents to read *Common Problems in Play Sessions* for the following week and mark the top two to three issues they have questions about or write in an issue they are challenged by that is not on the worksheet prior to their play session, and to read *Choice Giving 101* and *Advanced Choice Giving* and practice giving at least one choice outside of the play session (this is the first assignment to practice a skill outside of the session).
6. One to two parents are scheduled to be video-recorded.
7. Parents are reminded of the Rule of Thumb for this week.

Partial Transcript of CPRT Session 6

(Dr. L. notices that Kathy seems unusually quiet as she sits and waits for group to start.)

Dr. L.: How's your week been, Kathy?

Kathy: Last night Cody kicked me and I told him I wasn't for kicking, and then I didn't know what to say. It made me furious because he was mad when he kicked me. It was a bad time.

Dr. L.: So when he gets to the point of actually doing something, then you're not quite sure of what to do next, because you're so angry.

Kathy: Right, I told him I'm not for kicking, and then I was just furious. I figured, so I tell him to go kick something else, but then what's going to stop him from coming back and kicking me again, and again, and again?

Dr. L.: Seems like you're just not sure if it will work, especially when Cody is already so mad.

Kathy: That's right.

Dr. L.: And it may not work every time, especially if Cody knows you're furious with him. The reason that I want you to practice these skills only during your 30-minute play session is because it is a time when you are more in control of the situation. You purposefully chose a time for your play sessions when you would be less stressed and more relaxed, and this is a special time for Cody to play with all those neat toys. So you're more likely to be successful applying these skills during your play sessions. Kathy, I bet you are not the only one who has questions about limit setting. *(Several parents nod.)*

(Refocuses on group.) Let's talk some more about limit setting during your play sessions. A-C-T can be used at other times, but we are really most concerned about applying it in the special playtime. When your child picks up the crayon and looks at the wall, you know what's in his mind. He's thinking, "I wonder what it would look like on the wall," and you simply go through A-C-T. "*Looks like you'd like to mark on the wall, but the wall's not for marking on.*" Then the third step is to communicate some choices, which is to tell children what they can do. In this approach, we don't set out to stop the behavior. We set out to help the child complete what

they started, but in a way that is acceptable. So, "*The wall is not for marking on. The paper is for marking on.*" We always give a choice, so children can express their need. *(Dr. L. looks over at Kathy.)* "*I'm not for kicking. You can tell me you're angry.*" Or the trash can could be for kicking.

Kathy: OK.

Dr. L.: In limit setting, it's really important that you point to what the acceptable item is. The wall is not for marking on. The paper (pointing) is for marking on. I'm not for kicking. The Bobo (pointing) is for kicking. You point to what is acceptable, and that diverts the child's attention toward what is acceptable. In this approach, the objective is to help the child to learn to say "No" to self. Where we're headed with this approach is when your child is 13 or 15, and he is across town, not under your thumb, and he needs to stop himself when peers suggest he do something he should not do. He will need to say "No" to himself. Kim, did you have an opportunity to use A-C-T?

Kim: Yes, a little too late. My daughter decided my solid lean-back chairs needed designs painted on them, but it worked when I told her that she could color on the coloring book, but not on my chairs.

Sonya: There was something you said last week that really left an impression on me. When you were talking about our children being angry, and that doesn't just go away. It stays with them until they're able to get it out in some form or another. I noticed that a lot this week with Jenny. Until she had a chance to resolve her anger, she would act out in tiny little ways all over the place. It was a powerful little piece of information, and it's true with her.

Dr. L.: In this new approach, you give your children a chance to express the need or feeling.

Sonya: And, one more thing.

Dr. L.: Yes.

Sonya: Just in the tools you've given us so far, I was able to make a decision after watching some of this work. I had the courage to wean both of the girls off of their bottles. It was like parenting from hell, though. Before coming here, I didn't know how to redirect their behaviors or just say, it's not OK to scream and holler and throw your body all over the house. I feel a lot more confident in being able to handle the repercussions of no crutch and perhaps replacing it with something appropriate like a special doll or something.

Laura: These playtimes have allowed me to appreciate my son more than anything else.

Dr. L.: Can you add to that?

Laura: We were having a real hard time, and I didn't really like a lot of his behavior. I associated a lot of his behavior with him, and didn't like him, and the playtimes have brought a new love feeling for Dawson, especially a closeness. Just learning to play and enjoy him, 'cause being a single parent I'm always the one who has to discipline him, and I forgot to just enjoy and play with my children. The playtime allowed me to do that, and I have found a new joy.

Dr. L.: It's almost as though you're saying, "I've rediscovered how to be a loving mother," instead of having to always keep things straightened out and take care of things.

Laura: Yes, everything has to be in control, and perfect, and that makes for a perfect life. Now, I've found that I can leave everything scattered around me, and I can take care of myself, too.

Dr. L.: So, your life is different. You know, as I listen to you, Laura, one of the things that keeps occurring to me is you're saying "I'm more free now."

Laura: Yes, I was a neurotic mom.

Dr. L.: That is a difficult place to be.

Laura: Yes, but the thing I'm still having trouble with is being in the middle of a crisis and being able to step back out of the crisis.

Dr. L.: And be objective.

Laura: And be objective from it and know that I don't have to react, that I can step back and get in control of my own emotions, and then decide what to do.

Dr. L.: Nita, you were reacting to that, when Laura said step back.

Nita: When Jeff does those things, the first thing I do now is just tell myself, he is not really doing this just to get to me. Because I used to feel that way, and that's how I would react: "You are doing this on purpose to get me." When I take myself out of it, then I handle the whole situation a lot better. I'm a lot happier, and he's a lot happier, but if I've got myself in there, my own ego or something, then it's just get focused on that!

Dr. L.: Then it's a real struggle, and self-defeating.

Nita: Oh, yeah!

Dr. L.: I think I hear you all saying that you're becoming more understanding. When you talk about stepping back, and being more objective, you're taking yourself out of the situation and working a bit harder at understanding your child at that moment.

Nita: Yes.

Sonya: And when we get together in these meetings every week and go over new skills or new techniques or whatever, it's easier than when I'm in the middle of some sort of struggle with Jenny because I'm taking this training. If I wasn't coming here, I wouldn't be keeping track of any of my behaviors, and each situation would just be more frustrating. Now, I feel a lot more comfortable in stepping back a little bit. Last night Jenny was yelling "I want my Tootsie Pop!" and I was thinking, I did promise it to her after dinner, but it's already almost bedtime. Finally, I said, "I need to think about this for a second." She was real quiet standing there watching me, and then I told her, I think it would be OK for you to have juice instead, and then you need to brush your teeth again. She said

OK, the compromise was OK, and it was OK for me. I felt empowered.

Dr. L.: So you're starting to think about what you're doing, and that's giving you self-control.

Sonya: Knowing actions, instead of just reacting, that feels good.

Kathy: Cody keeps telling me to shut up. I tell him I'm not for telling to shut up, and that he can tell me he doesn't want to listen to me, but I'm not for telling to shut up, and he still does it quite a bit. He did it a lot last night, over and over and over again. He was with his dad this weekend. Maybe his dad told him to shut up a lot.

Dr. L.: Would it help if we saw some of your session right now, and that might give us a better picture of what you're having to deal with?

Kathy: It might.

(Parents view video.)

Dr. L.: (Stops video.) Right there, you need to set a limit. He's asking you to do something that you really don't want to do.

Kathy: That's right.

Dr. L.: He's asking you to use a word that you don't want to use. So, what would you like to say to him?

Kathy: "I don't want to say that."

Dr. L.: Sounds great to me.

Kathy: OK, but I thought I was supposed to do what he wants me to do in his whole playtime.

Dr. L.: There are limits. For some reason, setting limits firmly is difficult for you.

Emily: Kathy, if he wants to mark on the wall, you're not going to let him mark on the wall.

Kathy: No, that's true. I'm not.

Dr. L.: There are limits. This is not a completely free or permissive relationship.

Kathy: He can say what he wants. Well, not exactly what he wants.

Dr. L.: Within limits.

Kathy: But I have the choice of saying what I want also, or something like that.

Dr. L.: You're the adult.

Kathy: Yeah.

Dr. L.: You're the authority, and you're the person responsible for setting limits. Your child is not. We set the boundaries, and the child is free within those boundaries, but they're not free to go outside those boundaries, and marking on the wall would be going outside those boundaries. Hitting you would be going outside those boundaries. Having you say words that you don't want to say is going outside those boundaries. The key to limit setting is responding quickly, firmly, and decisively. When you start hesitating, how does a child read that, Emily?

Emily: That he will get what he wants. That she's going to give in, and if I beg or throw a big fit, I'll get it.

Dr. L.: I would guess that some of what we just saw on the video is pretty typical of Cody.

Kathy: Oh, yes.

Dr. L.: When Cody tells you to say words you don't want to say, you could say . . .?

Kathy: "I don't want to say that, Cody."

Dr. L.: And then what's the choice you could give Cody since you're not going to say that?

Emily: "Is there something else you would like me to say?"

Dr. L.: Instead of asking the question, you could say, "You can choose some other words for me to say."

(Continue viewing video.)

Dr. L.: (Stops video.) You gave him credit. You made a self-esteem-building response. He can feel powerful by doing something constructive, taking the handcuffs off you, and then when he hears, "There, you figured out how to get them off," he feels powerful in a positive way instead of feeling powerful by pushing you around.

(Continue viewing video.)

Dr. L.: (Stops video.) How do you feel about Cody pretending it's your birthday and spanking you?

Kathy: Well, he wasn't really doing it out of anger. He was doing it like a birthday, and it really didn't hurt.

Dr. L.: Does he do things like that at other times?

Kathy: When he spanks me out of anger and it hurts, then that makes me really angry. That is what I'd like to correct, but here he was just playing birthday.

Dr. L.: There may be some times when he doesn't know the difference between hitting you hard and hitting you easy.

Kathy: Yeah.

Dr. L.: Does he play this birthday game often?

Kathy: Yes, some.

Dr. L.: Maybe it would be a good idea to set a limit on spanking you during the special playtime. You could say, "I'm not for spanking. You can pretend the Bobo is me and spank the Bobo."

(Continue viewing video.)

Dr. L.: (Stops video.) Laura, do you think Kathy's capable of being firm?

Laura: Yeah.

Dr. L.: I do.

Kathy: I don't know if I can.

Nita: Yes, yes.

Laura: Because I've been mush, too.

Dr. L.: And?

Laura: And I'm stronger now, and the more that I set a limit, then the easier it is.

Emily: Kathy, I was mush with my first born. He is now 13, and I pay the price on a daily basis, with his mouth, with his attitude, with his lack of respect, because I did not correct it at a much earlier age. I thought, "Oh, another fit, give him what he wants." But it's not any easier later—it's not.

Dr. L.: During your special 30-minute playtime, you get a chance to work on those issues, and for 30 minutes it can be easier. It doesn't mean you must do it for 24 hours, but you work on it for 30 minutes, with a commitment to stick this out for 30 minutes.

Nita: Since you're not trying to do laundry or something else, it's easier to stand back and assess and understand what's going on during that 30 minutes than when you're also trying to do something else and interact with your child and address issues.

Sonya: And that 30 minutes is great because it gives me enough practice time, and I try it a couple of more times during the week without thinking. If I had to do this every single moment of my life, I probably would give in too many times. Any time I try it outside of special playtime, I figure that's gravy on the potatoes.

(Continue to view video.)

Dr. L.: (Stops video.) Kathy, would you have preferred not to taste that sand?

Kathy: Probably.

Dr. L.: Then, you can say, "I choose not to taste it."

Kathy: OK, but it seems to me if I didn't taste it, I wouldn't be doing what he wanted to do for that 30 minutes.

Dr. L.: That's not the rule. The rule is not that you have to do everything that he wants you to do. The rule is that he can do a lot of things he would like to do, and you will let him lead. That doesn't mean you do everything he wants.

Kathy: OK.

Dr. L.: You do some of the things he wants if it's appropriate, but if there are some things you don't want to do, you don't do them.

(Group gives Kathy supportive feedback. It is obvious she has serious personal boundary issues that require more help than a filial group can provide. This is a classic example of a parent who needs private counseling sessions with the filial therapist.)

Dr. L.: Let me share with you my Oreo® Cookie Theory about choice giving. The Oreo® Cookie Theory of choice giving requires a shift in attitude, creative thinking, and spontaneous reaction. The shift in attitude is a change from making decisions for the child to allowing the child to decide. For example, if a child doesn't want to take her medicine, taking the medicine is not a choice—that is a given. So the parent can say, "*You may choose to have orange juice with your medicine or you may choose to have apple juice with your medicine. Which do you choose?*" The question calls for a commitment on the part of the child, and once the child has made a choice, the child is more willing to follow through. Allowing the child to be a part of the decision-making process usually results in cooperation or willingness to compromise. Keep in mind that you must be willing to live with either choice the child makes.

The Oreo® Cookie Theory is also a new approach to discipline—not punishment, but discipline, helping a child to learn how to engage in making appropriate choices and learning self-responsibility. "If you choose to finish your homework by 4:00, you choose to get to play your computer game. If you choose not to finish your homework by 4:00, you choose not to play your computer game." This method of choice giving can be used in the special playtime to help your child learn self-discipline and self-control as the fourth step in the A-C-T model. You set the limit that walls are not for marking on, but your child keeps trying to mark on the wall. Now, what do you do? You've gone through the three steps three or four times, and your child is still trying to mark on the wall. (Parents brainstorm ideas of possible choices.) Now, let's watch the video on choice giving.

(Parents watch Dr. Landreth's *Choices, Cookies, & Kid*s video. This video can be obtained from the Center for Play Therapy, University of North Texas, P.O. Box 310829, Denton, TX 76203, or by visiting www.centerforplaytherapy.com.)

Dr. L.: (After facilitating discussion regarding video.) Let's practice generating some choices. You three are in a group and you three are in a group. Your assignment is to think of at least three things your children have done or might do and develop a choice for each of those situations. Then you can share your situations and choices with the rest of us.

(After parents have a chance to share the above assignment.) This week I would like for you all to give your child a choice. It may be during a special playtime or at some other time. "*If you choose to continue to try to shoot me with the dart gun, you choose not to play with it for the rest of our playtime together today.*" "*If you choose to try to mark on the wall, and the wall is not for marking on, you choose not to play with the crayon for the rest of the time today.*" That sets the item off-limits for the rest of the time—not forever, just for that time.

Kim: Do you think children understand the word "choice"?

Dr. L.: Yes, even at 2 years of age, they understand.

Kathy: But then when they do choose to give up the television or give up Mr. Rogers, how do you handle their anger towards that?

Dr. L.: You say, "*I know you're angry.*" You reflect their anger and accept it.

Laura: We can't accept the guilt of it, because it's something they chose.

Dr. L.: Yes, parents have a hard time accepting their children's pain.

Emily, we didn't get to hear about your play session. What was it like?

Emily: It was interesting.

Dr. L.: What does that mean, "interesting"?

Emily: He had all the little doll furniture and the dolls, and the plastic knife. He picked the knife up and said, "I'm going to stab the baby." He didn't wait for me to respond. He stabbed the baby, and then he went down the line, stabbed everyone, all five. That caught me off guard. I said, "Gee, you look real angry, why are you doing that?"

Dr. L.: You reflected his feeling. He knew you understood, so the question wasn't needed.

Emily: And he kept doing it. He took the plastic knife and started slashing furniture.

Dr. L.: Acting out his anger.

Emily: And then he threw the knife in the box, got on his hands and knees, started goo-goo and gaa-gaaing, got the bottle that was full of water, crawled into my lap, lay down like a baby, and said, "Rock me." So for the last 10 minutes of our special time, I rocked him.

Dr. L.: What a tender moment.

Emily: Yes, I think that time was significant in his life. (The remaining parents report on their special playtimes.)

Dr. L.: I want to show you all a few minutes of one of my play sessions emphasizing the use of self-esteem-building responses. As your child is doing something, you can build their self-esteem by giving your child credit. A self-esteem-building response is when you see your child doing something, and you give your child credit for it. I'd like for you to specifically work on building your child's self-esteem in your 30-minute playtime this week. That will be one of your assignments.

(Parents view video.)

Dr. L.: (Stops video.) OK, got the idea?

Kim: You didn't tell her what that number was.

Dr. L.: It can be whatever she wants it to be for 30 minutes. Later, in the kitchen tonight, it may need to be 5, but for this 30 minutes it can be whatever number she wants it to be. Give your child credit. You stacked those blocks as high as you wanted them to be. The child is counting, one, two, three: "*Sounds like you can count all the way to three.*" You just give your child credit for all the little things they do in your 30-minute session. That's one assignment, self-esteem-building responses; your second assignment is to give your child a choice this week. Have a good week. I'll see you next Monday.

Reference

Bratton, S., & Landreth, G. (2019). *Child-Parent Relationship Therapy (CPRT) treatment manual: An Evidence-Based 10-session filial therapy model* (2nd ed). New York, NY: Routledge.

CHAPTER 14

CPRT TRAINING SESSION 7: SUPERVISION AND SELF-ESTEEM-BUILDING RESPONSES

Overview

Refer to the Overview section at the beginning of Chapter 13 as a thorough review of the overall supervision process and important reminders that apply for Sessions 6 through 9. As in training Sessions 6 and 7, the major focus of this session is supporting and encouraging parents' skill development and confidence through group supervision and feedback; thus, the majority of the allotted time is devoted to this activity. Esteem building is the only new skill introduced this week.

Materials

Suggested materials include: *CPRT Session 7—Treatment Outline*; parent information form with pertinent notes; homework assigned in Session 6, including extra copies of any homework worksheets; and Session 7 handouts and homework, including: *Session 7 Parent Notes and Homework, Esteem-Building Responses*, *Parent Play Session Notes*, and *Play Session Skills Checklist*. Additional materials include: a display poster with *Play Session Dos and Don'ts*, *Choices, Cookies, & Kid*s video by Garry L. Landreth (if used in Session 6 and time didn't allow viewing the entire video), and optional video clip demonstrating self-esteem-building responses.

> *Note: All handouts listed above, as well as a training session outline for the therapist, additional supplemental parent handouts, and resources for this training session are found in the CPRT Treatment Manual, 2nd Edition, and accompanying Companion Website.*

Content and Procedure

As in Session 6, the major focus of this session is supporting and encouraging parents' skill development and confidence through group supervision and feedback; thus, the majority of allotted time is devoted to this activity. The only new skill introduced in Session 7 is esteem-building responses.

Review Homework

The session begins with parents sharing how their week has been. The therapist uses this time to ask parents to briefly report on their homework assignment to practice giving a choice outside the play session and to review the handouts, *Choice Giving 101* and *Advanced Choice Giving*, and finish viewing the *Choices, Cookies, & Kid*s video by Garry L. Landreth, if necessary. The skill of choice giving is an important tool for parents; therefore, allotting plenty of time to review and practice this skill is a priority. Continuing to review homework assignments, the therapist asks parents to get out the *Common Problems in Play Sessions* worksheet and addresses parent concerns (suggested answers to these common problems can be found in Common Problems in Play Sessions in Session 6 of the Therapist Notebook in the CPRT Treatment Manual, 2nd Edition.

Filial Play Session Reports

Parents report briefly on their home play sessions and their homework assignment to practice choice giving during a play session, if the occasion arose. **The therapist listens for opportunities to reinforce the skill of choice giving in the parents' sharing of play session happenings, providing additional strategies for successful choice giving, as needed.** The skill of limit setting remains a challenge for most parents; therefore, allowing time to reinforce and practice this skill continues as a training priority. Role-play and worksheets that provide limit-setting scenarios for parents to respond to are helpful supplemental strategies for helping parents master this skill.

Self-Esteem-Building Responses

Esteem building is the only new skill focus for training Session 7. Introduce the **Rule of Thumb: Never do for a child that which he can do for himself.** *When you do, you rob your child of the joy of discovery and the opportunity to feel competent. You will never know what your child is capable of unless you allow him to try!*

Parents help their children develop a positive view of self not only by providing their children with love and unconditional acceptance, but also by helping their children feel competent and capable. Parents help their children feel competent and capable by first allowing them to **experience** what it is like to discover, figure out, and problem solve. Parents show faith in their children and their children's capabilities by allowing them to struggle with problems, all the while providing encouragement (encouragement vs. praise is covered in detail in Session 8). For most parents, allowing children to struggle is hard, but it is a necessary process for children to truly feel capable. **The next step in helping children develop a positive view of self as competent and capable is learning to respond in ways that give children credit for ideas, efforts, and accomplishments without praising.**

Many parents and children have difficulty with this concept. Most parents do too much for their children, and in response their children have learned to depend on their parents to solve their problems, believing they cannot do it by themselves. The therapist needs to take time to role-play how parents respond when children say, "Here Mommy," (handing the playdough to mom) "take the lid off for me." Or, "Daddy, help me set the soldiers up." Parents need lots of practice in how to return responsibility to their children to do things they are capable of figuring out for themselves. Parents benefit from seeing a video demonstration illustrating the use of esteem-building responses or a brief live demo in which that skill is focused on.

Additional information about self-esteem and examples of self-esteem-building responses are found in Esteem-Building Responses in Session 7 of the Therapist Notebook in the CPRT Treatment Manual, 2nd Edition.

Filial Play Session Video Critique

This portion of the training session continues to hold the most importance for parents learning and integrating the skills. The therapist uses the focused supervision time of the video-recorded parents to not only emphasize the filial play session "Dos," but to also to point out examples and missed opportunities for making self-esteem-building responses. Emphasize to parents that **simply noticing and showing interest in their children's play is a powerful builder of self-esteem—that their actions can speak as loud as words!**

Role-Play

Allow 10–15 minutes at end of session for role-playing self-esteem-building responses, limit setting, and reflective responding.

Homework Assignments

1. Parents are reminded of the importance of conducting their play session at the same time and same place and to video-record their sessions.
2. Remind parents to take a few minutes to review *Play Session Dos & Don'ts* and *Esteem-Building Responses* prior to their play session.
3. Remind parents to practice giving at least one self-esteem-building response during their play sessions and one self-esteem-building response outside of the play sessions. They are to write down what their children did and how they responded.

4. Parents are reminded after conducting the play session to complete the *Parent Play Session Notes* and *Play Session Skills Checklist* and bring it to the group the following week.
5. Each parent is asked to write a note to their child of focus, as well as to other children in the family, pointing out a positive characteristic or a quality the parent appreciates about the child. Ask parents to write down the following sentence: "Dear ____, I was just thinking about you and what I was thinking is you are so ___________," (thoughtful, responsible, considerate, loving, etc.). "I love you, ______ [Mom, Dad]." If time permits, the therapist can help parents generate some ideas. Providing parents with a list of positive character qualities is beneficial. Suggest that parents mail their notes; children seldom get mail, so this makes the note an extra special treat. If the child cannot read, arrange for someone else in the home to read the note to the child when it arrives in the mail, if possible; if not, the parent would read the note. Parents are to continue this assignment each week, identifying a different character quality for the remainder of the CPRT training, varying how the note is delivered; for example, placing it in the child's lunchbox, taping it to the mirror in the bathroom, placing it on the child's pillow or under the child's dinner plate, etc.
6. One to two parents are scheduled to be video-recorded.
7. Parents are reminded of the Rule of Thumb for the week.
8. Close by reading *The Struggle to Become a Butterfly: A True Story (see Session 7 handout in the CPRT Treatment Manual, 2nd Edition).*

Partial Transcript of CPRT Session 7

(After parents shared how their week had been, including briefly reporting on their homework assignment to make two self-esteem-building responses in the play sessions and to practice giving a choice outside of the play sessions, Dr. L. went over the handout on Common Problems in Play Sessions. This part of the transcript was omitted, because the answers to the questions contained in that worksheet can be found in Session 6 of the Therapist Notebook in the CPRT Treatment Manual, 2nd Edition. *The transcript begins with parents reporting on how their play sessions went, with the therapist*

using parents' reports to look for opportunities to review and reinforce skills, particularly focusing on the skill of choice giving.)

Dr. L.: Emily, what was your play session like this week?

Emily: Pretty normal. I haven't seen any aggressive behavior since that one time with the knife when he stabbed and cut everything. Actually, that one time was enough for me, because it was pretty scary.

Dr. L.: So maybe he needed to get some anger out, and he did.

Emily: Yeah, I guess. (pause) But he still likes playing with the dart gun, shooting the darts and asking me to get them for him.

Dr. L.: How do you feel about having to retrieve the darts for him?

Emily: I think it's fun.

Dr. L.: So it doesn't bother you.

Emily: No, not at all. As a matter of fact, I'm not sure he has ever asked me to get the darts. It's just something I started doing. He shoots them and I go get them. That's just the way it is.

Dr. L.: And for 30 minutes, he's in charge. Maybe then he doesn't have to get angry or be aggressive to try to be in charge at other times. You have already met that need.

Emily: That's true. He has been angry a lot less lately. He still likes the Band-Aids. He uses every one I put in the box every week. He puts them in a criss-cross pattern one on top of the other and makes a big patch out of them on my hand. He thinks that's lots of fun. He played with the playdough a bunch, just rolling it into balls and stuff and made some pretty creative things. Our playtime is in my bedroom, and he got some things out of the bathroom like a comb and a brush, and a bottle of lotion. He pushed them down into the playdough and made different imprints. Then he would feel the different imprints. He spent a lot of time doing that.

Dr. L.: His play this time seems to have been a bit different: calmer, quieter, more subdued, and a fun time for both of you. You followed his lead. I do have one suggestion. **The special playtime is just for the part of the room where you set the toys. The rest of the room and other items in the room are off-limits so this can be a consistent and predictable time for Chris.** He might want to play with some items in your bedroom that you wouldn't want him to play with, like a lamp or clock. He might have taken the top off the lotion bottle and poured some out, and that would make a huge mess. During the special playtime, he is to play only with the toys you have in the play kit. You can practice reflective responding and set a limit by saying, "*I know you would like to play with stuff from the bathroom, but this is our special play area right here in this part of the room, and these toys are the only things that are to be played with during our special playtime.*" How do you react to that, Emily?

Emily: I can do that—makes sense to me. But what do I do next time if he wants to play with those same things, and he says, "Last time you let me?"

Dr. L.: You can say, "*I know I didn't say anything last time, but I should have said, 'Those things are not for playing with during our special playtime.'*"

Dr. L.: Nita, what was your play session like? Describe it to us.

Nita: Jeff keeps up a running monologue. I just sit there and watch him, and he keeps up this running monologue. I have very little opportunity to say anything. He's very, very pleased with the playtimes.

Dr. L.: So he's doing what he wants to do for that 30 minutes, a lot of talking.

Nita: He says things like, "I'm doing this like this, and then you see I put this like this. You see this, Mom." I say, "Yes, I see that."

Dr. L.: That's his way of including you. When children talk about their play, "Now, this guy is going to do this, then he's going to jump in here," that's the child's way of including you in his play, without you actually being a physical participant.

Nita: Sometimes Jeff wants me to go outside and play and I tell him, I just can't. I am just so tired. I just really don't feel good, and he'll say that's OK, because I know at special playtime it'll be just you and me, anyway.

Dr. L.: So the playtime is a very special time for him and a place where he gets his needs met.

Nita: And he will tell me things like, "Wesley and I do this at Nanny's house." But when I ask him, "What did you do at Nanny's house?" he just says, "I played." But during the playtime, he'll say, "Wesley did it like this at Nanny's house." He tells me about things I could never get out of him otherwise.

Dr. L.: Sounds like some important things are happening. He's sharing his life with you.

Nita: I just thought of something. We're still having trouble when it's over. He understands it's over. He says, "That's OK, Mommy, you go wash your face," or whatever. I just go ahead, put the toys in the box, and put the box away. Then, sometimes he hits me and kicks me because he wants to play more.

Dr. L.: You're not for kicking. So, give him a choice. If you choose to kick me, you choose to—what choice could you give?

Nita: Go to bed without a story.

Dr. L.: I'd rather not take a bedtime story away from him. That's important sharing time.

Nita: He likes using the telephone a lot.

Dr. L.: OK, if you choose to kick me, you choose not to use the phone for the rest of the day. If you choose not to kick me, you choose to get to use the phone.

Nita: That's what I'll do.

Dr. L.: How about the rest of you—what kind of choice would you give your child in a similar situation? Remember that the consequence you establish needs to be something your child will not like giving up, but just like the example of not using forfeiting a bedtime story, in general, the consequence should not take something away that is a special time in your relationship or in your child's relationship with other important people, like grandparents.

(Parents discuss choice-giving ideas and continue to report on play sessions).

Dr. L.: Debbie, tell us a bit about your session before you show your video.

Debbie: It was OK, but Rachel didn't want to leave. She started screaming, and I had to carry her out of the playroom. It was awful!

Dr. L: Let's see what happened.

(Note: Debbie is the parent we are following more closely from intake through follow-up; Dr. L. uses Debbie's play session happenings to focus the training on self-esteem-building responses, limit setting, and reflective responding.)

Dr. L: We're going to use Debbie's play session with Rachel to work on self-esteem-building responses. I want all of you to notice when you think Debbie uses a self-esteem-building response—when she gives Rachel credit for deciding, figuring out, knowing, etc.

(Group watches video.)

Child: (Looks at Debbie, laughs, runs to Bobo, hits it, and then runs to kitchen cabinets.) What is this? A kitchen. (Opens cabinet doors and then runs back to easel.)

Child: (Looks at Debbie, moves to toy shelves, and plays with cash register on floor by the sandbox.)

Debbie: You're making those numbers go up. (Sits in chair next to the table.)

Dr. L.: (Stops video.) What kind of response did Debbie just make?

Sonya: She gave Rachel credit.

Kim: A self-esteem-building response.

Dr. L.: Yes, Debbie's statement "You're making those numbers go up" empowers her child.

(Starts video.)

Child: Look Mommy!

Debbie: Wow!

Child: (Sits next to sandbox.) I'm going to take my shoes off.

Debbie: You're going to take your shoes off?

Dr. L.: (Stops video.) Debbie, that was an accurate reflection of content, but what did your tone of voice say?

Debbie: I didn't hear anything.

Dr. L.: (Replays last comment.) What did you hear that time?

Debbie: My tone of voice turned it into a question.

Dr. L.: Yes, that says you don't understand.

(Starts video.)

Child: Yeah, and socks and stuff before I go in there.

Debbie: You take your shoes and socks off before you go in the sand.

Child: Yeah. Look what I can do, Momma. (jumps in sandbox)

Debbie: You're making your fingers go right through that . . . your toes go right through that sand.

Dr. L.: (Stops video.) Your tracking comment shows you are noticing what Rachel does.

(Starts video.)

Child: (Sits down in sandbox.) Look what I can make, Momma. I can make something. I just need these. (Puts pebbles in Debbie's hand.) I don't think . . . (silently stares at bottom of the sandbox) Why do they put that much in here?

Debbie: Hmm . . . why do they?

Dr. L.: (Stops video.) Debbie, you are being very empathic. Rachel is wondering, and you are wondering with her.

(Starts video.)

Child: (Pours sand into a bucket.) I'm getting it all over my new outfit.

Debbie: You're getting it all over your new outfit.

Dr. L.: (Stops video.) Group, what did Debbie just communicate to Rachel?

Emily: That being messy is OK.

Sonya: She's being very accepting.

Dr. L.: And understanding. (Starts video.)

Child: (Takes pebbles from Debbie's hand and puts them on top of the sand mold.)

Debbie: Oh . . . you're putting these on top.

Child: Ah!

Debbie: (Laughs.)

Child: (Holds her hands toward Debbie, nonverbally suggesting Debbie should put the pebbles back in child's hands. Child puts the pebbles on top of the bucket, which is full of sand.) Ahhh! (Child picks up bucket and tosses it in the air. Sand flies up at Debbie.)

Debbie: I'm not for throwing sand at.

Dr. L.: (Stops video.) Group, what kind of response did Debbie just make?

Group in unison: Limit setting.

(Starts video.)

Child: But Momma! (Walks away from sandbox, looks at other toys, then picks up machine gun and points it in Debbie's direction.)

Debbie: I'm not for pointing the gun at. You can point it at the Bobo or you can point it at the wall. (Debbie points at alternative targets.)

Dr. L.: (Stops video.) Excellent job setting a limit, and you pointed toward an acceptable alternative.

(Starts video.)

Child: (Starts shooting in the air. Child is excited by the sound the gun makes and puts the gun closer to her ears while shooting, then puts the gun back on the shelf, touches a knife and two dart guns, but does not play with them. Child finds a box on the shelf and shows it to Debbie, mumbling excitedly. Debbie smiles and walks to child and kneels down next to her. Child picks up doctor kit and brings it to the art table.) I got a doctor bag, Momma. Let's play doctor.

Debbie: You want to play doctor.

Child: Yeah, over there, we'll play it. (Points to chalkboard, is busy checking the doctor kit and clearing space.) Lay down over there. Lay down, Momma.

Debbie: Where?

Dr. L.: (Stops video.) What does that one word "where" do for Rachel?

Laura: It keeps her in the lead.

Dr. L.: Yes. (Starts video.)

Child: (Points to floor.) That place . . . you know, where you are standing. Lay down. (Child sits on a chair facing Debbie, then starts looking inside the doctor kit.)

Debbie: Oh . . . lay down here? (Sits on the floor.)

Child: Yes. (Glances at Debbie.) Lay down.

Child: (Goes through doctor kit, picks up stethoscope, and turns to Debbie.) Let's play doctor, Momma.

Debbie: Are you taking those out of there?

(Debbie catches herself before anyone in the room can respond blurts out. "Oops, asked another question." Others laugh; video is not stopped.)

Child: (Takes out a second stethoscope.) This is a special one. (Puts it on her head.)

Debbie: A special one . . .

Child: (Offers two boxes of bandages to Debbie.) Do you want the little ones or the big ones?

Debbie: I don't know . . . hmmm . . . what do you think?

Child: (Looks at box of little ones.) Oh . . . that's for fingers.

Debbie: That's for fingers.

Child: Lay down, Momma.

Debbie: Where? Show me.

Child: Just lay.

Debbie: Oh, OK. (Lies down on floor.)

Dr. L.: (Stops video.) Rachel obviously knows what she wants.

Debbie: Yeah, she always does.

(Starts video.)

Child: (Goes to Debbie with stethoscope on her ears. Child tries to lift up bottom of Debbie's shirt.)

Debbie: (Holds her shirt down.) No! My clothes are for staying on right now. You can check my ears . . . my nose . . . my mouth . . . (*Blurts out "No," then makes quick recovery to set limit and provide alternative choices.)*

Child: But this is for looking into you.

Debbie: (Sits up and looks into Rachel's face.) I know, but my clothes are for staying down right now. I know you want to, but . . . (*Shows understanding.*)

Dr. L.: (Stops video.) Great job recovering; your first impulse was an old behavior—"No"—but you quickly recovered, set a limit, and provided an acceptable alternative of several choices. Then you came back to the first step in A-C-T by saying, "I know you want to."

(Starts video.)

Child: (Pushes Debbie down.) Lay down, Mommy! (Said with frustration.)

Debbie: You can check my eyes and my nose and my mouth. (Lies down.) OK?

Child: (Checks Debbie's eye with stethoscope, runs to the doctor kit on the art table, puts the stethoscope down, and picks up syringe.)

Debbie: (Sits up.)

Child: Lay down, Mommy! ***(Pushes Debbie down.)***

Debbie: Oh . . . Oh . . . OK . . . (Lies down.)

Child: Let me give you a shot. (Gives shot to Debbie and opens bandage box.)

Dr. L.: (Stops video.) Debbie, or some of the rest of you, how do you think Rachel is feeling right now?

Emily: Like she's in charge—that she gets to boss her mom around.

Dr. L.: Yes, she looks like she's really enjoying being in charge for these 30 minutes. She can't be the rest of the week, but Debbie, during these 30 minutes, you can grant Rachel in fantasy something she can't do the rest of the week: boss you around. Remember the Rule of Thumb we talked about last week—this is a perfect example of "Grant in fantasy what you cannot grant in reality."

Rachel can't smack her baby brother at home, but she can pretend the baby doll is her brother and smack it during her special playtime.

Emily: So, that's like when Chris was angry and was going around stabbing all the toys with the play knife? He certainly couldn't do that in real life.

Dr. L.: Exactly, You were granting him in fantasy to do something to get his anger out that he couldn't do in reality.

(Starts video.)

Child: (Places bandage on Debbie's arm where she gave the shot.)

Debbie: You're putting that right there on my arm. (Sits up.)

Child: (Gets blood pressure instrument from the doctor kit and puts on Debbie's arm.)

Debbie: You're putting that right there on my arm.

Child: Lay down Mommy! Why do you keep getting up?

Debbie: (Lies back down.)

Dr. L.: (Stops video.) How's Rachel feeling right now?

Debbie: I think she's frustrated with me because I keep getting up.

Dr. L.: So you could say . . .

Debbie: You're frustrated with Mommy. You want me to stay laying down.

(Starts video.)

Child: (Takes Debbie's blood pressure and goes back to the table, takes a plastic reflex hammer from the doctor kit and taps Debbie's arm hard with it.)

Debbie: Ouch! (Gently reaches out in an attempt to grab the reflex hammer.)

Child: I know what it's for, Mom.

Debbie: I know that's what it is for, but Mommy is not for hitting. (This time she realizes she did not personalize her response and corrects.) I'm not for hitting.

Child: But this one's just for a little bit, this is for a little bit . . . (Goes back to the doctor kit and gets eye examiner.) Lay down, Mom. (Looks into Debbie's eyes with examiner, goes back to the table.) And OK, Mom, you're all good. You can't do it because you don't know how. (Puts all the doctor instruments back in the kit.)

Dr. L.: (Stops video.) Rachel sure seems to know a lot about what doctors do—how could you give her credit for that?

Nita: When she says that at the end, "You don't know how," could you say something like, "But you do, you know how to doctor"?

Dr. L.: Sounds good to me, gives Rachel credit, builds her self-esteem.

(Rachel goes over to dollhouse and picks up doll.)

Child: How do you take this off Momma? (Trying to undress doll.)

Debbie: Hmm . . . you got it, it was kind of hard, but you did it.

(Kathy starts to say something, so the video is stopped.)

Kathy: I would have probably reached over and taken the clothes off for her—the doll is so small, and I didn't think she could get it off. But, Debbie, you waited, and she did it. You could tell she was happy that she got it off by herself.

(Stops video.)

Dr. L.: That's a good place to stop, another good example of a self-esteem-building response. You were giving Rachel credit for figuring out how do that all by herself. And you could tell she was proud of herself.

Debbie: I was really surprised that she could that. I would never have let her have a big hammer like that. I would have been afraid that she would hurt herself.

Dr. L.: So what did you learn about Rachel?

Debbie: That she was capable of hammering a nail without hurting herself. She was being careful. I really wasn't afraid, because she was being careful.

Dr. L.: You wouldn't let her have a hammer unsupervised. That wouldn't be appropriate. But during this 30-minute special time, you can allow her more freedom, and you know you're right there to keep her safe.

Emily: I think that Rachel knew that you thought she could do it. You could tell. That was really empowering.

Dr. L.: Any other feedback for Debbie?

Nita: Debbie really did well at allowing Rachel to play with what she wanted and just following along.

Kathy: And she did a great job of setting limits—something I have a lot of trouble with! (Smiles.) Especially when Rachel wanted to pull her sweater up to doctor her. I wouldn't have known what to say. I'd probably let her and then remember I was on video and yank it down. (Everyone laughs.)

Dr. L.: Since, we're talking about limit setting, let's shift focus and work on the Limit Setting worksheet we didn't get to last week. We'll work some more on self-esteem-building response a little later. Did everyone find it? It looks like this. OK. Susan picks up the dart gun. Aims it at your head. How did you respond?

Kathy: I'm not for hitting.

Dr. L.: I'm not for shooting.

Kim: Susan, I'm not for shooting.

Dr. L.: Kim, you added something different there, a really important word.

All: Her name.

Dr. L.: What's important about that?

Sonya: I'm talking to you.

Dr. L.: Exactly. You get your child's attention in a hurry when you say their name.

Kim: Susan, I'm not for shooting. If you choose to shoot at me, you choose time out for 5 or 10 minutes.

Dr. L.: Sounds a little long, Kim. How about if you take the middle part of that out and read it. "Susan, I'm not for shooting."

Kim: "You can shoot at the Bobo."

Dr. L.: The choice does not need to be given until you have gone through the limit setting three or four times. And then you can say, "*If you choose to shoot me with the gun, you choose not to play with the gun.*" But that's not needed until later. Give your child a chance to comply first. Emily, what did you put down?

Emily: I don't have anything written down.

Dr. L.: In your mind, what do you say?

Emily: "Susan, I'm not for shooting."

Dr. L.: Um-hum. And then we want to give an alternative. "You can shoot the Bobo." And what do you do with your hands?

Kathy: You point to it.

Dr. L.: So the child's eyes follow to what is an acceptable alternative. Look at number 4 on the sheet. Paul is very angry with you, calls you names, and tries to kick you. What did you say?

Emily: The first thing that popped into my mind when I read this was to slap him across the head.

Dr. L.: Giving up your initial reaction and responding more calmly, Emily, you'd say . . .

Emily: Paul, I can understand that you're very angry right now, but I'm not for calling names or kicking.

Dr. L.: Yes, you're not for calling names. There is no choice on that. Go through the whole thing again.

Emily: Paul, I can understand that you're very angry with me right now, but I'm not for calling names or kicking.

Dr. L.: And, then, we still need to help him do what he needs to do. And that is?

Emily: Hit the bop bag.

Dr. L.: The Bobo is for kicking. The important thing is that you end your statement by telling your child what he can do. I might even offer this, "You can tell me you're angry. You can say, 'I'm angry at you.'"

Laura: It's interesting that we adults go through life trying to find out what our choices are in buying a car, in doing lots of things. The more choices we have, the more freedom we feel like we have to choose what is best for us.

Dr. L.: Yes, and it's important for children to find out what their choices are and to learn how to make decisions. When you make a decision, you are then responsible. So you're helping your child learn what it feels like to be responsible. I want to show you a short video of a child with me in the playroom. I want you to count how many times you hear me make a self-esteem-building response. **A self-esteem-building response is when you give your child credit for knowing or doing.** "You made that stay together."

(Parents view video.)

Dr. L.: (Stops video.) How many did you hear?

Kathy: I got eight.

Emily: I got 12.

Dr. L.: **When children feel better about themselves, what difference does that make in their life? They do better. They're more self-confident, they follow through. Lots of important things happen.** Now, let's do some role-playing. Let's work on two things. Limit setting: children, you all do some things that will cause your parent to set limits. "I'm going to paint on the wall," or "I'm going to cut this," or "I'm going to break this." And let your parents set a limit. Also, parents, you practice making self-esteem-building responses.

(Group pairs up to practice responses.)

Dr. L.: That's all for today. Your homework is to practice giving a self-esteem-building response outside of the play session and at least one during your play session. Write down what your child did and how you responded and bring it next week. Who will volunteer to come to the clinic to video your play sessions? OK, Laura and Emily. See you all next Monday.

Reference

Bratton, S., & Landreth, G. (2019). *Child-Parent Relationship Therapy (CPRT) treatment manual: An Evidence-Based 10-session filial therapy model* (2nd ed). New York, NY: Routledge.

CHAPTER 15

CPRT TRAINING SESSION 8: SUPERVISION AND ENCOURAGEMENT VS. PRAISE

Overview

Refer to the Overview section at the beginning of Chapter 13 as a thorough review of the overall supervision process and important reminders that apply for Sessions 6 through 9. As in training Sessions 6 and 7, the major focus of this session is supporting and encouraging parents' skill development and confidence through group supervision and feedback; thus, the majority of the allotted time is devoted to this activity. Encouragement is the only new skill introduced this week and builds on the training on esteem-building responses covered in Session 7.

Materials

Suggested materials include: *CPRT Session 8—Treatment Outline*; parent information form with pertinent notes; homework assigned in Session 7, including extra copies of any homework worksheets; and Session 8 handouts and homework, including: *Session 8 Parent Notes and Homework*, *Encouragement vs. Praise*, *Parent Play Session Notes*, and *Play Session Skills Checklist*. Additional materials include: a display poster with *Play Session Dos and Don'ts* and optional video clip demonstrating play session skills, specifically self-esteem-building responses and encouragement.

> *Note: All handouts listed above, as well as a training session outline for the therapist, additional supplemental parent handouts, and resources for this training session are found in the CPRT Treatment Manual, 2nd Edition, and accompanying Companion Website.*

Content and Procedure

Review Homework

The session begins with parents informally sharing about how their week has been. The therapist uses this time to ask parents to briefly report on their character quality note-writing activity, remembering to caution parents not to expect an overt response from their children. Parents are reminded to continue the note-writing activity over the next few weeks. This time is also used to ask parents to report on their homework assignment to practice giving a self-esteem-building response outside the play session (if parents bring it up during session responses, ask them to share those responses when they report on play sessions in a few minutes).

Filial Play Session Reports and Video Critique

Parents report briefly on their home play sessions and their homework assignment to practice self-esteembuilding responses during their play sessions. The therapist listens for opportunities to reinforce this skill in the parents' sharing of play session happenings, providing additional strategies as needed. Review of self-esteem-building responses continues to be a focus during focused supervision of the video-recorded parent. The therapist encourages parents to give each other feedback (parents are generally ready by Session 8 to move into peer supervision). As the video-recorded parent's session is reviewed, the therapist stops the video after an obvious CPRT skill has been demonstrated and asks parents if they have any feedback for that parent. This strategy encourages parents' sharing of feedback and keeps the focus on parents' strengths.

Caution parents that the newness of the special playtime and the toys may begin to wear off and their children may seem uninterested or bored. The playtime is still important. Continue to insist on having the playtime.

Encouragement vs. Praise

The concept of encouragement, and how it differs from praise, is introduced in training Session 8. When possible, the therapist uses the focused supervision time to spontaneously introduce the concept by pointing out examples of encouragement in play session happenings of the video-recorded parent. The therapist introduces the **Rule of Thumb: Encourage the effort, rather than praise the product**, either in response to a play session happening that fits this Rule of Thumb (as demonstrated in the transcript below) or when reviewing the skill. Parents are given a handout, *Encouragement vs. Praise*, that explains the rationale for using encouragement over praise and delineates how to use encouragement in different situations, both during and outside of play sessions. This handout is used during the session as a visual aid to helping parents understand encouragement and how to use the skill, and later as a review for homework. Most parents have difficulty grasping the concept of encouragement and how it differs from praise. Society, particularly schools, places a strong emphasis on praise as the preferred way to motivate children to do what authorities want them to do.

Praise: Although praise and encouragement both focus on positive behaviors and appear to be the same process, praise actually fosters dependence in children by teaching them to rely on an external source of control and motivation rather than on self-control and self-motivation.

Encouragement: Focuses on internal evaluation and the contributions children make; facilitates development of self-motivation and self-control. Encouragement focuses on effort and can always be given; children who feel their efforts are encouraged, valued, and appreciated develop qualities of persistence and determination and tend to be good problem solvers.

In summary, encouragement is (a) valuing and accepting children as they are (not putting conditions on acceptance), (b) pointing out the positive aspects of behavior, (c) showing faith in children so that they can come to believe in themselves, (d) recognizing effort and improvement (rather than requiring achievement), and (e) showing appreciation for contributions. **The therapist emphasizes that encouragement shows faith in children and fosters self-esteem, self-motivation, confidence, and creativity in children by focusing on effort, improvement, and contributions.** On the other hand, praise limits children's creativity, self-confidence, and self-motivation by teaching them to depend on others' views and opinions to determine their own self-worth. *(Refer to Chapter 6 in this text and Encouragement vs. Praise in Session 8 of the Therapist Notebook in the CPRT Treatment Manual, 2nd Edition, for additional discussion and strategies for teaching encouragement.)*

Homework Assignments

1. Parents are reminded of the importance of conducting their play session at the same time and same place and to video-record their sessions.
2. Remind parents to take a few minutes to review *Play Session Dos & Don'ts* prior to their play sessions.
3. Parents are reminded after conducting the play sessions to complete the *Parent Play Session Notes* and *Play Session Skills Checklist.*
4. Remind parents to practice giving children a choice outside of play session and report back.
5. Ask them to write down one thing in play session that didn't go well and write down one thing they did in play session that went really well.
6. Write down one issue they are struggling with most outside of play session time. It may be one they have brought up before, or they may have already solved that one on their own and have a new issue they want help with.

7. Read over the handout Encouragement vs. Praise, and practice giving child encouragement one time outside play session, reporting back on how that went.
8. One to two parents are scheduled to be video-recorded.
9. Remind parents of the Rule of Thumb for the week.

Partial Transcript of CPRT Session 8

(Parents shared about their week, reported on making self-esteem-building responses, described their character quality note writing, and reported on giving a choice outside the playtime.)

Dr. L.: Well, how have your playtimes gone? Laura, we'll see your video in a few minutes, so we'll hear from you then.

Kathy: We had a pretty good one.

Dr. L.: Tell us some specifics. What happened in the playtime?

Kathy: He wanted to play with some different things this time. He has usually been playing with the punching bag and that kind of stuff, but this time he got the furniture out and started arranging that. He didn't ask me to do anything with him. Sometimes when I tell him I see what he's doing, he says, "Mom, quit talking," or "Mom, I know that already. I know what I'm doing already."

Debbie: Yeah, Rachel said, "I don't want you telling me what I'm doing." She got real agitated with me for making tracking comments.

Dr. L.: Such responses may mean your children feel that you're tracking a little too closely. Sometimes, that may be your child's way of pushing you a little bit to find out "Can I get away with this? Can I tell you I don't like that?" It may not really bother them so much at all. It's just a way of pushing you to find out how you're going to react. If you sense that is going on you can say, "*Oh, the way I'm talking now bothers you.*" It doesn't mean you're going to change, it just says, "I have recorded what you said." The other possibility is maybe your child doesn't want you to change. They would like for you to be the way you used to be. Why?

Debbie: It's comfortable.

Kathy: Change is uncomfortable for them.

Dr. L.: Do you experience any of that, Emily?

Emily: No, I haven't gotten anything so far but real positive results from the playtimes. As a matter of fact, my child is really different since we started doing this.

Dr. L.: Tell us about that.

Emily: He's not nearly as demanding. The temper tantrums are gone. He's just different. He doesn't argue as much. I usually tell him, "These are your choices." He never picked the right one. He doesn't do that anymore. It may be because I follow through in the sessions now.

Dr. L.: So you're more consistent now.

Emily: Probably. He doesn't test me as much now.

Dr. L.: So, he doesn't have a need to test you as much.

Emily: Maybe he feels he doesn't have to kick me or bite me to get my attention anymore because we have the special playtime.

Dr. L.: So, you're meeting his needs, and you're doing it, not someone else.

(Emily describes playtime.)

Dr. L.: Listening to you, I can tell it's fun for you, too.

Emily: It is. I love that time together. I really do.

Dr. L.: Then Chris surely must know that you like being with him, that you enjoy the time. If you put yourself in Chris's spot, and your mom likes being in the play session with you, looks forward to it, and has fun while you're together, how would Chris feel?

Emily: Pretty special. Loved.

Dr. L.: Loved, and that he's important. That's a special gift you're giving. Sounds like a real active time, too. Sonya, tell us about your session.

Sonya: They're getting more and more interesting. Now, she wants to help set up the toys before time to start. She takes everything out of the box and sets it where she wants it, and then pretends like she's starting: "Oh, here's some toys," and then she comes in and plays. She's exploring the more aggressive toys now. I get the feeling that maybe she feels like it's safe to do that now. Before, she never touched the gun or the knife, or the oven mitt that looks like a dragon. Now, that's her pet. She gives it a different name every week. She feeds it Tinkertoys. And even though it's scary looking, she says, "He's nice."

Dr. L.: He's a nice dragon, and she is experiencing being in charge of the playtime.

Sonya: Uh-huh. She likes the Band-Aids, too. She always Band-Aids the dolls. I'm amazed watching her. She's 3 years old, and she takes the Band-Aid out of the wrapper, and it will be sticking to her fingers, but she can get it all undone by herself. It's so frustrating for me to sit there. I want to say, "Honey, let me do that for you."

Dr. L.: You want to take control.

Sonya: Yes, but once I see her achieve, it feels so good. I say, "You did that all by yourself." And she says, "I know." (Sonya smiles.) You could tell she felt good about it.

Dr. L.: So you knew that your response was heard, that Jenny felt empowered. By being patient and allowing her a chance to figure things out for herself, you gave her the opportunity to feel good about "doing all by herself." And your response let her know that. Folks, one of the best things we can communicate to our children is that they are competent. Tell a child she is capable and she will believe she is capable. Tell her or show her enough times she can't do it, and sure enough, she can't.

Emily: So, if we do it for them, we're telling them they can't do it.

Dr. L.: You got it! Sonya, tell us some more about your play session.

Sonya: The big deal for her the past couple of times is she ties the bop bag up. Last week she put the Lone Ranger mask on the bop bag and said that was the mean daddy. She spent most of the session tying up the mean daddy. She took pieces of tape, taped him all up, and shot him. She wanted me to stick him with the knife and I told her I wouldn't like to do that. And she said, "OK, I will."

Dr. L.: So you were able to convey your feeling in such a way that she still felt free to go ahead and do what she wanted to do. She didn't feel, "Oh, I'm not supposed to do this."

Sonya: Yeah.

Emily: That kind of surprised me when you said, "So she took the knife and did it." I expected her to say, "Why don't you want to do that, Mamma?"

Sonya: I just told her I wouldn't like to do that. It didn't feel good. That's the first time she brought up her dad in the playtime, and I really wanted to find out more about this mean daddy, so I stepped out of the nondirective play role and asked her about the mean daddy. She didn't respond and I went, "Oops," that's not going to work.

Dr. L.: You learned something important about playtime. Questioning doesn't work.

Sonya: Um-hum. She just went on with something else. It's a real important time for her and me, and it's getting more fun as we do it. I can't wait to see what she explores next. She's starting to use the toys in different ways. Now when it's time to pick up, she says, "I'm going to help you." And she starts picking up the toys, and I'm thinking, "What is this?" I have to negotiate deals with her all the time to get her to pick up.

Dr. L.: So, what have you learned about her?

Sonya: Well, she is capable of picking up her toys.

Dr. L.: She is capable of being helpful. Isn't that amazing that she will volunteer to pick up in the playtime but not where you would like for her to?

Sonya: It's just absolutely amazing. I have found in using the A-C-T limit setting a lot of times all I have to do is say, "You look very angry," or "I understand that you want to do that," and that's all I have to do for her to decide that it's not a big deal anymore.

Dr. L.: That's the end of it. She stops herself because you allow her to stop herself.

Sonya: I don't have to count one, two, three, or four anymore. And another thing, now, when she says, "I don't like you. You're not my friend anymore," I haven't been feeding into that. I just check, is she angry or frustrated? Usually she's angry. I just say, "Sounds like you're very angry because I won't do what you want me to do," and it works great.

Dr. L.: At that moment, your child knows that her message has been received by you and that you understand. She doesn't have to escalate to get her message across.

Sonya: She seems to really cherish the fact that this is a special time just for me and her.

Dr. L.: So, she feels important.

Sonya: Uh-huh. I think I'll probably just keep doing the playtimes way after the training.

Dr. L.: So, they have become important to you, also. Debbie, did you have a playtime this past week?

Debbie: A short one. Rachel really wasn't interested. I think she's really angry with me. She's not really saying it, but she's demonstrating it really heavily, and she doesn't want playtime to be very long.

Dr. L.: Tell us what happened.

Debbie: We got into the playtime, and she wanted to play. She seemed very distracted. Even outside playtime, she won't pay attention to me because she's angry with me. She really is. There's other things going on.

Dr. L.: All the more reason for you to have the playtime even though she's not quite sure she wants to be there with you.

Debbie: So, make her stay in the playtime?

Dr. L.: You can take a compromise position when she wants to leave after just a few minutes. You can say, "*We have 20 more minutes, and then it will be time to stop.*" If that doesn't work, and in a minute or two she says, "But I want to leave now," then try compromising. "*We have 20 more minutes, let's do this. Let's take 10 more minutes to be together in our special playtime, and at the end of the 10 minutes, you can decide if you want to have the rest of the playtime, or if you want to end it.*" So, she still gets to feel in control. When things are not going well in your child's life, or in your life, that may be all the more reason to have the special playtime and to stick it out even if she's angry at you. Can you try that?

Debbie: Sure.

Dr. L.: Kim, how was your session?

Kim: It was great.

Dr. L.: What made it great?

Kim: He played with toys he had never even picked up before. I want to ask you something. If he names things wrong during playtime, I can't correct him, right?

Dr. L.: What do you think my answer is?

Kim: No. But I can't let him get away with thinking incorrect labels are correct.

Sonya: Like what?

Kim: Like the house. He knows what's right. But it's like he's waiting for me to tell him he's wrong. I just sat there and didn't correct him.

Dr. L.: So you passed the test. Maybe he's wondering, "Can it be what I want it to be, or will Mom tell me, 'No, it's got to be a house?'" You passed the test.

Kim: But outside the playtime, I should tell him that's not what that is.

Dr. L.: Outside the 30-minute playtime, you can be his teacher and give the right answers.

Emily: But inside that 30-minute playtime, you're stupid.

Dr. L.: And it can be whatever they want it to be.

Kathy: It's hard to stop yourself.

Sonya: Or to say, "It looks like you want that to be the refrigerator or you want that to be the stove."

Dr. L.: Yes, change is difficult. Kim, what else did he do?

Kim: He just played. He talked a lot. He doesn't usually talk.

We've been trying to stimulate his verbal ability, and in the playtime, he was just rattling on and on. I told my husband when he got home, I didn't talk hardly at all in the playtime because Toby was just rambling on.

Dr. L.: Sounds like he surprised you in a lot of ways, and you're really pleased.

Kim: Oh, yeah. He's come a long way from not wanting to play at all.

Dr. L.: And it was a fun time.

Kim: Oh, yeah. It was great.

Dr. L.: Well, we've heard from everybody. Laura, let's see the video of your playtime. Do you want to tell us anything about your session ahead of time?

Laura: It was different than what I expected as far as what his interests were. (She describes different toys her son played with.)

Dr. L.: Well, let's see what happened.

(Parents watch video.)

Dr. L.: (Stops video.) Dawson quickly got involved. You made the kind of nonevaluative response that we've talked about. Instead of saying, "That's a pretty picture," you responded to his effort, "Working real hard on that." That's an example of another important **Rule of Thumb** we are going to talk more about today, **"Encourage the effort instead of praising the product."** You can always find something to encourage in your children, but praise can only be given to your child when he does something that meets some external standard. In this case, Laura, you gave Dawson credit for working hard on his picture. This kind of encouragement fosters creativity—praise limits creativity and freedom of expression.

Kathy: So we're not supposed to tell our children that their drawings are pretty?

Dr. L.: Not during this 30-minute playtime. We'll come back to this later. Let's watch more of Laura and Dawson.

(Parents watch video.)

Laura: (Stops video.) I put a limit on him there, right? By stopping him from mixing the colors.

Dr. L.: It would be OK to mix the colors. If you could redo what we saw right here, physically, not what you said, what would you do differently? Did you see yourself?

Laura: I leaned toward him with my hands to stop him.

Dr. L.: Yes, and you'd do what next time?

Laura: I won't try to touch him physically to stop him. I'll just tell him.

Dr. L.: Because the message is, if you start to reach out, "I don't believe you will stop yourself."

Laura: I didn't touch him or grab him. But I started to reach.

Dr. L.: And we want our children to stop themselves without any kind of threat. Here comes Mom's hand. I'd better . . .

(Parents view video.)

Dr. L.: (Stops video.) Dawson has your full attention. I haven't seen you even look away from him. He has your absolute attention.

Debbie: And he's taking care of himself.

Dr. L.: Yes, he is.

Laura: He washed each brush. He cleaned the sink afterward, and he cleaned the play dishes that were in the sink.

Dr. L.: Such responsibility. I gather from your reaction that's pretty unusual for him.

Laura: Yeah. I was shocked to see him clean each brush and put it back, and he even cleaned the whole sink after all that.

Dr. L.: You're discovering some new attributes of Dawson. Why is it that your children will take this kind of responsibility in this 30 minutes?

Laura: Because it is their choice. It wasn't because Momma was standing there telling him to do it. And him standing there saying, "I'm not going to do it."

Debbie: No battles.

Dr. L.: And when your children are free to make some of these kinds of decisions, they naturally move toward taking care of themselves and the situation without a lot of hassle.

Laura: Yeah, boy, do we know that.

Dr. L.: **What an important discovery that in the playtime when you're not the teacher, you're not the boss, and you're not correcting, your child's self-direction comes forth.** The only way you could have discovered that is in this kind of free playtime.

(Video continues.)

Dr. L.: (Stops video.) My, such patience, Laura. Not once did I hear you say, "Now hurry up. You've been washing your hands there a long time now. Now hurry up." You all give Laura some feedback. What did you see, and what did you hear?

Kim: You stayed right with him. He knew you were interested.

Sonya: I agree. You didn't overtrack what he did. You let him lead. And you reflected what he was feeling.

Emily: You were so patient and relaxed, real comfortable, real calm. Looked like you've done this for years.

Kathy: I liked your facial expressions. Your response built up his self-esteem.

Debbie: Your reflections were so good. You didn't take over, and you allowed him to struggle to figure things out.

(Dr. L. passes out the handout Encouragement vs. Praise and reviews the similarities and differences between the two. Examples of encouraging responses for use in different situations are reviewed and parents are given a homework assignment to practice encouragement with their children.)

Dr. L.: OK, let's stop, and I want to remind you we have two more sessions. For homework, I'd like for you to reread the handout I just gave you and work on the use of encouragement. Write down one time you made an encouraging response to your child this week. Come back next week and report on what your child did or said and how you responded. I also want you to practice choice giving again this week, so write down one time you gave your child a choice and what happened. Also, would you make a note right after your session this week on anything that happens in your special playtime that doesn't go very well for you or a time when you're not quite sure what to do or say, and also write down one thing that went really well.

Next week we will be discussing how to use some of these skills outside of play session—so think of an issue that you'd like help with and write that down. So, you have a lot to do this week—four assignments:

(1) practice encouragement, (2) practice choice giving again, (3) write down something in your play session you'd like to have some help with and one thing you're really proud of, and (4) one issue outside of your play session that you'd like some help on. See you next Monday.

Reference

Bratton, S., & Landreth, G. (2019). *Child-Parent Relationship Therapy (CPRT) treatment manual: An Evidence-Based 10-session filial therapy model* (2nd ed). New York, NY: Routledge.

CHAPTER 16

CPRT TRAINING SESSION 9: SUPERVISION AND GENERALIZING SKILLS

Overview

Refer to the Overview section at the beginning of Chapter 13 as a thorough review of the overall supervision process and important reminders that apply for Sessions 6 through 9. Supporting and encouraging parents' skill development and confidence, as well as their struggles, through group supervision and feedback continues as the chief aim, with the majority of training in Session 9 spent in group supervision and support, rather than didactic instruction.

No new skills are introduced; rather, the focus is on advanced application of CPRT skills and on generalizing the play skills to happenings outside of the play session, specifically those concerns that parents have introduced over the past 8 weeks. The use of the A-C-T model of limit setting outside of play sessions receives extra emphasis, as this is the hardest skill for parents to master in everyday happenings.

Materials

Suggested materials include: *CPRT Session 9—Treatment Outline*; parent information form with pertinent notes; homework assigned in Session 8, including extra copies of any homework worksheets; and Session 9 handouts and homework, including: *Session 9 Parent Notes and Homework, Advanced Limit Setting: Giving Choices as Consequences for Noncompliance, Generalizing Limit Setting to Outside the Play Session, Parent Play Session Notes*, and *Play Session Skills Checklist*. Additional materials include: a display poster of *Play Session Dos and Don'ts*, an optional video clip demonstrating specific play session skills parents are most struggling with, and, most importantly**, the written list of concerns that parents have expressed over the past 8 weeks.**

> *Note: All handouts listed above, as well as a training session outline for the therapist, additional supplemental parent handouts, and resources for this training session are found in the CPRT Treatment Manual, 2nd Edition, and accompanying Companion Website.*

Content and Procedure

Although training Session 9 follows a similar format to Sessions 6 through 8—sharing how the week went, reporting on home play sessions, and focused supervision of the videotaped parent(s)—this session differs in the amount of time spent in group processing of the parents' week. The majority of homework assignments from last week focused on the use of skills outside of the play sessions; therefore, focusing more time and energy into the sharing of happenings outside of playtimes is warranted. The amount of time spent will vary depending on the needs of the group. The more advanced the group, generally the more they will generalize skills outside the play sessions; therefore, more time is spent on applying skills to everyday activities. Typically by Session 9, parents are demonstrating greater awareness of their own feelings and reporting greater sensitivity to their children's feelings; therefore, the therapist uses the parents' discussion of happenings outside of play sessions to facilitate parents' sharing of their feelings, as well as their recognition of their children's feelings. This informal sharing provides many opportunities for parents to continue to practice how to more effectively respond to their children's feelings, wants, and needs, without accepting all behavior.

Review Homework

Homework assignments to practice encouragement and choice giving are reviewed and reinforced as parents share how their week has been. The therapist should be prepared for a lively debate and discussion about encouragement vs. the use of praise. The concept of praise, along with reward and punishment, is so ingrained in parents' thinking that they typically challenge the suggestion that praise should be limited in their interactions with their children.

Filial Play Session Reports and Video Critiques

Parents report briefly on their home play sessions and their homework assignment to write down one thing that went well and one thing they need help with. The therapist listens for opportunities to facilitate peer feedback to reinforce CPRT skills in the parents' sharing of play session happenings, following the strategy employed in training Session 8, to stop the video after **an obvious skill has been demonstrated** and ask parents if they have any feedback for that parent. The therapist's goal is to facilitate parents' growth and learning to a higher level of awareness. The ability to recognize demonstrated skills and give accurate feedback to others is not only empowering, it requires a higher level of learning for parents than simply being able to demonstrate the skills in their play sessions.

Parents are reminded of the importance of being consistent in their interactions with their children while allowing their children to struggle with responsibility for their own behaviors. **It is not the parent's responsibility to make the playtime fun or interesting for the child or to entertain the child.** The child is in the lead and is responsible for what she does for 30 minutes. Most parents have difficulty with this. As seen in the following interaction between the therapist and a parent during training Session 9, parents often believe they are responsible for their children's happiness—and unhappiness.

Dr. L.: Kim, I heard you say something I want to check on. I think I heard you say that you have a hard time keeping Toby interested.

Kim: Yes, he has a short attention span, and when we first started, the toys were new.

Dr. L.: **For 30 minutes, it is not your responsibility to keep Toby interested.**

Kim: But, I wait all week for the playtime, and then he doesn't have fun.

Dr. L.: So *you're* disappointed . . .

The therapist uses these kinds of sharings to generalize CPRT play session skills to outside the playtime, in this case, to emphasize that the **parents are not responsible for their children's happiness.** It is not their job to make sure their children are always occupied, interested, busy, or happy. Remind parents that if they take responsibility for their children's happiness, their children will never learn to do that for themselves. Although no new play session skills are introduced, the therapist may introduce strategies that will help parents with specific problems. Additional strategies can be introduced, as needed, as long as the strategy is consistent with the basic child-centered philosophy that CPRT training is based on.

Because limit setting continues to challenge most parents, it is helpful to briefly cover limit-setting strategies for noncompliance.

Generalizing Skills to Outside the Play Session

Although by this point in this session the therapist has already addressed some parent concerns and how the CPRT play session skills can be used to respond more effectively, be sure to allow time to go over your written list of parents' concerns from the past 8 weeks. Begin by checking to see which ones are still troublesome. It is our experience that many of the "problems" are not problems anymore! Prioritize concerns to address by those shared by the most parents. When discussing the generalization of play session skills to problem areas, tell parents the **Rule of Thumb is: Don't try to change everything at once!**

A specific concern expressed by some parents in our CPRT groups is how to respond to their children who are feeling anxious or insecure about new happenings in their life, e.g. going to a new daycare or preschool, parents' divorce, first visit to dentist, doctor, or play therapist. In addition to encouraging parents to reflect their children's fears and concerns, rather than problem-solve, we have found a storytelling procedure called *structured doll play* helpful to parents to prepare their children for new experiences. The transcript at the end of this chapter provides a detailed example of how Dr. Landreth explained *structured doll play* in response to a parent's concern for her child. The e-Resource section which accompanies the CPRT Treatment Manual, 2nd ed. contains a detailed 2-page handout, ***Structured Doll Play for Parents***, that can be provided to parents on an as-needed basis.

The therapist should allow time to go over generalizing limit setting to outside the play session and what to do when limit setting isn't working outside of play sessions. Begin by reviewing the three-step A-C-T model:

1. ***A***cknowledge the feeling.
2. ***C***ommunicate the limit.
3. ***T***arget alternatives.

Next, go over an outside-of-play session example of the A-C-T method of limit setting, followed by **"If–Then" choice giving** to establish consequences for noncompliance of the limit. Detailed instructions for implementing this process are in the handouts *Advanced Limit Setting: Giving Choices as Consequences for Noncompliance* and *Generalizing Limit Setting to Outside the Play Session* in Session 9 of the Therapist Notebook in the CPRT Treatment Manual, 2nd Edition. After processing these handouts, provide parents with a practice worksheet with additional examples. This is a difficult skill to learn. Parents feel foolish using *choice* and *choose* so frequently. Follow with a discussion of how to modify choice giving and establishing consequences with older children. Remind parents of the **Rule of Thumb: Give big choices for big kids and little choices for little kids.**

No matter how skilled the parent is at using limit setting, it will not always work. Parents need to know that! Allow time to discuss what to do when the A-C-T method of limit setting doesn't work (a supplemental worksheet is provided in the *CPRT Treatment Manual, 2nd Edition*).

1. Look for natural causes for rebellion.
2. Remain in control, respecting yourself and the child.
3. Set reasonable consequences for disobedience.
4. Never tolerate violence.
5. If the child refuses to choose, you choose for him.
6. Enforce the consequences: Don't state consequences that you cannot enforce. If you crumble under your child's anger or tears, you have abdicated your role as parent and lost your power. **GET TOUGH!** Introduce the **Rule of Thumb: Where there are no limits, there is no security. Consistent Limits = Security in the Relationship**. When you don't follow through, you lose credibility and harm your relationship with your child.
7. Recognize signs of more serious problems: As parents feel more confident in their newfound skills, they are typically eager to tackle every problem they are having with their children. Help parents **choose one issue to focus on**—for example, bedtime problem, aggressive behavior, hitting, getting ready for school, etc.—and report back the following week on which issue they have selected to focus on.

Homework Assignments

1. Parents are reminded of the importance of conducting their play sessions at the same time and same place.
2. Remind parents to take a few minutes to review *Play Session Dos & Don'ts* prior to their play session.
3. Parents are reminded after conducting the play session to complete the *Parent Play Session Notes* and *Play Session Skills Checklist*.
4. Parents are asked to notice the number of times they touch their children in interactions outside the special playtime

(hugging, patting on the head, a touch on the arm, etc.). Ask them to actually try to keep count during the week.

5. A related assignment is to play-wrestle with your children. Research shows that when asked what activity they remembered most in playing with their parents when they were children, both male and female adults in their late 20s identified wrestling as the activity they remembered and had the most fun doing. (Example: In a two-parent family with small children, mom and kids can sneak up on dad and try to get him down on the floor—accompanied by lots of fun and laughter.)
6. Parents are asked to choose one issue they are struggling with (outside of the play session) to focus on and report back the following week on how they can use their play session skills to respond to the issue.
7. One to two parents are scheduled to be videotaped.
8. Remind parents of the Rules of Thumb for the week.

Partial Transcript of CPRT Session 9

Dr. L.: How has the week gone for you?

Laura: I tried to bring David, my 6-year-old, to the clinic here for play therapy this week, and he refused to stay; it was a really bad time. I was real angry at him when we left. But I didn't vent a lot of things on him that I would have at other times in the past. On the way home in the car, he said, "Well, Mommy, you were a kid once too, and I just didn't want to go into the room with that lady." I blew it for a moment by saying, "Yes, I was a kid too, but I didn't have parents that cared enough about me to try to help." I was still angry at him, but I didn't say some things that I usually would have said.

Dr. L.: So you didn't dump on him.

Laura: No, except for that one statement.

Dr. L.: That's progress. You controlled your emotions.

Laura: Yes, that is progress for me.

Dr. L.: Laura, if you could go back through that episode of bringing him here, and he didn't want to stay, what would you do differently?

Laura: I guess it has to be OK, but it's hard to believe a 6-year-old should be allowed to make a decision about whether or not he, uh . . .

Dr. L.: Needs help or not.

Laura: Yeah, but I don't know what to do except let him decide.

Dr. L.: For some reason, he's anxious about going into the play-room with the therapist, or he's anxious about you leaving him.

Laura: OK. Tell me what to do. We're supposed to go back Wednesday at 6:00.

Dr. L.: Today is Monday. Before he goes to bed tonight, and again tomorrow, I would like for you to try a procedure I call structured doll play. (To the group) This is a procedure all of you can use when your child is anxious about something or your child is worried about something, like being left with a babysitter, going to the dentist, going to school, or going to a birthday party for the first time. Laura, sit down with David, and say to him, "I want to tell you a special story about David going to play therapy." For this story, we need a toy or stuffed animal that can be David, one that can be Mom, and one that can be Mrs. Brown (the play therapist)." Let David choose the items. "And, we also need a car." David chooses, and the story begins. "David is playing in his room, and Mom says, 'Dinner is ready'." You use the chosen characters to act out the story as you tell it. "David sits down at the table, and everyone eats. Then Mom washes the dishes. OK, it's time to get in the car and go to see Mrs. Brown. Here David goes and here Mom goes," as you show the characters going to the car. "Mom helps David buckle his car-seat, **click**, and then Mom buckles her seatbelt, **click**." Be sure to use lots of noise props in telling the story. Make motor noises, **brrrmmm brrrmmm**, as you drive. "Here we are. Mom locks the car, **Click,** and David and

Mom walk across the parking lot to the building where the playroom is. David and Mom go in, and Mrs. Brown says, 'Hi", and you start a conversation between David and the Mrs. Brown back and forth. "David goes down the hall with Mrs. Brown to the playroom. The playroom has lots of neat stuff to play with," show the figures walking down the hall, "and Mom waits right here in the waiting room. Mom looks at her watch and thinks to herself that David will be in the playroom for 45 minutes (look at your watch) and then Mom begins reading a book. And then Mom hears footsteps coming down the hall; so Mom gets up and looks down the hall and sure enough there David is coming down the hall. Mom says, 'Hi, we can go home now.' David and Mom put seatbelts on, **click-click,** and drive home, **brrrmmm, brrrmmm**. 'Now we're home. Let's get a snack.' David and Mom go in the kitchen and have chocolate chip cookies and milk. David says, 'yum, these are good cookies, Mommy." And the story ends with a hug and big kiss **(smaaaack)** as you show the characters hugging and kissing. Be sure the kiss is a loud **smaaack**. Children like that. And the story ends. The story should not take longer than 5 minutes to tell.

The reason this kind of story is important is because your child will remember what he has seen and how the story ended. If you just tell your child what to expect, he won't be able to visualize what is going to happen. Your child will remember what he has seen and that it ended OK. So, Laura, you will tell your son this story Monday night and Tuesday night. It would be great if you could also tell him the story Wednesday afternoon before you take him to the playroom. This will help him to get ready for the visit.

Some of you are having trouble with your child at bedtime. You can use the same kind of story to prepare for bedtime. You tell your child a story about what is going to happen in the process of going to bed and end the story with, "Mom gives David a big kiss (smaaaack), Mom tucks David in bed, and Mom goes to her room to work; so Mom is in her room and David is in his bed.

Before mom goes to bed, she comes back and checks on David. 'Yep, he's asleep,' and Mom gives David a big kiss so he knows that his mom came to check on him." That's reassuring to your child to know you will be there after he goes to sleep.

Dr. L. Laura, your son may be afraid you aren't going to be there when he comes out of the playroom.

Kim: Yeah, that he would be there all by himself with a stranger.

Laura: When I got ready to leave for work Sunday, David went running out to the car, got in, and locked the doors because he didn't want me to leave.

Dr. L.: Let's work on getting him ready for his playtime Wednesday, and then we'll work on helping him get ready for you to leave for work. You had an assignment last week to use choice giving at least one time this week. Did anyone give a choice this week?

Kathy: I did at the movies. We went to a movie, and Cody kept flopping around in his seat, kicking the back of the seat in front of him, so I took him out in the lobby and told him, "If you choose to kick the seat and bother people, then you choose for us to leave the movie." It worked. He stopped kicking.

Dr. L.: You took charge, Kathy, and Cody brought himself under control. There is another half to the choice giving though.

Laura: If you choose not to kick the chair, you choose to get to stay and watch the movie.

Kathy: Well, he was real good for most of the movie, but then he started kicking again, so I said, "I see you have chosen to leave the movie," and we left.

Dr. L.: So you followed through, and Cody experienced the consequence of his choice. Kim, did you give a choice this week?

Kim: Toby has a really low frustration level, and he will get hysterical about little things and that has gotten a lot better, but we're still working on that; so we used the choice giving a lot this week. He will throw things in anger, and I won't allow that, so I give him a choice. But it's sad, because I have to take toys away.

Dr. L.: (interrupts) Excuse me, I'm not sure I heard you accurately. I think I heard you say, "I have to take away his toys."

Kim: (interrupts) He chooses to get the toys taken away.

(Laughs.)

Dr. L.: Oh! Do you hear the difference?

Kim: Yeah.

Dr. L.: Yes, that's his choice. So, Kim, you can sit there and tell us with great calmness, "Would you believe he chose to give up his favorite toys 3 days in a row?" (Group laughs.)

Kim: That's true. My two kids share toys, and the other day Toby was playing with his sister's doll, and he threw it. That was real hard taking it away from my daughter because it's hers, but I can't let her play with it if I have taken it away.

Dr. L.: She can play with it because it's hers.

Kim: That doesn't work because they share everything.

Dr. L.: What else does Toby like to do?

Kim: I can't take TV away because they both watch TV.

Dr. L.: Is there just one room in your home? (Group laughs.)

Kim: No, there are lots of rooms. (Laughs.)

Dr. L.: Oh, you have more than one room. (Group laughs.)

Kim: Yeah.

Dr. L.: (Long pause.) So . . .

Kim: What do I do?

Dr. L.: How old is Toby?

Kim: Four and a half. Oh, he chooses to stay in his room a lot.

Dr. L.: The doll is your daughter's and Toby chooses not to play with it; you use the next step, "If you choose to keep trying to play with the doll, you choose to go sit in your room for 5 minutes. If you choose not to try to play with her doll, you choose not to go to your room for 5 minutes."

Kim: So you think it's wrong to take the doll away.

Dr. L.: If the doll was his, then that would be an appropriate choice, but taking the doll away punishes her.

Kim: Oh, I see.

Dr. L.: OK. You had an opportunity to use choice giving.

Kim: And it works. It really does. Oh, I started having playtimes this week with my daughter, like we talked about. She is so different from Toby in the playtimes.

Dr. L.: How did it work out?

Kim: She really liked it. The problem has been that the baby gets a lot of attention, and because he has special needs, Toby gets lots of attention; she has felt left out. I could see a difference in her behavior this week because of the special playtime. Her behavior was better. It was neat to see how she is different from Toby in the way she plays with the toys.

Dr. L.: So you learned something about her.

Kim: Oh, yeah. Everything we learn here is seeping into real life outside the 30-minute playtimes, and the whole family is different now.

Dr. L.: Great report.

Debbie: I have a question about bedtime. At what point do I start the choice giving, after she gets up?

Emily: When you put her to bed tonight, because she has already been getting up a lot every night. If you choose to get out of bed, you choose to give up TV in the morning.

Dr. L.: There are two parts to choice giving. If you choose not to stay in bed, you choose not to watch TV in the morning. If you choose to stay in bed, you choose to watch TV in the morning. Be sure to use both sides of the choice. The word "choose" must be used four times.

Emily: I don't think I've been doing that.

Laura: I haven't either.

Kim: Yeah, me too.

Laura: I've been saying, "You choose this or you choose this."

Debbie: And then that's where the spanking comes in.

Laura: I've learned lately that I go to spanking when I don't know what else to do. I've lost total control, and I think I can control my children by using physical strength and it doesn't work.

Debbie: My use of spanking has decreased by 99 percent since this class started. I use to spank her for everything because I didn't know what else to do.

Dr. L.: Great progress.

Debbie: But I still have this urge to clobber her sometimes.

Dr. L.: But you're controlling yourself.

Laura: I feel like I'm overcoming that, and it's a powerful feeling.

Debbie: It's just that bedtime is so exasperating. That's the only time now that I feel physically angry at her.

Dr. L.: Bedtime has been a problem for some time, and you get really angry at Rachel; you need to intervene in a different way. You have two things you're going to do. You're going to tell her the going to bed story first and then go through the choice giving.

Kathy: Cody was sleeping in my bed when I first started coming to this class, but now he's sleeping in his room.

Laura: When I come home on Saturday nights, my kids are usually in bed, and after 16 hours at work, I'm not a real happy person. (Group laughs.) Well, this past Saturday night when I came home, they weren't in bed, and they wanted my attention. I wasn't physically or emotionally ready to give them any attention.

Dr. L.: How did you handle that?

Laura: Because of what I have learned in my playtimes with Dawson about detaching and being objective, I was able to be calm, detach from my day, and reflect their feelings. "I know you want to spend some time with me, and you would like to stay up, but this is not the time for staying up longer. It's time to be in bed."

Dr. L.: And what happened?

Laura: They went to bed and didn't get back up, and I visited with the couple that was babysitting the kids.

Dr. L.: So you handled it.

Laura: Yeah, I thought, wow! (Group laughs.)

Dr. L.: You did it!

Laura: Yes, without getting angry. That's an awful feeling to be so angry at your child. I know what you feel, Debbie, and it's awful.

Dr. L.: So you're not alone with that, Debbie.

Laura: And it's hard not to hit sometimes, but I can learn a new way.

Dr. L.: It seems to me, Laura, you're saying, "I have learned a new way."

Laura: Yes, I think so. For such a long time I was afraid of my own feelings, even to touch my kids for hugs and kisses.

Dr. L.: And now?

Laura: Now, I'm not afraid, since I've been coming to this class.

(Other parents discuss issues they are struggling with outside the play sessions. The group shares what didn't go well in their play

session and what went well. Dr. L. gives home assignments and reminds group next week will be the last training session.)

Reference

Bratton, S., & Landreth, G. (2019). *Child-Parent Relationship Therapy (CPRT) treatment manual: An Evidence-Based 10-session filial therapy model* (2nd ed). New York, NY: Routledge.

CHAPTER 17

CPRT TRAINING SESSION 10: EVALUATION AND SUMMING UP

Overview

Parents briefly report on their play sessions and one or two parent play sessions are viewed. Basic CPRT principles are reviewed, and parents are asked to share what part of the training has been the most helpful and what parts they continue to have the most concerns about. The last part of the training time is spent with parents sharing their evaluation of the experience, how they and their children have changed. Parents share their perceptions of changes they have observed in other parents. Therapist shares notes of parents' original descriptions of their children as points of reference for parents to evaluate progress. The partial transcript at the end of this chapter vividly illustrates typical parent comments regarding their changes in perceptions of their children and themselves. **Parents are encouraged to accept and own their part in contributing to changes in their children's lives.** This is usually a very rewarding and empowering experience for the parents. Parents are encouraged to continue the special playtimes. Parents and/or children needing additional help are scheduled for such help.

Materials

Suggested materials include: *CPRT Session 10—Treatment Outline*; parent information sheet with notes **including parents' descriptions of their children from Session 1**; homework assigned in Session 9, including any homework worksheets; and Session 10 handout, *Rules of Thumb and Other Things to Remember.*

> *Note: All handouts listed above, as well as a training session outline for the therapist, additional supplemental parent handouts, and resources for this training session are found in the CPRT Treatment Manual, 2nd Edition, and accompanying Companion Website.*

Content and Procedure

As is true of the first nine training sessions, Session 10 is a jam-packed time. Lingering concerns of parents need to be addressed and suggestions offered. Supervision of play sessions is continued. Basic skills may need to be reviewed. Parents need to debrief the experience and prepare to disengage from the group. Parents evaluate the experience and share their perceptions of how they and their children have changed. Time must be taken to emphasize the importance of the special playtimes and encourage parents to continue to have their special playtimes. Arrangements need to be made for those parents who want to begin having a special playtime with a child other than their child of focus. If older children are to be involved, appropriate toys and materials will need to be discussed. The specifics of plans for follow-up sessions will need to be presented.

Support and encouragement are the rule of the day throughout this last session. The cohesiveness of the group is usually fully evident in this last session through increased parent interaction, and the leader may often find it helpful to stay in the background as parents process their feelings and reactions. **Typically, parents are generous with their support and encouragement for other parents and may playfully tease each other, modeling the type of humor exhibited by the leader in earlier sessions. This playful, accepting, fun attitude modeled by the**

leader throughout the training sessions reduces the threat of "There must be something wrong with me, or I wouldn't need to be here," and helps parents to relax, thus aiding the learning of a new parenting role.

Wrap-Up of Parent Concerns

Parents are asked if they have any lingering concerns about the special playtimes or other issues they would like to share. These questions project an attitude of continuing concern on the part of the leader for parents in the group. The following interaction in the CPRT group we have been following was facilitated by these questions:

Kathy: At what age can you tell a child that there's something serious going on, like my sister has breast cancer, and she could die? I don't know how much to tell Cody (6 years old) about why I'm so on edge.

Dr. L.: You're really worried about your sister, and all the facts aren't important for Cody to know. What is important is the general message: your concern, your worry, because she is very sick and is in the hospital. Those messages can be understood by Cody.

Kathy: He has found out stuff he wasn't ready for. I was on the phone telling a close friend when Cody found out his dad was in jail. He went around announcing to the world, "Daddy's in jail."

Laura: Yeah, I know. Dawson reacted kind of like that, and I told him we weren't with his dad because he hurts us. I didn't go into the details of how he hurt us. He just needed to know that because he hurts us, we're not with him.

Dr. L.: So you told him as much as he was ready for.

Laura: Yes. (To Kathy) So you could do the same and say your sister is really sick. You don't have to explain what's wrong with her.

Dr. L.: I have a feeling that by asking the question, you're beginning to feel Cody should be told something.

Kathy: Yeah, I know he should know something. I don't know how much to burden him with right now.

Dr. L.: I hear you saying almost the same thing Laura said last week when her concern was, "Gee, I don't think I should go home and burden my child with my feelings," when she was feeling stressed to the limit because her music teacher had really dumped on her.

Laura: Yeah, I'd still like to hit him over the head with my guitar. (Group laughs.)

Dr. L.: A safe place to start is with yourself, your own worry, that your sister is very sick and she is in the hospital. How does that sound to you?

Kathy: I get worried about Cody going into depression because he's a very moody child.

Dr. L.: As you handle your feelings by sharing some of them with him, perhaps that will help him learn to handle his. If he seems bothered, you could suggest he draw a picture for her.

Sonya: I have been thinking I need to have a playtime with my second daughter. I feel like I'm ignoring her.

Dr. L.: Your other daughter, Jenny, doesn't seem to be ready to stop her playtimes; so how do you feel about a special playtime once a week with each of your daughters? I think you are ready to take that on.

Sonya: That's what I was thinking of doing.

Dr. L.: Ok, you can let us know in our follow-up meeting how that works out.

(*Since this interaction is included here, it is not repeated in the transcript at the end of this chapter.*)

Depending on the size of the group, the discussion time on these topics will need to be limited. Avoid getting bogged down in new concerns of major significance that may not be of interest to the rest of the group. Keep the interaction moving and focused.

Supervision, evaluation, and follow-up are the primary concerns of this session.

Review Homework

Parents give a very brief report on what they noticed about the number of times they touched their children and their reaction to the wrestling time. Parents also report on issues they are struggling with and CPRT skills they can use.

Supervision

As in previous sessions, parents report on their play sessions and a parent-child play session is viewed. Continuing supervision in the last session is important because parents need all the feedback they can get, and issues emerge in supervision that might not otherwise be explored. At this stage in the group process, parents are usually quite adept at modeling the leader's approach to supervision by overlooking mistakes and responding to positive behaviors and skills. Our experience is that at this point in the training, most parents do a very satisfactory job of demonstrating the skills that have been taught.

How Child Behaviors Have Changed

The therapist shares her notes of parents' original descriptions of their children as points of reference for parents to evaluate progress. This sharing usually facilitates accounts of dramatic changes and tremendous insight on the part of the parents as in the following interaction. *(This CPRT training group is not the group we have been following throughout this book. This interaction is included here because the parent-child play session results are so dramatic and unusual.)*

Dr. L.: Ten weeks ago, as you were talking about your child of focus, I wrote down your descriptions. I'd like to read these descriptions, and then you give us an update on what your child is like now. Jan, in our first session, you said Jennifer does a lot of attention seeking, especially at bedtime. She has severe headaches and gets attention because of her medication and medical problem. She doesn't get along very well with other children. She's been like a little adult. She argues a lot. She has several seizures a day and the medication doesn't help. You said, "I think she has learned to cause her own seizures to get attention." Has any of that changed?

Jan: Yes. She had only one seizure in the past 4 weeks and has complained of a headache only 3 or 4 times in the past 4 or 5 weeks. (Group applauds.)

Dr. L.: What a dramatic change! That is a super report.

Jan: She was having as many as 10 seizures a day on some days.

Dr. L.: What has made the difference, Jan?

Jan: Well, I think a lot of it, ah . . . well, I've probably made some difference by the way I respond to her. I know the playtimes have really helped her.

Dr. L.: Yes, you have made a difference in your child's life.

Jan: She seems happier now. And there's a lot less stress at home.

This is a remarkable description of behavior change, especially when considering the short time span of only 10 weeks. However, this description is not atypical of descriptions given by parents when they report behavioral changes in the tenth session. In the first CPRT training session, Erin described her 2-year-old daughter as a strong-willed child. She reported that they often engaged in power struggles, and that from the moment that her daughter was born, she found it difficult to connect with her. In the tenth session, Erin stated, with tears in her eyes, that she finally loves her daughter. She had stopped punishing her and was able to spend more quality time with her. (This report and the following parent reports in this section are not from the CPRT training group we have been following in this book.)

In Session 1, Michal reported that she rocked her 4-year-old daughter to sleep in her stroller every night in order to avoid bedtime arguments. In the tenth session, Michal reported that her daughter now went to sleep on her own and that their relationship was much more calm and loving. She also stated that her relationship with her two teenagers had improved and was now based on attitudes of understanding and respect.

In Session 1, Jeanie expressed fear of her 7-year-old son's anger and aggression. She wept as she described his behavior problems in school, her inability to control his behavior at home, and her shame. After two play sessions, she reported progress in her son's behavior and how excited he was that she was taking a class to learn how to play with him. In the tenth session, Jeanie beamed with excitement as she said her son was no longer angry or out of control, there were no behavioral problems at school, and she was no longer afraid of her son. She particularly benefited from the homework assignment in which she wrote her son a note saying she appreciated his honesty and mailed it to him. He was excited about the note and asked her hopefully, "Is it true?" The note had such an impact on her son that she decided to e-mail the exercise to all of her friends as well as the school counselor.

Tenth-session parent reports from the group of parents we have been following through the previous nine sessions are described in the partial transcript of CPRT Session 10 at the end of this chapter.

How Parents Have Changed

Asking parents how they are different now, how they have changed, or how their feelings about their children have changed facilitates opportunities for insight and can result in parents feeling more empowered. **Parents need an opportunity to formulate new descriptions of themselves.** Succinctly summarizing parents' descriptions of themselves helps them to recognize their changes and their accomplishments. It can also be helpful to ask parents to compare and contrast what is currently occurring in their families to what was happening 10 weeks ago, and what is currently happening in the play sessions to what happened in the first special playtime. The objective is to send parents away feeling empowered.

Important changes in parental behavior and attitudes can be seen in the following excerpts:

Dr. L.: Group, how are you different now?

Kim: I believed that parents had to be in charge of every single thing that kids did. I expected my children to make decisions and to behave kind of like adults. Now I see my children as so much more. They're not an extension of me. They are different. They are unique. Now my son knows I'm going to love him for who he is, and that I still love him and trust him even if he doesn't make the right choices.

Sonya: I was a sergeant-of-arms with my daughter, and we usually got into power struggles. Our interactions were like open-heart surgery crisis-type. I mean, screaming and crying and slamming doors. My anger was abrupt and quick, and we yelled and hollered at each other at least four or five times a day. Now, I know a lot of her behavior is kinda normal, and I'm more accepting of her. Filial has taught me how to set limits without getting angry to make my point.

Debbie: I used to yell at my daughter all the time. I don't do that anymore, so there's less stress. I spend more time with her now. I feel more in control. Even when I make a mistake, and things go wrong, I know I can do it differently next time.

Laura: I had a lot of my self-worth tied up in trying to make my children happy. I tried real hard not to do things that would make them mad at me. I felt completely responsible for their happiness. My children had to obey me so other people wouldn't think I was a bad mother. I learned in the play sessions that I don't have to fix things for my child. This one principle has changed my thinking and attitude about parenting. I have learned to acknowledge my children's feelings without having to fix them or do things for them. I can be there and offer what I have to offer, and I don't have to fix it.

Kim: I've discovered I don't have to be the perfect mom. I've been trying to be the perfect mom and provide everything for my child, meet all his needs, and I don't have to do that.

Dr. L.: And that feels good to you.

Kim: Yes, it does! It's a relief.

Dr. L.: Debbie, you're shaking your head.

Debbie: Yeah, I feel less stressed and a lot better about myself and the way I am responding to my daughter. I know I can handle the problems now. Before I didn't think I could; so I wouldn't even try.

Kathy: I feel closer to my son. I don't love him anymore, but I feel closer. I listen to him better now. I don't turn him off.

Emily: I'm more ready to be a parent now. I haven't had special playtimes with my other children, but I respond differently to them. I have realized that these situations with my children don't have to be resolved immediately, that it often takes time to work through the process.

(*This interaction is not repeated in the transcript at the end of this chapter.*)

It is also reinforcing to ask parents how they think other parents in the group have changed or how they are different. They often are aware of changes not recognized by the parent of focus. It is difficult to maintain positive changes in behavior and attitudes if there is no awareness of the changes that have occurred. Since behavior is a function of self-perception, helping parents' perceptions of themselves to "catch up" with where they are now is key to sustained behavioral change. It is important that parents go away from this last session with a reinforced new perception of themselves.

Parents Evaluate the Experience

Parents are asked to share their reactions to the CPRT training and what part of the training has been most helpful to them. Sharing on this topic provides opportunities for review of basic skills that can serve as a reminder to parents of skills they will need to continue to focus on and utilize with their children. Parents can also be asked to share how what they have learned has been transferred or generalized to other children in the family. A mom shared about her increased confidence in a note, "I never dreamed parenting could be so easy and so very rewarding!!!"

Increased confidence seems to be a key factor for parents, as is seen in the following reactions:

Sonya: I would do this training forever even if I was perfect doing the techniques, because of the support of everyone in this group. And not just that, but also because we have Dr. Landreth sitting here, who is supposed to know everything. And he takes the pressure off when he doesn't know the answer by just saying, "I don't know." I need to know if I'm going to screw my kid up. I'll really miss that.

Laura: It's just nice having an outlet, somebody you can talk to that knows what you're talking about. A person who knows and understands and touches on your feelings. Somebody who cares about you.

Debbie: The special playtimes started out being for my daughter, but now they are for me, too. I came from a really bad family background, and I don't have a good parenting role model; so you (Dr. L.) have become my parent role model figure. I need more of this.

Kim: I wish this could be a once a week session until the kids are all grown! The supporting atmosphere with positive suggestions, comments, and stories in a safe, caring, nonjudgmental atmosphere is so wonderful. We didn't analyze what we were doing wrong, so there was no guilt trip.

Emily: Recently, my family experienced some problems, and I was truly grateful for the skills I learned here because I think they helped keep some difficult times from going into disastrous times. When things got out of hand, I was aware of how automatically some of the new skills came to mind.

(*This interaction is not included in the transcript at the end of this chapter.*)

This last training session is typically characterized by an air of camaraderie, and telephone numbers are usually exchanged with parents offering to help each other with projects or babysitting.

Continuing the Special Playtimes

When CPRT groups complete their 10 sessions of training, about half of the parents tend to stop having special playtimes. The reasons vary. Parents become involved in other projects that they placed on hold while they were in CPRT training. They no longer have the group or the leader to answer to. Their children's behavior has improved, so they no longer feel a sense of urgency to get something done. The importance of encouraging parents to continue having their special playtimes cannot be overemphasized. The 10 sessions of CPRT training are considered to be minimal, and children who have more severe problems certainly necessitate more extensive training to equip parents with the skills required in such cases. However, in all cases, parents should be encouraged to continue having their special playtimes. Introduce the following **Rule of Thumb: Good things come in small packages.** *Explain to parents that they should not wait for big events to enter into their children's worlds—that entering into their children's lives in small ways is what really matters. Continuing to have a weekly 30-minute special playtime is one way for parents to enter into their children's lives and create special moments between them and their children in a relatively small amount of time.*

Dr. L.: Even though summer school is out and vacation is about to begin, I want to encourage you to continue your special playtimes. They are valuable, because **what you do for 30 minutes in the special playtime usually doesn't occur at other times in your home.**

You have no tasks to complete during that time.

You focus completely on your child.

You are a mirror for your child's emotions.

Your child is allowed to take the lead.

Your child directs himself and assumes responsibility.

For 30 minutes, you are not your child's teacher.

You are encouraging, supportive, and accepting.

You don't offer any suggestions or solve any problems.

You don't criticize any behavior.

Now that we have concluded the first training phase, it's important that you continue your play session each week, then when we meet in September, you can report on how the month has gone with your playtimes.

Kathy: Cody wants the playtimes to be longer and to have three playtimes each week.

Dr. L.: Thirty minutes is enough time. You all have busy schedules, and you may not be able to be consistent if you have longer sessions and more sessions each week. Also, your child doesn't need three playtimes each week. One will be enough. It is better to be consistent in having one play session each week than to be inconsistent in trying to have three.

The therapist discusses the importance of continuing the home play sessions, and parents are asked to sign a contract committing to continue the play sessions for x number of weeks. The therapist tells the parents, "If you stop the play sessions now, the message is that you were playing with your child because you had to, not because you wanted to." Parents will usually commit to continue the play sessions at least until the follow-up training session around 4 to 6 weeks later. Parents may also set up their own continuing support group with time for the children to play and the parents to talk. One of the parents should take responsibility for coordinating the group's meeting time and place. The filial therapist concludes the session by providing parents with the handout, *Rules of Thumb and Other Things to Remember* (see Session 10 of Therapist Notebook in the CPRT Treatment Manual, 2nd Edition, as a reminder of main points covered over the past 10 sessions. We have also had this handout made into a refrigerator magnet to provide a handy resource for parents, or you can laminate the handout and add a stick-on magnet).

Follow-Up Session

We have had some success scheduling one-month follow-up sessions for updating, dealing with play session problems, answering questions, etc. The therapist sends parents a postcard reminding them of the follow-up training session. Providing child care at this session is important for the reasons described earlier, but also because the children like to revisit the clinic with "all those neat toys." The session begins with the parents sharing their experiences in their play sessions since the last meeting, focusing on changes in themselves and their children. The therapist uses their comments to reinforce the CPRT skills and principles taught earlier. The therapist affirms the parents' progress by asking them to give examples of their successful use of the skills. A primary focus of this session is on helping parents generalize their skills outside the play sessions. Parents are encouraged to give each other suggestions, a process that can be very empowering for them as they help each other with their difficulties. Parents may choose to continue to meet on their own for support. If there is enough interest, another follow-up training session can be scheduled to be held in about 3 months.

Updating of parent skills can also be provided for by scheduling an advanced CPRT training group for parents who have completed previous CPRT training. In advanced CPRT training, skills are reviewed, the play process is examined in more depth, parent–child issues are updated, and much more time is spent than in the previous training on applying skills outside the play sessions. The therapist sends a personal invitation to CPRT "alumni" spanning several years, inviting them to sign up for the advanced CPRT training. The importance of advanced CPRT training was described by a parent:

> I have been having some major problems with my child, and I knew things would get better if I would start having play sessions again. I just couldn't get started having them, though. Coming to these training sessions meant I had to make a commitment to have playtimes, and my child's behavior has improved dramatically.

Partial Transcript of CPRT Session 10

(Parents shared about their week, reported the number of times they touched their child, and excitedly described their play-wrestling experiences with their children.)

Dr. L.: Ten weeks ago, as you were talking about your child of focus, I wrote down your descriptions. I'd like to read these descriptions, and then you give us an update on what your child is like now. Debbie, you said Rachel was sensitive, strong-willed. I get angry. I totally reject her, I spank her, and it doesn't work. She's bossy and demanding. She throws temper tantrums. I'm wishy washy. What's that like now?

Debbie: She still throws her tantrums, but they are more controlled.

Dr. L.: What are your reactions to her now?

Debbie: My reactions are more calm. When I see her throw herself on the floor, my reactions are no longer, "What do I do?" Now they are, "OK, let's try something." It's OK. This is what I've got to do. Knowing what to do has helped me take all the undercurrent out of my reactions to her. Giving choices has been the key. She has direction now.

Dr. L.: Choices allow her to use her own resources.

Debbie: Giving choices places the responsibility back on her. She's more than capable of deciding what she wants to do.

Dr. L.: So you're a different person with her.

Debbie: I think so. It just makes it easier to put the responsibility back on her. Now, I know what to do, and that solved 90 percent of the problem, instead of spanking or doing something else that doesn't work.

Dr. L.: What is the spanking like now?

Debbie: I don't spank anymore. The only time I have spanked her is when she is in direct harm.

Dr. L.: So most of the behaviors you were concerned about have changed.

Debbie: Yes.

Dr. L.: How about your own reactions; you said, "I get angry and totally reject her."

Debbie: That is what I am really working on, not physically pushing her away. I realized that I constantly pushed her away rather than embrace her. Pushing her away makes her more and more hyper. Putting responsibility back on her keeps me from getting angry. I think the feeling of being out of control is where the anger comes from.

Dr. L.: So you feel in control now, and it seems to me that you are saying, "I am more loving with her."

Debbie: I am. And in turn, her loving attributes come out.

Dr. L.: Because of what you do.

Debbie: She's even mirroring choices. For so long I feared the terrible 2s and terrible 3s because I just didn't know what to do. I have really prayed for a class like this for a long time to teach me what I need to know, because I come from a highly dysfunctional family. I needed basic tools.

Dr. L.: You sound very satisfied with yourself now, and you do have some tools.

Debbie: Yes, but I have to choose to use them because there are times when I would like to throw her out with the trash. (Group laughs.) I have a relationship with her now, not a dictatorship.

Dr. L.: All because of what you are doing.

Debbie: But because of the tools I've been given.

Dr. L.: But you are the one that uses them.

Laura: Debbie, he's trying to give you a compliment, but you're not letting him.

Debbie: I think every one of us here wants to be good parents, but until this class, we didn't know how.

Sonya: We didn't know what to do.

Debbie: We've all been taught children are told what to do, and they have to do it.

Emily: "Be seen and not heard." That's how we were raised. I was scared not to do what my parents said to.

Laura: I don't think it was so much fear as it was respect.

Emily: I didn't have that respect. I did for my Dad. He only gave me one spanking in my whole life. He was always there to reason with me.

Kathy: I still don't have a close relationship with my parents.

Debbie: Haven't we grown up thinking, "My parents did this wrong and that wrong, and I don't want to do that to my children"?

Emily: I think for a really long time I blamed Mom, that was so wrong of her to do that, but then I had to resolve within myself that she probably did what she was taught, what she learned from her parents. And she did the best she knew how to do.

Sonya: Mom was so off the mark, but I know she meant well.

Debbie: Before this class, I could see Rachel being 14 and being messed up.

Dr. L.: What I hear all of you saying is, your children are going to grow up, and they will say different things about you as parents, that you parented in a way they will want to parent. Sonya, you said of Jenny that she is trying to show me something, and I'm not sure what it is. I don't use physical discipline; you were already giving some choices and so forth. But your main concern was that you were sensitive to the fact that she was trying to show you something.

Sonya: She's angry, she's real angry. I thought a lot of it was sadness, and I found out through the things we did here in class that she was angry. And what I learned to do through these classes was to set up a safe situation for her. That poor Bobo, he gets taped up and knifed. I think the first three or four playtimes she never even touched the knife, the gun, or any of the aggressive looking toys. I have learned how to read her face. When she cried, I thought she was sad, so I would say, "Oh, are you sad?" and she seemed so confused by what I was saying to her. Now, she will say, "I'm angry." So often I just didn't know what was going on with her, and I think that even though I'm not comfortable with physical discipline, the verbal yelling and screaming I did hurt her emotionally as much as if I had spanked her. I'm glad I don't have to do that anymore. I do know what else to do. I feel empowered. She's even giving her little friends choices now. I can tell she is feeling more comfortable with being able to say what she needs, and the special playtimes made the difference. I really needed to set up a time for her to know that she can be and do and say whatever she needs to, and know that she is safe, and there never was that time. I'll continue to do the special playtime; it's really important. I feel a lot better, I do.

Dr. L.: Sonya, you have made a huge difference in your child's life, and you're really sold on the special playtimes. Laura, you said of Dawson: lots of anger. He has resented my times with the baby. He's very demanding. He wanders off, he's a real challenge. He pushes the limits. I have a real hard time following through. He demands my time. How are those behaviors now?

Laura: Kara is very independent, she doesn't need much of my time, so there's not that much competitiveness there. They seem to be better friends; his resentment toward her seems to be less. He doesn't wander off. I think there are other things that have helped that. He does have a physical boundary. He knows the limits and he has a choice; if he gets beyond the boundary, then he has to come back inside the house.

Dr. L.: How about his being very demanding of you?

Laura: I think it has been resolved. I don't feel as stressed about it as I did.

Dr. L.: How about this statement: you said, "I have a hard time following through."

Laura: We are doing better with that, too. He doesn't test the limit as much anymore, either. When he is in time out, he stays there now.

Dr. L.: So you are different in some ways, and he's different.

Laura: Yes, there are a lot of changes in our lives. I'm just excited about the depth of what we are really giving to our kids. I've done a lot of research on myself, and my inner child and where I came from. I know that allowing children to make choices, learn self-discipline, and allowing them to express themselves is wonderful.

Dr. L.: I'm aware of changes in you. You are more relaxed, open, more shows in your face now than when this training began.

Laura: Yeah, it's not so frightening to talk about those skeletons in the closet anymore. Here, there is acceptance from other people who are having the same struggles.

Dr. L.: I hear you saying "Thank you" to these people in the group.

Laura: It just feels good. When I first came in here, I wanted you to make me feel better, but it's something much bigger than that.

Dr. L.: The bigness of it is what's in each of you.

Sonya: We feel better about ourselves.

Dr. L.: So you react differently to your children, and they like themselves better.

Laura: Yes, I think that has a lot to do with Dawson. He likes himself better. Our interactions are so much better now. Before, he was going to go out the window no matter what, and it was a struggle every time. Now we don't have exchanges like that anymore. He doesn't go out the window anymore. He realizes now he will get to go out later.

Dr. L.: And who has made the difference?

Laura: A lot of things.

Dr. L.: I'm not going to let you off the hook, Laura. Who has made the difference?

Laura: I have.

Dr. L.: You have, yes, you are doing things differently. I heard you say, "I've been working on myself, I'm learning about my child." You have made the difference. That's true of each one of you. You can't give someone else credit, Debbie. Each one of you did it.

Debbie: I'll accept that. (Group laughs.)

Dr. L.: Kim, you said of Toby, "He was premature, has ADD, delayed speech. He's in speech therapy, has low self-esteem. He's very affectionate, real sweet, easily frustrated, and impatient with himself." Has any of that changed?

Kim: Oh, yeah. A lot. It's a result of what my husband and I have been doing and all the outside help. Even Toby's speech is getting better, so he's feeling more confident about himself. His interactions with his sister are just so much better. Yesterday, he told me Michelle hit him, and he told her, "I'm not for hitting." I know he got that from our playtimes. It's helped a lot.

Dr. L.: How are you feeling about him, now?

Kim: Oh, a lot better. I was the youngest and was spoiled rotten. I never had any limits. Setting limits was the hardest thing for me. I wanted my children to like me so much, to be their friend. I wanted my children to know that they were loved all the time, and it was hard to discipline them. But I've learned that disciplining them is loving them. Now I'm not afraid to go to restaurants. (Laughter.) Now, they are so much more in control. I came here to help my little boy, but the choice giving has helped my little girl, too. I felt frustrated. I felt like I was failing. I knew that my child wasn't where he needed to be developmentally, and now I've realized it wasn't my fault, but I can help him.

Dr. L.: It's pretty hard to do things the way they need to be done when you feel like you are already failing. Your creativity is stifled, and so the solutions and good things you're already capable of don't come out, because you are so frustrated. One important thing I hear you saying is your perception of yourself has changed.

Debbie: When I started coming here, I had Rachel in day care full time because that's where I wanted her to be. My reaction was, "Oh, good. She's going to school. I can't get her there fast enough." Now, I put her in school just one day a week because I want to be with her. This training has made a big difference in her.

Emily: When we started this class, you wanted us to concentrate on one child during this 10-week period, but everything you have taught us, we've been able to apply to all of our children, no matter their age. It works for all ages.

Kim: I've even caught myself using these skills at work when things are difficult.

Debbie: Yeah, it works with husbands too. "You can choose meatloaf or chicken, which do you want?" (Laughter.)

Dr. L.: I appreciate so much the eagerness with which you all have tried these skills. It's easy to suggest that you try this or this would be helpful, but you all are the ones who have to make it work. And you have made it work.

(Other parents report on changes. See instructions for Session 10 for continuing the play sessions and plans for follow-up.)

Dr. L.: My students, who have been watching these sessions from the observation room, would like to come in and ask you some questions, if that is OK with you all.

Group: Sure, we don't mind.

(Students enter. Introduces students and they ask questions.)

Student: How do you feel now that you have gone through this training?

Sonya: Relieved. I like the word empowered, that I am not going to permanently damage the psyche of my child. (Laughter.) I feel empowered to make the right choices. I have been given the ability to choose. I can do a little extra work and do it this way, or I can scream and yell at my kid. I can make choices today. I had pretty limited options before.

Kim: Now the children answer to me, rather than me answering to them. My days are much easier. Everything that goes wrong is not my fault.

Student: Do you feel like your philosophy of child rearing or ideas of what your child might need from you are any different now than when you started the course?

Debbie: Definitely. I used to be really scared of children in the beginning. Yesterday, I taught a 4-year-old Sunday school class, and I wasn't terrified sitting there. Now, I know more about what they want. I feel good about myself when I'm dealing with children.

Student: How has having the support of the whole group helped rather than just doing the training one on one with Dr. L.? What has it been like having each other to bounce ideas off of?

Emily: I think Dr. Landreth could sit there and tell us all day that there are other parents like you who are struggling, to try to make us feel better, but knowing that there are other people we can see, hear, and touch makes a big difference.

Dr. L.: It's a really frustrating and scary spot to be in when you think, "I'm the only one."

Kathy: And now we know we're not. At 8:30, thousands of parents all across the country are trying to get their child into bed just like me! (Laughter.) It has changed my attitude.

Student: What have you learned specifically about yourself?

Sonya: I'm capable. Before it was frustrating not knowing what the options were. I thought I had to know how to be a parent just because I had a baby. That's how it was for my mom, and I thought I should know, too. It has been nice to find out that I am capable, and that I can do all these things.

Emily: It's parent training, but it's also a support group here.

Student: What do you think was the most difficult concept or skill that was taught?

Emily: Tracking has got to be the most unnatural thing, because you can see what the child is doing, but to verbalize it was the most difficult thing. I just felt so stupid. It's very awkward. Now it's not, but it was 10 weeks ago.

Kim: For me, it was not being able to direct my child's play or tell him what to do or what things are. That was hard, to let it be what he wanted it to be. If the number is a three, it's hard to say, "That can be whatever you want it to be."

Sonya: Choices, but also sitting back and letting the child lead. I kept wanting to give directions. We covered how to give choices to problems, but when there is a unique situation, I have to stop and really think about a choice I could give that makes sense.

Student: Did any of you at any point think that this training was not working, and wanted to drop out?

Group: No.

Sonya: The first time I was here, I was thinking, this is not what I thought it was, especially when I came in here and saw all these toys. I wanted some more specific behavior things. But after the first assignment, I was hooked.

Debbie: Dr. Landreth started out restricting what we did to the 30-minute playtime knowing our use of these skills would spill over into the rest of our week. (Laughter.)

Student: Were there any skills or techniques that you didn't agree with?

Kim: At first I disagreed with the no praising, but then when I tried it in the 30 minutes, I saw and understood why I shouldn't praise him. Now, I don't say "Good job" anymore. I expand that and give my child more by saying,

"You worked hard on that." Now he knows I see exactly what he is doing. It builds his self-esteem.

Debbie: Leaving off the praise makes you really focus on what the child is doing instead of just making a general praise statement. Now, Rachel will say, "Tell me what I am doing, Mama."

Sonya: I took an Active Parenting class, and it just didn't help me like this one did. This is really working. Jenny is 3 years old and she tracks herself: "I'm doing this all by myself," she says. She even tells me how I'm feeling.

Student: What was your favorite part of the training?

Laura: The special one-on-one playtime; I didn't know what I was missing.

Debbie: All of it, especially the sharing time. Each point made sense, and Dr. L. structured it so well, giving us a little at a time so that it all fell into place.

Kim: It was all so easy to understand. I always remember the stories or catch phrases when I'm trying to think of what to do.

Student: What about the video-recording of your playtimes? Do you see that as a positive part of your learning process?

Emily: I thought it was real helpful, and also that there were people here to critique you. Every time I watched the video, I heard myself saying, "Didn't you?" I knew I didn't need to be saying that. It was real helpful. Every week I watched my first session to see what I was doing differently in that week's session. Was I more relaxed or tracking better? The feedback here was wonderful. I was told all these great things I did and then there was one thing I needed to improve on.

Dr. L.: Is this a good place to stop? Again, I really appreciate your courage to allow all these people to watch our sessions, and your courage to go home and try all the things I asked you to do. It has been a very rewarding time for me to see you all get excited about what was working.

I have had fun being with you, and it was because of you that I had fun. Thank you.

Reference

Bratton, S., & Landreth, G. (2019). *Child-Parent Relationship Therapy (CPRT) treatment manual: An Evidence-Based 10-session filial therapy model* (2nd ed). New York, NY: Routledge.

CHAPTER 18

ADAPTING CPRT FOR PARENTS OF TODDLERS

Mary Morrison Bennett and Kara Carnes-Holt

Training and supervision in traditional Child-Parent Relationship Therapy (CPRT) is highly recommended before facilitating the adapted models of CPRT. CPRT-Toddler requires knowledge of child development, group experience, and understanding of toddlers. The authors highly recommend therapists do additional reading and training regarding this population to address caregiver questions and concerns. In this chapter, we will use the terms parents and caregivers interchangeably.

Unique Needs of Families of Young Children

Toddlers are fun, energetic, and interested, in everything. Their growing personality, vocabulary, and skill development is exciting and fun; you never know what is coming next. They explore their world and want to experience each moment (Schaefer & DeGironimo, 2000). Parenting a toddler can be demanding as parents often find themselves chasing their toddler, physically intervening when setting limits, and setting the same limit over and over. Most parents of toddlers are at the beginning phase of parenting and often still determining their parenting philosophy. Many families desire to do things similarly to how they were parented while others want to do things differently. Sometimes it is hard for both parents to be on the same page due to the difference in their upbringing. Regardless, caregivers are likely experiencing moments of confusion and frustration and need encouragement, support, and empathy.

The CPRT-Toddler therapist should be prepared to provide empathy and understanding to the weary caregivers with whom they work. Therapists will need to be especially empathetic with caregivers' perspectives. As parents in the group share their experiences, the therapist will sensitively reflect feeling and connect group members to facilitate support among members.

New Babies

When parents of toddlers decide to have a second child, adjustment to the second child is stressful for both parent and toddler. Struggles with the toddler that were hard before the baby was born are now exponentially more difficult. The toddler's world is turned upside down with the birth of a sibling. Often toddlers need to be held more and experience regression in some areas. Andrew (18 months) suddenly started crying every day when his parents announced it was bath time. The CPRT therapist encouraged limit setting and choice giving. "*I know you really don't want to take a bath, but it is bath time. You can choose to hop like a bunny or hiss like a snake to the bath tub, which do you choose?*" CPRT therapists equip parents with tools to provide the sensitive responses toddlers need. Helping parents feel heard and supported by modeling empathetic understanding is critical for parents to do the same for their children. **CPRT skill training is based on the philosophy that experiential learning is the most effective.**

Technology

Technology is a tremendous part of our environment, culturally it has changed the way we interact with others and the way we accomplish tasks in life. Many parents are concerned about "screen time," and the numbers of screens in a child's life are numerous, including television, tablets, computers, smartphones, and watches.

Screens truly are everywhere, and families who are interested in limiting screens face a difficult challenge. Professionals disagree about the amount of screen time that is appropriate for children (Elkind, 2007). The American Academy of Pediatrics (AAP, 2011) recommends no screen time for children under the age of 2 years and for children older than 2, the AAP recommends a maximum of 2 hours per day of screen time. As technology changes, recommendations may change. CPRT therapists should stay abreast of current AAP recommendations on technology. Parents get differing messages regarding screen time as many apps or games are advertised as educational, yet parents also hear of the AAP recommendations. *Child development specialists report children learn best from unstructured play which allows them to problem solve, role-play, and interact with the environment with their hands* (AAP, 2011; Elkind, 2007). If technology is brought up in the CPRT-Toddler group, the therapist can reflect parents' feelings and allow them to come to their own conclusions regarding how they want to handle technology. However, it does seem appropriate for the therapist to introduce parents to recommendations of groups such as the AAP. It is important to emphasize there is no place for technology during special playtime. Toys or electronics that entertain with sounds and buttons do not allow for emotional expression or connection between parent and child.

CPRT-Toddler Rationale

Adapting CPRT for toddlers (ages 1½ to 3 years) can assist parents in developmentally appropriate expectations and the creation of secure attuned relationships with their young child. Understanding children and their developmental stages and tasks is essential when creating interventions that are appropriate to the level of development and comprehension of the child (Weiner & Robinson-Kurpuis, 1995). According to Siegel and Hartzell (2004), relationships that provide experiences of connection, safety, and understanding promote secure attachments. Therefore, it is essential that parents of toddlers learn the therapeutic skills necessary to meet their child's need to form a secure attachment. CPRT-Toddler directly addresses the training and development of these therapeutic skills.

Toddler Development

The first three years of life are full of significant development in all areas for young children. Rogers (1951) proposed that all children are born with the innate desire to grow and learn to connect with people and their environment. Perry and Szalavitz (2006) concluded that the experiences children encounter can enhance or deter their development and that parents and other primary caregivers play an important role in influencing a child's development. The most important thing parents can offer children is contained in the natural, unhurried, and sensitive responses that come from "being with" their child (Thompson, 2001).

The CPRT-Toddler therapist will explain to parents pertinent developmental issues as they apply the parents' concerns. Example: Toddlers are entering a phase where they desire more independence; they want to "help" parents complete tasks. Toddlers desire to experience the moment and adults desire to complete the task. Dad is folding laundry; Harper (2½ years) wants to help and proceeds to pull each pair of folded pajamas off the couch so she can look at them. Needless to say, Dad feels exasperated and Harper is delighted as she studies each pair of flowered PJs. A CPRT-Toddler therapist might encourage Dad to reflect Harper's delight and set a limit that the clothes are not for touching, but she could play with these towels. Erikson (1963) explained this desire for independence in his psychosocial stages of development. Children ages 1–3 years are in the autonomy vs. shame and doubt phase. During this phase, the toddler gains some self-control and desires to be separate from the caregiver. The good news is, the resulting psychosocial strength is will. This push/pull that parents experience is confusing, as one minute the child wants help and the next minute she is shouting, "No! I can do it!"

According to Loevinger's (1997) theory of ego development, children aged 2–5 years are in the "impulsive" stage of ego development, their emotional range is small, and their focus is on immediate needs as well as needs only impacting them directly. This immediacy can be a challenge when parents need their child to get dressed and leave for school, but the child is concerned about arranging cars on the shelf and school is not his immediate need. When the CPRT therapist explains this is typical development for children this age, parents are able to set their expectations more appropriately, which ultimately positively impacts their relationship with their child. This is also a great opportunity for parents to set a limit, "Malik, I know you want to play cars, but now is time for getting dressed. You can choose to put your shorts or shirt on first, which do you choose?" Consistent with the CPRT A-C-T model of limit setting, this response shows understanding by Acknowledging that Malik wants to play with the cars, Communicates the limit and Targets a choice.

Children with advanced verbal skills may be confusing to parents. Two-and-a-half-year-old Ford is very verbal; he can tell detailed stories about going to the bathroom, but he cannot seem to use the potty on his own. His mother feels frustrated and confused. CPRT therapists reflect parents' confusion and explain that children can only develop in one area at a time. While Ford is busy expanding his vocabulary, his brain cannot also focus on the learning required for toilet training (Wood, 2015). This explanation may help his parents be more empathic and patient with the toilet training. Therapists will need to anticipate these types of challenges caregivers face and reflect feeling as well as provide them with information regarding development, so they know what they are experiencing is characteristic of this stage.

Parents of children who are more physical, coordinated, and often taller may wonder why their child does not have an expansive vocabulary. It is critical that the CPRT-Toddler therapist have an understanding of emotional, cognitive, and physical development of young children in order to alleviate parents' anxiety and help them set up appropriate expectations of their child. (See suggested reading list in the CPRT-Toddler chapter of the CPRT Treatment Manual, 2nd Edition, for additional resources.) Managing expectations is a critical component of parenthood.

Child development has been extensively studied, and it has been determined there is a typical pattern of development, that given time, most children will progress through the stages of development, often at predictable times (NAEYC, 2009). Although the stages of development are sequential, children move through them at their own pace. Caregivers may be concerned about their child who is not moving through the developmental stages as quickly as they would like or not doing the same tasks as their nephew at that age. Caregivers may ask, "Is my child normal?" It is the therapist's responsibility to be attentive to these parents and help them understand the importance of developmental tasks and respecting their child's pace (Ray, 2016).

One general piece of development knowledge we have found helpful for parents is the concept of disintegration. As children develop, they may unexpectedly seem to regress in a particular skill, just before the integration of new skills. Caregivers may report the child is falling apart and suddenly cannot do things they previously could. Then once integration is complete, the child has several new skills (Davies, 2011). This is because the human brain can only concentrate on one thing at a time. If a child is growing in one area, all the brain's energy is going toward that growth and cannot attend to other areas of development (Wood, 2015). Gesell (Gesell Institute of Child Development, 2011) referred to stages as either being periods of equilibrium or disequilibrium. Periods of equilibrium are described as calm, confident, and compliant while periods of disequilibrium are described as explosive, fearful, and self-focused. Caregivers also benefit from knowing to expect horizontal growth versus vertical growth. Some parents create a hierarchical view of development and value some skills more than others, such as verbal skills commonly associated with an increased intelligence, which is simply not the case. Assisting caregivers in understanding that children develop in different areas at different rates helps them to understand their child more.

Order in the environment, in relationships, and in the child's daily schedule provides security and predictability for young children. There are often tremendous tears when the child's order is disrupted. Many parents worry they are creating a *monster*, a child who requires things to be the same everywhere (Schaefer & DiGeronimo, 2000). As caregivers express frustration regarding this issue, the therapist reflects their frustration and explains that children are building an understanding of their world. Montessori (1995) referred to this as a sensitive period; the child is extremely sensitive when order is disrupted. Often parents want to do things to disrupt the child's order, thinking they are helping the child learn to be flexible. However, this only disrupts the child's thought process and does not allow the child to understand how the world works in their head. When parents understand that once the child has a solid understanding of the world, she will then be ready for disruptions and will handle them better, they usually calm down and are more patient with the process.

Emotional Development

Toddlers experience intense emotional highs and lows, as do their parents in trying to be sensitive to their child's needs (Loevinger, 1997; Schaefer & DiGeronimo, 2000). Toddlers often experience intense emotions, which are expressed through tantrums and crying, as they do not have the words to communicate what they are feeling. The enormous meltdowns 2½-year-olds often experience over seemingly minor issues are confusing and exhausting for caregivers. Emotional expression is more focused in fear or frustration in the second year of life. As children approach three years of age, deeper feelings such as pride, shame, embarrassment, and even guilt are expressed (Elkind, 2007). An advanced 2-year-old can begin to understand the difference in socially acceptable and unacceptable behaviors (Elkind, 2007). This information is helpful to caregivers, who may begin to wonder if setting limits with their child is effective at all.

Caregivers may suspect children are being defiant when in reality young children lack the verbal skills to express the intense emotions they are experiencing (Siegel & Bryson, 2012). As toddlers become more goal directed and assertive in expressing their desires, caregivers increase their expectations of compliance. Toddlers commonly demonstrate refusal before they consider complying, negotiating, compromising, or stating their preferences in other ways (Thompson, 2001). These new relationship skills can be challenging to parents and can result in parents feeling frustrated and confused by their child's behavior. Eleanor's (2½ years) grandfather reported that every time he gave a direction, Eleanor refused. He was concerned that Eleanor had a defiant spirit. After reflecting his frustration with Eleanor, the therapist then shared with Eleanor's grandfather that this is typical and an aspect of development as Eleanor learns to be more independent. It was also helpful to share with him that tantrums are often the result of frustration and not always willful disobedience.

Brain Development

Brain development during the toddler stage has a primary focus of integration of numerous functions, such as perceptual, cognitive, and language, and child-led play is an important component in this process (Davies, 2011). The brain develops over time with constant repetition and exposure, and each experience can reinforce positive or negative behaviors (Perry & Szalavitz, 2006). During the toddler stage, a high degree of brain plasticity is present that supports learning and flexibility and the ability to reorganize and respond to a variety of experiences and environmental conditions. Early experiences for young children are highly influential regarding how the brain structures. For example, emotional development is strengthened when caregivers use emotional language such as mad, happy, and sad when interacting with a young child (Woolfolk & Perry, 2015). Simple reflections to toddlers such as "*You feel excited grandma is coming!*" or "*You are angry that your favorite toy broke*" assists with optimal brain development, as opposed to trying to solve the problem or excessive questioning.

Secure attachment develops in the midst of an attuned relationship that facilitates repeated experiences of love, safety, and trust. The rapid development of the amygdala primarily takes place in children ages 0–36 months (Perry & Szalavitz, 2006). The amygdala is a part of the basal ganglia and is involved with emotional regulation, often referred to as controlling the fight/flight and freeze responses. For example, Tommy becomes frustrated with all of the toys on the floor and yells at his 20-month-old son, David. David sits on the floor and refuses to move. It can be helpful to parents to recognize this behavior is most likely a freeze response rooted in fear and not simply defiance. Often when parents receive this knowledge about the brain, it helps the parent to be more emotionally responsive to the child. **The skills taught in CPRT such as reflection of feeling can assist in the crucial development of self-regulation. Therapeutic and relational responsiveness, the focus of CPRT, assists in the parent/toddler attachment dance that promotes the development of a healthy stress response system.** Often parents of very young children may have difficulty seeing the value of reflecting feeling to a child who is not verbal. Susan reflected feelings to her son even as an infant, which was good practice for her and her son. Susan would say, "*I know you are frustrated*" or "*I know you don't want your diaper changed.*" Once her son was 18 months old, each time he started throwing a fit he would say, "*I know, I know, I know,*" indicating he had gained enough self-awareness to know he was feeling out of control and these were the words used to reflect that feeling.

Attachment Development

Infants born into this world are dependent on their primary caregiver for survival. The core of the attachment relationship is a matching and attuned relationship. Attachment is the "reciprocal, enduring, emotional, and physical affiliation between child and a caregiver. The child receives what she needs to live and grow through this relationship, and the caregiver meets her needs to provide sustenance and guidance" (James, 1994, p. 2). CPRT-Toddler focuses on promoting a relationship that is consistent with the "Be-With" Attitudes and is emotionally responsive. For example, the skills of reflecting feelings in statement form communicates to toddlers on an emotional level and allows toddlers to feel heard and understood. A secure foundation of a safe, predictable, and dependent relationship provides the needed socio-emotional framework for individuation and independence (Schore, 1994). This attachment relationship develops the framework for the child's perception of the world, relationships, and self-concept.

Healthy attachment enhances the child's ability to feel safe and secure and to self-regulate. The primary caregiver's ability to meet the basic needs of an infant in a genuinely nurturing and consistent manner is basic to the formation of a secure attachment. It is unrealistic to expect parents to be in complete attunement all of the time (Tronick, 2007). CPRT-Toddler focuses on teaching caregivers how to be sensitive to windows of time, such as a special playtime, to practice skills with toddlers such as esteem building, feeling refection, and basic noticing of the child's actions. These skills assist with the ongoing development of a securely attached relationship and assists parents with becoming more emotionally attuned to their child. **Secure attachments are thought to develop from an attuned and predictable relationship such as the CPRT-Toddler special playtimes**, in which the child has repeated experiences of feeling understood, connected, and protected by the parent. In the special playtime, the caregiver is emotionally responsive and consistent in the parent-child interactions. This secure attachment provides the resources for the child to develop meaningful interpersonal relationships in the future (Siegel & Hartzell, 2003).

Physical Development

Young children are growing at a rapid pace. It is common to hear parents marvel as they talk about how it seems their toddler changed overnight. Gross motor skill development often present for toddlers includes the ability to hop on one foot, walk backwards, and catch a rolled ball. Fine motor skills include turning pages one at a time, unscrewing lids on jars, and making snips with scissors (Woolfolk & Perry, 2015). Between ages 2 and 3 years, most toddlers develop sufficient bowel muscles and bladder control for toilet training (Davies, 2011).

The gap between the toddler's wants and abilities regarding physical development can often be a source of frustration (Davies, 2011). Sometimes parents are frustrated by the pendulum swinging between the toddler's desire to be fiercely independent one moment and the next moment seeking overdependence from the caregiver. For example, Sarah (3 years) may insist on putting on her own clothes but begs her mother to feed her. It is important for caregivers to remember toddlers utilize perceptual, motor, motivational, and cognitive systems regarding motor development and learning (Woolfolk & Perry, 2015). Many of the tasks that parents see as simple are requiring numerous systems at work for a young child. In CPRT-Toddler, parents are taught to reflect Sarah's wish of wanting mom to do it for her today and return responsibility to her by responding, "*You want me to feed you; you can feed yourself.*"

Cognitive Development

A toddler's cognitive development is woven into the development of his sense of self and he demonstrates a strong interest and desire to learn about his body as well as his physical and social world (Davies, 2011). Play is a holistic avenue that allows children to explore their developing identity without judgment or external expectations. **Toddlers are able to understand language well before they can speak, which is why reflective responses communicating the "Be-With" Attitudes are valuable skills for parents of toddlers.**

According to Woolfolk and Perry (2015), toddlers are able to arrange words into short sentences with more advanced messages to express their thoughts, feelings, and wants. Therefore, in order to support ongoing language development, it is important to use reflective responses with children. Making statements such as "*You stacked the blocks on top of each other*" facilitates the child's vocabulary and language comprehension. The CPRT skills of tracking the child's actions, reflecting content and feeling during special playtimes, are supportive of toddler cognitive development.

During this time, toddlers are also seeking emotional support from caregivers. They develop cognitive expectations such as seeking comfort from a caregiver when they are hurt (Davies, 2011). For example, Penelope (2½ years) falls and skins her knees and immediately seeks out her mother at the playground for comfort and security. During toddler development, children begin to understand the perspectives of others, and they primarily learn by observing and imitating (Woolfolk & Perry, 2015). Penelope is learning how to express empathy and care for others as she watches and experiences how her mother is caring for her during this time.

Play of Toddlerhood

Play is a critical aspect of childhood. Play allows children to express emotion, gain mastery, and make meaning of their lives. Imaginative play of young children is fun and exciting; however, it often does not make sense to adults. Children around 15 months old may spend most of their special playtime handing toys to the adult or pouring and dumping the same container of items. Children this age are learning how things work together and interact (Davies, 2011). Caregivers may not know that children under three years of age have difficulty differentiating imaginative and real life. Jason (2 years) talks for his tow truck during play, and he genuinely believes the tow truck talks. For several weeks, my 3-year-old son has been talking about the princess coming and finally, today, she came! Turns out she was a puppet, and she finally came for her visit. We were all really excited.

When Grady (2 years) was playing trains with his dad, he said to his train, "Aren't you having fun staying home and playing with your daddy?" Dad responded in a similar train voice, "Yeah, I love playing with daddy." Clearly in this situation, Grady was having fun playing with his daddy and expressed that through his play rather than telling him directly. The CPRT-Toddler therapist may need to help caregivers to stay in the metaphor with children and get into character, talk as the toy, give the train a voice (Woolfolk & Perry, 2015).

Changes in play are also indicative of the toddler's rapid cognitive development. At approximately 18 months, toddlers enter the cognitive development state of mental representations that includes development of symbolic thought and deferred imitation. Play behaviors that often indicate this developmental stage include anticipation of objects, role-playing imaginary activities, and play involving make-believe beings (Woolfolk & Perry, 2015). "Decentered symbolic play" occurs at 19 to 22 months and involves pretend actions with toys such as making car noises and moving the car along the floor. Children 20 to 25 months are able to sequence their pretend play with multiple steps such as getting the fire truck, driving it to the house, and rescuing the people (Woolfolk & Perry, 2015). The next play developmental stage, 24 to 30 months, is "internally directed symbolic play" where objects have intentions such as the shoe is a telephone to talk with the caregiver. "Behavioral role plays" manifest around 30 to 36 months and involve the toddler pretending to be someone or something else like teacher, doctor, or caregiver (Woolfolk & Perry, 2015). CPRT-Toddler teaches parents how to enter into these developmental play stages as a therapeutic play partner with their children. (A detailed description of this process is in the CPRT-Toddler chapter in the CPRT Treatment Manual, 2nd Edition.)

Multicultural Considerations

There has been a rapid increase in the number of minority children in the United States (Ceballos, Parikh, & Post, 2012). Traditional Western values that promote early independence may be challenging to some parents that participate in CPRT. Attachment-based parenting is widely practiced in numerous cultures, and CPRT leaders need to be sensitive to various parenting styles and child expectations. It is important to remember that timing and sequence of motor development varies according to culture due to the cultural norms for caring for children and encouraging independence (Woolfolk & Perry, 2015).

Sensitivity is especially needed, for example, when using the CPRT Rule of Thumb "Never do for a child what a child can do for themselves." While the intent of this rule is to foster the child's independence and sense of confidence, it is important to also consider this guideline within a multicultural framework. In many cultures, parents may hand feed their children for longer than what is typical in Western culture. The CPRT therapist will need to be sensitive to cultural norms in the context of culture, attachment, and relationship dimensions.

Another way for CPRT leaders to consider cultural factors is to contemplate the inclusion and exclusion of particular toys. Many families live within a system that includes multiple generations in the home, while some families have external individuals such as nannies care for their children. The CPRT therapist needs to be flexible in helping families represent their child's world through toys. Dolls of various skin tones and generations may be suggested as well as play food that reflects the diet of that family. Musical instruments that are included could be reflective of the family's culture as well. CPRT therapists should be aware of cultural differences in families and use this opportunity to help the family connect to their culture and facilitate their child's cultural expression.

Modifications for Child-Parent Relationship Therapy-Toddlers

It is important that CPRT therapists closely follow the CPRT-Toddler chapter in the CPRT Treatment Manual, 2nd Edition (Bratton & Landreth, 2019) for specific adaptations in handouts and session outlines for CPRT-Toddlers. There are some general adjustments that need to be made to the special playtime. Due to the short attention span of children ages 18 months to 3 years, the length and fluidity of location of special playtime for toddlers is a significant deviation from the standard CPRT model. The younger the child, the shorter the special playtime should be. For children closer to 18 months, having special playtimes three times a week for approximately 10 minutes each time is recommended. For children 2 years old, 15 minutes twice a week is needed, and the closer the child is to 3 years old, 20 minutes once a week.

The concept that the parent is "dumb" and does not have answers during the play session is not as appropriate for toddlers. Parents may need to label toys; however, parents should avoid teaching. CPRT therapists should stress the focus of this time is the Child-Parent play rather than the child's learning. Toddlers frequently ask what something is, and parents will need to supply an answer. Developmentally, toddlers do not have the capacity to expand their imagination for the item to be anything they want it to be. However, as the child gets closer to 3 years of age, her imagination develops, as do her verbal skills, and the parent may not need to label as often.

The toy kit is a significant modification for this developmental stage. For children 1–2 years of age, parents may consider using bath time or water playtime as their special playtime. Children love to splash, and parents can reflect, "*You made that splash*," "*Splashing is fun*," "*You know how to pour water into the cup.*" Toys recommended for the toy kit are described in the CPRT-Toddler chapter in the CPRT Treatment Manual, 2nd Edition. Parents should use their discretion in choosing toys. Some children put toys in their mouth at this age, and others do not. Therefore, toys with small parts should be avoided.

In limit setting, the younger the child, the shorter the limit needs to be; therefore, parents may only reflect the child's feeling rather than wishes and desires during the first step of limit setting. Parents may also need to physically direct the child to another activity rather than pointing when targeting an alternative. Limits set outside the session will require a lot of practice with toddlers. It is critical that parents understand that at this stage of development, their children are exploring their world and that involves testing limits regularly. Often parents feel frustrated that limit setting is not working. Encourage parents that this is typical for toddlers and that limits may need to be set many times (sometimes hundreds of times) before toddlers begin regulating their own behavior.

The Rule of Thumb "Big choices for big kids, little choices for little kids" needs modification and additional explanation for the toddler population. Although parents are often eager to find a solution to children's behavior, understanding child development is key when utilizing choice giving. Very young children will be able to understand basic choice giving such as "Do you choose to wear the blue shirt or red shirt to daycare today?" Caregivers should use advanced choice giving with caution and consider implementing more complex choice giving as the child approaches the age of 3. The additional Rule of Thumb "Grant in fantasy what you cannot grant in reality" may provide a wonderful time to visit with parents about the importance of nurturing creativity and imagination in young children. The CPRT-Toddler chapter in the CPRT Treatment Manual, 2nd Edition, contains additional instructional adaptations and adaptations to the handouts.

Conclusion

Child-Parent Relationship Therapy-Toddler model is designed to enhance the parent-child relationship between parents and their young children. In learning these skills, parents can have a greater understanding of their toddlers and learn to see the world through their child's eyes and therefore increase empathy and understanding of how their child experiences the world. CPRT therapists have a unique opportunity to support parents in developing their relationship during this critical time of development.

References

American Academy of Pediatrics (AAP). (2011). Policy statement: Media use by children younger than 2 years. *Pediatrics, 128*(5), 1–7.

Bratton, S. C., & Landreth, G. L. (2019). *Child-Parent Relationship Therapy (CPRT) treatment manual: An Evidence-Based 10-session filial therapy model* (2nd ed). New York, NY: Routledge.

Ceballos, P. L., Parikh, S. B., & Post, P. B. (2012). Examining social justice attitudes among play therapists: Implications for multicultural supervision and training. *International Journal of Play Therapy, 21*, 232–243. doi:10.1037/a0028540

Davies, D. (2011). *Child development: A practitioner's guide* (3rd ed). New York, NY: Guilford Press.

Elkind, D. (2007). *The power of play: How spontaneous, imaginative activities lead to happier, healthier children.* Cambridge, MA: Da Capo.

Erickson, E. (1963). *Childhood and society.* New York, NY: W. W. Norton.

Gesell Institute of Child Development. (2011). *Gesell developmental observation-revised examiner's manual.* New Haven, CT: Gesell Institute of Child Development.

James, B. (1994). *Handbook for treatment of attachment-trauma problems in children.* Lexington, MA: Lexington Books.

Loevinger, J. (1997). Stages of personality development. In R. Hogan, J. Johnson, & S. Briggs (Eds.), *Handbook of personality psychology* (pp. 199–208). San Diego: Academic Press.

Montessori, M. (1995). *The absorbent mind.* New York, NY: Holt.

National Association for the Education of Young Children. (2009). *NAEYC Developmentally appropriate practice in early childhood programs serving children from birth through age 8*. Washington, DC. Retrieved from www.naeyc.org/files/naeyc/file/positions/PSDAP.pdf

Perry, B. D., & Szalavitz, M. (2006). *The boy who was raised as a dog and other stories from a child psychiatrist's notebook*. New York, NY: Basic Books.

Ray, D. C. (2016). An overview of child development. In Dee Ray (Ed.), *A therapist's guide to child development: The extraordinarily normal years* (pp. 3–13). New York, NY: Routledge.

Rogers, C. (1951). *Client-centered therapy: Its current practice, implications and theory*. Boston: Houghton Mifflin.

Schaefer, C. E., & DeGeronimo, T. F. (2000). *Ages and stages: Tips and techniques for building your child's social, emotional, interpersonal and cognitive skills*. New York, NY: John Wiley & Sons.

Schore, A. N. (1994). *Affect regulation and the origin of self*. Mahwah, NJ: Erlbaum.

Sigel, D. J., & Bryson, T. P. (2012). *The whole-brain child*. New York, NY: Bantam Books.

Siegel, D., & Hartzell, M. (2003). *Parenting from the inside-out: How a deeper self-understanding can help you raise children who thrive*. New York, NY: Jeremy P. Tarcher/Putnam.

Thompson, R. A. (2001). Development in the first years of life. *The Future of Children, 11*(1), 20–33. Retrieved from http://search.proquest.com/docview/220152495?accountid=5683

Tronick, E. (2007). *The neurobehavioral and social-emotional development of infants and children*. New York, NY: W. W. Norton.

Weiner, N., & Robinson-Kurpuis, S. E. (1995). *Shattered innocence: A practical guide for counseling women survivors of childhood sexual abuse*. Washington, DC: Taylor & Francis.

Wood, C. (2015). *Yardsticks: children in the classroom ages 4–14* (3rd ed). Turners Falls, MA: Center for Responsive Schools.

Woolfolk, A., & Perry, N. (2015). *Child and adolescent development* (2nd ed). New Jersey: Pearson.

CHAPTER 19

ADAPTING CPRT FOR PARENTS OF PREADOLESCENTS

Peggy L. Ceballos, Kristin Meany-Walen, and Kara Carnes-Holt

Child-Parent Relationship Therapy: Preadolescent Model

Preadolescence is a developmental phase in which youth are transitioning from childhood into adolescence and might be referred to as early adolescents, preteens, or tweens. A specific age range is not agreed upon by developmental experts but generally consists of ages between 9 and 13 (Meany-Walen, Carnes Holt, Ceballos, & Michero, 2014). Typically regarded as either children or adolescents, this stage of development has been neglected in much of the developmental literature. However, recently, developmental experts have acknowledged and outlined some of the unique characteristics of this age group and how to respond to those changes in ways that foster growth and maturity (e.g., Center for Disease Control [CDC], 2016).

The emerging literature supports that a strong parent-child relationship during preadolescence serves as a protecting factor against behavioral problems (Lederman & Mian, 2003) and facilitates optimal development for preadolescents (Papalia, Olds, & Feldman, 2007). Despite the importance of the parent-child relationship at this age, most parents report feeling unprepared to deal with the changes that their preadolescents go through (Baril, Cromer, & McHale, 2007). Similarly, preadolescents feel misunderstood by their parents, which leads to disruption in the parent-child attachment (Bulanda & Majumdar, 2008). In response, Child-Parent Relationship Therapy (CPRT) can serve to strengthen the parent-child relationship during this important developmental stage. CPRT provides parents with skills to develop and maintain an open communication and a relationship within which preadolescents feel safe and understood.

Developmental Characteristics of Preadolescents

During preadolescence, maturing children experience social/emotional, physical, and cognitive changes in a relatively short period of time. These rapid and intense changes may parallel those that take place during toddlerhood (Vernon, 2009). Notably important, parents remain a vital part of preadolescents' social sphere, although autonomy and peer influence start to take a greater role (Papalia et al., 2007). Following is a description of the expected changes in each of the developmental areas (cognitive, physical, and socio-emotional).

Social/Emotional

A basic human need is belonging and acceptance (Maslow, 1962). For young children, parents fill this need; however, as children mature, peers begin to serve this role, which typically starts during preadolescence (CDC, 2016). Preadolescents begin to feel as if nobody, particularly parents, understands them and their feelings, and they increasingly align with others who have similar experiences, mainly peers. Preadolescents begin to spend more time with friends outside of the home, and they become increasingly reliant on peers for support, problem solving, and a sense of belonging as compared to childhood (Kretschmer, Sentse, Kornelis Dijkstra, &

Veenstra, 2014). As such, peer groups that emphasize athletics, music, arts, or other areas of interest begin to overtly develop. Although preadolescents start to take interest in extra-curricular activities, they may start to dislike school and feel increased stress as the amount of school work and academic challenges increase (CDC, 2016). They often teeter between conformity and competition, and they may set high expectations for themselves. The balancing act of polarizing expectations and experiences might increase their shift in moods and self-esteem (CDC, 2016).

A major consideration for preadolescents social-emotional development is what Elkind (1980) described as an *imaginary audience*, wherein people believe that others are constantly watching and judging them. *Imaginary audience* is common among preadolescents, and it impacts how this age group view themselves and how they believe they are perceived by others. According to CDC (2016), the socio-emotional pressures that preadolescents experience coupled with the strong sense of *imaginary audience* might increase their susceptibility to mental health concerns such as depression, anxiety, or eating disorders. Thus, they may also begin to feel pressure and experiment with alcohol, tobacco products, drugs, sex, or other risky behaviors.

Physical

Preadolescents' bodies begin to grow upward and outward as they become taller and stronger. They may start puberty, experience voice changes, and have an increase in body odor. Their bodies begin to appear more similar to that of adults—growth of pubic and underarm hair, and widening of shoulders in boys and hips in girls (CDC, 2016). Girls may also experience their first menstrual cycle and develop breasts, and boys may start to grow facial hair, although boys typically mature later in life than girls (Papalia et al., 2007). However, as compared to late childhood, both sexes exhibit a better demand of their body as evidenced by increased coordination. As these changes occur at rapid speeds and at rates different from their peers, preadolescents may feel inferior or self-conscious about their changing bodies (CDC, 2016). A combination of age, gender, timing of puberty, and hormonal development increase the heightened emotional reactions characterizing preadolescence (Papalia et al., 2007).

Cognitive

Evidence suggests that the right hemisphere of the brain, often referred to as the creative and emotional side of the brain, experiences a significant growth spurt and pruning process during this period (National Institute of Mental Health [NIMH], 2011). Simultaneously, significant growth in the frontal lobe begins to occur, which is responsible for reasoning, regulating emotions, planning, and controlling impulses (Papalia et al., 2007). Thus, while preadolescents begin to practice making rational/safe decisions, they are also flooded with hormones and processes which make them appear hypersensitive or self-critical (NIMH, 2011). They may make impulsive choices that serve their immediate gratification without analyzing the long-term consequences of their decisions (Schwartz, 2008).

According to Piaget (1969), children use preoperational and concrete operational thinking to navigate and understand their worlds. During late childhood and early adolescence, children begin to have access to formal operational thinking (Piaget, 1969). This new cognitive development allows them to engage in abstract reasoning, characterized by an increased ability to think hypothetically, consider opposing views, and apply learning from one context to another (CDC, 2016). Even though growing children are able to use abstract thinking skills, they often revert back to concrete thought during times of emotional or cognitive stress (NIMH, 2011). Whereas abstract thinking generally starts during this age period, preadolescents are still developing their advanced reasoning skills and are not able to make all intellectual leaps, such as making guesses about another person's intentions. They are beginning to think beyond their own experiences and hypothesize about how another person might feel in various situations, consider moral reasoning that does not fit in right-wrong perspectives, and recognize cause and effect series of events (NIMH, 2011). During these years, preadolescents also begin to develop their own moral compass and verbally express their feelings (CDC, 2016).

CPRT Enhances the Parent–Preadolescent Relationship

As is true of CPRT with young children, the primary focus of CPRT for preadolescents is enhancing and strengthening the parent–preadolescent relationship by equipping parents with basic

Child-Centered Play Therapy skills that have been proven to be necessary and effective dimensions in facilitating the development of positive parent-child relationships. CPRT is based on the rationale that the relationship between parent and child is the essential and curative therapeutic dimension for improving and correcting children's problems and preventing the development of future problems (Landreth & Bratton, 2019). Research indicates that having open communication between parents and preadolescents based on respect, acceptance, and empathy serves as a protective factor to reduce risk-taking behaviors (Coatsworth, Duncan, Greenberg, & Nix, 2010). Additionally, research by Qu, Fuligni, Galvan, and Telzer (2015) found that the quality of the parent-child relationship during the adolescent years serves as a mediating factor in the development of the ventral striatum, a part of the brain that serves to control one's sense of reward. The results of this research indicated that "adolescents who reported decreases in their positive parent-child relationships . . . showed longitudinal increases in ventral striatum activation over time, which were associated with increases in . . . risk-taking behavior" (p. 32). These findings highlight the importance of parent-child attachment for preadolescents' healthy development and support interventions such as CPRT that focus on strengthening the parent-child relationship.

Because preadolescents experience emotional swings and moodiness, parents might be inclined to become strict and demanding, or disengaged and allow their growing children to have a tremendous amount of freedom (Mbua & Adigeb, 2015). Not surprisingly, parents commonly report being most concerned about their parenting abilities when their child entered preadolescence and felt at a loss as to how to properly communicate with them (Baril et al., 2007). CPRT leaders help parents understand the developmental needs of their children as a way to normalize behavior and to help parents find more appropriate ways of responding to their children (Landreth & Bratton, 2019).

CPRT is an intervention that helps parents and preadolescents remain emotionally close as they navigate the new independence that is part of this developmental phase. The skills taught in CPRT help parents empathize with their preadolescents and strengthen their communication skills. According to Coatsworth et al. (2010), it is important for parents to demonstrate the ability to self-regulate and provide a relationship where preadolescents feel accepted, supported, and emotionally connected with their parents. These are the attitudes CPRT teaches through the four messages: I am here, I hear you, I see you, and I care (Landreth & Bratton, 2019). Additionally, in CPRT, parents learn reflective responding skills that enhance communication as parents learn to listen more attentively with empathy and understanding rather than with judgment. Although abstract thinking skills are developing during the preadolescent years, preadolescents often revert back to concrete thought (NIMH, 2011). CPRT provides parents with the skills needed to communicate in a developmentally appropriate manner. Using play, craft projects, and other activities during designated parent/preadolescent special times together allows preadolescents to move back and forth between verbal and nonverbal communication while providing opportunities for parents to actively respond.

It is recommended that parents of preadolescents communicate their expectations and show an understanding for the changes the child is experiencing (CDC, 2016). Negotiating a balance in which the preadolescent and the parent feel heard and validated facilitates a relationship wherein both parties compromise. This mutually satisfying experience is a central dimension of the CPRT preadolescent model. The CPRT limit-setting and choice-giving skills (Landreth & Bratton, 2019) facilitate preadolescents' engagement in decision making, a pivotal skill to practice during this developmental phase as preadolescents are becoming more independent, learning to take more responsibility, and accepting the consequences of their own decisions. These skills can also diminish the power struggle that many parents of preadolescents may experience.

The special times and the emphasis on creating family rituals within CPRT are designed to help parents and preadolescents share moments that strengthen the parent-child attachment. A supportive parent-child relationship acts as a buffer to a child's low self-esteem during this developmental phase (Ackard, Neumark-Sztainer, Story, & Perry, 2006). Children with higher self-esteem are more likely to make safe and positive decisions throughout preadolescence (Chowdhury & Pancha, 2011). According to Hemphill and Littlefield (2006), treatment outcomes are more successful when parents believe they have the skills necessary to handle their children's behaviors. Although the underlying philosophical principles of CPRT apply equally to relationships between preadolescents and their parents as they do to parents of small children, several modifications must be made to ensure the training is developmentally responsive.

Modifications for CPRT

Special Times

Because the word play can sound too childish for preadolescents, it is preferable to change the name *special playtime* to *special time*, which conveys to preadolescents that parents understand they are not children anymore. Similarly, instead of using toys during special times, parents can use more age-appropriate materials and activities such as crafts, cooking, baking, outdoor activities such as fishing or hiking, and games that allow for interaction to occur (e.g., puzzles, playing cards). Since it is important for preadolescents to develop their independence and have a role in decision making, preadolescents can be involved in deciding the weekly activities they want to engage in with their parents. As in CPRT with young children, the parent follows the preadolescent's lead. Parents can help guide the decision making by providing choices of activities that promote interactions. CPRT leaders should ensure parents are not limiting the choices of activities to expected gender roles, so preadolescents can feel free to choose an activity that is of personal interest (Meany-Walen et al., 2014). It is appropriate to let preadolescents change the activities from week to week, as developmentally, preadolescents may go back and forth between play and other activities they consider more age suitable. It is also appropriate for time in the special time to vary depending on the activity. Typically, the special times range from 45 to 90 minutes. Because the activities change weekly and at times take place outdoors, parents are not expected to video-record their special times every week. CPRT leaders can encourage parents to conduct a couple of indoor special times that can be easily recorded for supervision purposes. Following is an example of how a CPRT leader can help a parent choose appropriate activities while encouraging the preadolescent to be a part of the process. This example also exemplifies the incorporation of skills during the special times:

> Maya, who is 11 years old, had recently moved in with her grandparents. Her grandmother, Jewel, took the CPRT class. Following Session 2, Jewel reported that Maya said she was not as interested in "toys" and "playing" anymore. The CPRT leaders explored with Jewel

> special activities that she could do with Maya to build the relationship: sew a pillow, bake a cake, or build a bird house for the garden. Maya was very excited about these options and chose to sew a pillow for her new bedroom. Jewel took Maya to the store to select the fabric and pattern and reflected her feelings of excitement during this process, such as "*You're excited about decorating your new room*," and encouraged decision making with statements like "*You chose the fabric that you want for your new room.*" Jewel also used self-esteem-building statements during the pillow making process such as, "*You figured out how to trace the pattern onto the fabric for your pillow*" and used encouragement when Maya asked if she liked the fabric, "*What is important is that you like the fabric you chose and your room is going to be just like you want it.*"

A parent who participated in a CPRT preadolescent group stated that the special times helped her open communication again with her 13-year-old daughter. Following the first special time, this mother said, "It had been a long time since I was able to have a meaningful interaction with my daughter. The special time helped me feel connected to her again." This comment demonstrates how the special times can strengthen the parent-child relationship.

Appropriate Homework Assignments for Parents

The homework assignments found in the CPRT Treatment Manual, 2nd Edition are designed to enhance the parent-child relationship (Bratton & Landreth, 2019). For example, the Sandwich Hug, writing a positive note to the child, or bringing parents' favorite picture of their child of focus to the group are examples of homework assignments designed to help parents reconnect emotionally with their children. CPRT leaders can replace these homework assignments with ones that are developmentally appropriate for preadolescents. Following is an example of how a parent adapted writing a positive note to his preadolescent:

> Rafael, 12 years old, is really worried about a math test that he has at school today. Instead of sending him a

note of encouragement to school in his lunch bag, Paulo (Rafael's father) sent him a quick text message on his phone that stated, "*You are working so hard at school, thinking about you today as you take your math test.*"

Skills

Reflective skills can be used in the same way they are used for play sessions to convey the "**Be-With**" Attitudes (Landreth & Bratton, 2019). Due to the developmental differences between younger children and preadolescents, parents are cautioned not to use tracking as frequently (Meany-Walen et al., 2014). Preadolescents are particularly self-conscious and feel as if everyone is watching them, thus, tracking too much can intensify this perception and make them feel uncomfortable.

Cognitively, preadolescents are able to engage in higher levels of abstract thinking than younger children. Similarly, a major part of their social development is to advance towards independence from parents (CDC, 2016), which calls for their ability to make choices and own the consequences of their decisions. Thus, the last step of ACT limit setting can be modified to allow preadolescents to be part of the problem-solving process. Instead of parents targeting an acceptable alternative, they can invite preadolescents to **Explore** alternatives (in place of Target alternatives in the A-C-T model) and collaboratively decide on possible alternatives to the undesirable behavior. Following is an example:

Samantha, 10 years old, is having a conflict with her mother about wanting a snack before dinner. Claire, mother, may utilize an adapted version of limit setting regarding this conflict:

A: Samantha, I know you are hungry right now and would like to have a candy bar,
B: but candy bars are not for eating before dinner.
C: Let's look in the kitchen and see if we can find a healthy snack for you to eat now.

According to Landreth (2012), choice giving provides children the opportunity to practice problem-solving and decision-making skills and helps to decrease power struggles in the parent-child dyad. Since two developmental tasks during preadolescence are to learn to problem solve and make independent decisions (Sprenger, 2008), choice giving provides an opportunity for parents to facilitate optimal development of these skills. According to Nyarko (2012), preadolescents whose parents facilitate opportunities for them to engage in discussions regarding alternative behaviors have a more positive self-concept. Central to parents' success when using choice giving is to have alternatives that are age-appropriate (Landreth, 2012). Thus, CPRT leaders can help parents of preadolescents to brainstorm developmentally appropriate choices. Following is an example of how this can be done:

> "*James, I understand that you are disappointed that I can't drive you to the movies tonight. You can choose to rent a movie and invite some friends over or maybe we can think together of some people who could pick you up tonight and drive you to the movie theater.*" Parents of preadolescents who have participated in CPRT groups have commented on how helpful choice giving is to decrease power struggles at this age. For example, a parent in a CPRT group stated, "*Since I have been using choice giving I am not engaging in as many fights with my son (14 years old).*"

In CPRT, parents are taught to use encouragement to facilitate children's self-esteem and self-motivation (Landreth & Bratton, 2019). Because preadolescents are working through developing their self-concept as separate from their families (Kretschmer et al., 2014), the use of encouragement facilitates for preadolescents successful completion of these tasks. CPRT leaders help parents brainstorm opportunities where encouragement can be used in an age-appropriate way. Examples can include the use of encouragement with academic-related tasks, sports or extra-curricular activities, and social tasks such as making friends. For example, "*Madison, you were really running fast on the soccer field tonight. I noticed that you keep working hard on your foot work with the soccer ball.*"

Returning responsibility helps children develop a sense of competence and facilitates development and their independence in an age-appropriate way (Landreth, 2012). This is particularly important during preadolescence, as having a positive self-concept is associated with preadolescents' positive developmental outcomes and less engagement in risk-taking behaviors (Chowdhury & Pancha, 2011). CPRT leaders can help parents of preadolescents identify new tasks that preadolescents can be responsible for in their daily lives as they get older. For example, at this developmental age, preadolescents can take charge of more household tasks and be responsible for their daily schedule (e.g., initiating homework time). The following case exemplifies how a parent can return responsibility to her preadolescent: Carly asks her mom to choose a new bedspread for her. Carly's mom can respond, "*You can decide what kind of bedspread you want. We can go look online to get some ideas.*"

CPRT Research with Preadolescents

Although no research has been conducted to investigate the effectiveness of CPRT with parents of preadolescents, several CPRT research studies have included children ages 9 and 10. These studies have found that CPRT has had a positive impact on children's behavioral problems and on parental empathy (Carnes-Holt & Bratton, 2014; Topham, Wampler, Titus, & Rolling, 2011; Yuen, Landreth, & Baggerly, 2002). Similar results are reported in CPRT studies conducted with minority populations, such as Native Americans (Glover & Landreth, 2000), Germans (Grskovic & Goetze, 2008), Koreans (Lee & Landreth, 2003), and Israelis (Kidron & Landreth, 2010), that have included children 10–12 years old as participants. Because the focus on these studies was on the effects of CPRT with younger children, the average age for children participants was 5, and the authors did not address if any type of adaptations were made to accommodate parents of preadolescents in their groups. The review of literature corroborates the need for future quantitative research to investigate the effects of the proposed CPRT adaptations on preadolescents and their parents. Similarly, qualitative research is needed to better understand how the proposed adaptations meet the needs of this population.

Conclusion

The physical, cognitive, and social-emotional developmental changes that occur during preadolescence can negatively affect the parent-child relationship. Research findings have shown that this trend can be altered by improving the quality of parent-child relationships during preadolescence. Positive parent-preadolescent relationship has been associated with fewer problem behaviors (Klahr, Rueter, McGue, Iacono, & Burt, 2011) and better academic outcomes (Ackard et al. 2006). In response, experts in the field have called for parent training that focuses on strengthening the parent-child attachment during the preadolescent years (Coatsworth et al., 2010; Hemphill & Littlefield, 2006). CPRT is a viable intervention that can help parents of preadolescents develop and maintain a strong relationship with them, while helping parents gain the skills that can promote positive developmental outcomes for preadolescents. The modifications presented in this chapter serve to help CPRT leaders provide the training in a developmentally appropriate manner to parents of preadolescents.

References

Ackard, D. M., Neumark-Sztainer, D., Story, M., & Perry, C. (2006). Parent-child connectedness and behavioral and emotional health among adolescents. *American Journal of Preventive Medicine, 30*(1), 59–66. Retrieved from http://dx.doi.org/10.1016/j.amepre.2005.09.013

Baril, M. E., Cromer, A. C., & McHale, S. M. (2007). Process linking adolescent well-being, marital love, and coparenting. *Journal of Family Psychology, 21*, 645–654.

Bratton, S. C., & Landreth, G. L. (2019). *Child-Parent Relationship Therapy (CPRT) treatment manual: An Evidence-Based 10-session filial therapy model* (2nd ed). New York, NY: Routledge.

Bulanda, R. E., & Majumdar, D. (2008). Perceived parent-child relations and adolescent self-esteem. *Journal of Child and Family Studies, 18*, 203–212.

Carnes-Holt, K., & Bratton, S. C. (2014). The efficacy of child parent relationship therapy for adopted children with attachment disruptions. *Journal of Counseling and Development, 92*(3), 328–337.

Center for Disease Control. (2016). *Child development: Middle childhood (9–11 years of age)*. Retrieved from www.cdc.gov/ncbddd/childdevelopment/positiveparenting/middle2.html

Chowdhury, U., & Pancha, A. (2011). Posttraumatic stress disorder in children and adolescents. *Community Practitioner, 84*(12), 33–35.

Coatsworth, J. D., Duncan, L. O., Greenberg, M. T., & Nix, R. L. (2010). Changing parent's mindfulness, child management skills and relationship quality with their youth: Results *from* a randomized pilot intervention trial. *Journal of Child and Family Studies, 19*, 203–217. Retrieved from http://dx.doi.org/10.1007/s10826-009-9304·8

Elkind, D. (1980). Child development and counseling. *Personnel and Guidance Journal, 58*, 353–355. Retrieved from http://dx.doi.org/10.1002/j.2164

Glover, G. J., & Landreth, G. L. (2000). Filial therapy with Native Americans on the Flathead Reservation. *International Journal of Play Therapy, 9*(2), 57–80.

Grskovic, J., & Goetze, H. (2008). Short-term filial therapy with German mothers: Findings from a controlled study. *International Journal of Play Therapy, 17*(1), 39–51

Hemphill, S. A., & Littlefield, L. (2006). Child and family predictors of therapy outcome for children with behavioral and emotional problems. *Child Psychiatry and Human Development, 36*, 329–349. Retrieved from http://dx.doi.org/10.1007/s10578-005-0006-1

Kidron, M., & Landreth, G. (2010). Intensive child parent relationship therapy with Israeli parents in Israel. *International Journal of Play Therapy, 19*(2), 64–78.

Klahr, A. M., Rueter, M. A., McGue, M., Iacono, W. G., & Burt, S. A. (2011). The relationship between parent-child conflict and adolescent antisocial behavior: Confirming shared environmental mediation. *Journal of Abnormal Child Psychology, 39*, 683–694.

Kretschmer, T., Sentse, M., Kornelis Dijkstra, J., & Veenstra, R. (2014). The interplay between peer rejection and acceptance in preadolescence and early adolescence, serotonin transporter gene, and antisocial behavior in late adolescence: The TRIALS study. *Merrill-Palmer Quarterly, 60*, 193–216.

Landreth, O. (2012). *Play therapy: The art of the relationship* (3rd ed). New York, NY: Routledge.

Landreth, G., & Bratton, S. (2019). *Child-Parent Relationship Therapy (CPRT): An Evidence-Based 10-session filial therapy model* (2nd ed). New York, NY: Routledge.

Lederman, R. P., & Mian, T. S. (2003). The Parent-Adolescent Relationship Education (PARE) program: A curriculum for prevention of STDs and pregnancy in middle school youth. *Behavioral Medicine, 29*, 33–41. Retrieved from http://dx.doi.org/10.1080/08964280309596173

Lee, M., & Landreth, G. L. (2003). Filial therapy with immigrant Korean parents in the United States. *International Journal of Play Therapy, 12*(2), 67–85.

Maslow, A. H. (1962). *Towards a psychology of being*. Princeton: D. Van Nostrand Company.

Mbua, A. P., & Adigeb, A. P. (2015). Parenting styles and adolescents' behaviour in central educational zone of cross river state. *European Scientific Journal, 11*(22), 354–368.

Meany-Walen, K. K., Carnes Holt, K., Ceballos, P., & Michero, E. (2014). Child-Parent relationship training: A model for preadolescents. *British Journal of Play Therapy, 10*, 6–19.

National Institute of Mental Health. (2011). *The teen brain still under construction*. Retrieved from www.nimh.nih.gov/health/publications/the-teen-brain-still-under-construction/teen-brain_141903.pdf

Nyarko, K. (2012). The influence of peer and parent relationships on adolescents' self-esteem. *IFE Psychologia: An International Journal, 20*, 161–167.

Papalia, D. E., Olds, S. W., & Feldman, R. D. (2007). *Human development* (10th ed). New York, NY: McGraw-Hill.

Piaget, J. (1969). *The mechanisms of perception*. New York, NY: Basic Books.

Qu, Y., Fuligni, A. J., Galvan, A., & Telzer, E. H. (2015). Buffering effects of positive parent-child relationships on adolescent risk taking: A longitudinal neuroimaging investigation. *Development Cognitive Neuroscience, 15*, 26–34.

Schwartz, K. D. (2008). Adolescent brain development: An oxymoron no longer. *Journal of Youth Ministry, 6*(2), 85–93.

Sprenger, M. (2008). *The developing brain: Birth to age eight*. Thousand Oaks, CA: Corwin Press. http://dx.doi.org/10.4135/9781483329758

Topham, G. L., Wampler, K. S., Titus, G., & Rolling, E. (2011). Predicting parent and child outcomes of a filial therapy program. *International Journal of Play Therapy, 20*(2), 79–93.

Vernon, A. (2009). *Counseling children and adolescents* (4th ed). Denver, CO: Lave.

Yuen, T., Landreth, G., & Baggerly, J. (2002). Filial therapy with immigrant Chinese families. *International Journal of Play Therapy, 11*(2), 63–90.

CHAPTER 20

ADAPTING CPRT FOR ADOPTIVE FAMILIES

Kara Carnes-Holt and Kristie K. Opiola

Child-Parent Relationship Therapy for Adoptive Families

Each year approximately 136,000 children are adopted, adding to the 2 million adopted children in the United States (Kreider & Lofquist, 2014), with 59% adopted from the foster care system and 26% adopted from other countries (The Child Welfare Gateway Center, 2012). Potential maladjustment risks related to adoptions are present. Long waits for placements, inconsistent caregivers, and associated adverse experiences increase adopted children's risk of interpersonal trauma and insecure attachment (CCAI, 2011; Perry & Szalavitz, 2006). Such problems can be particularly challenging for adopting parents, who were not expecting intense emotional and behavioral struggles. Abuse, neglect, and deprivation have damaging effects on children, and the earlier children experience physical or relational harm, the greater the impact on their overall development (Perry & Szalavitz, 2006; Purvis, Cross, & Sunshine, 2007).

Facilitators of Child-Parent Relationship Therapy (CPRT) for adoptive families are recommended to have training and supervision in the traditional CPRT approach before utilizing and adapting the model for adoptive parents. Furthermore, CPRT therapists need knowledge and expertise in the needs and unique challenges of working with adopted children and their families. Adoption authorities encourage mental health providers to seek specialized training for working with adopted and malattached children and emphasize that parents should play a key role in the therapeutic process (Brodzinsky, 2013; Perry & Szalavitz, 2006).

Adopted Children

Children who have experienced frequent changes in caregivers, recurring neglect, and abuse can experience difficulty feeling safe in relationships with others (Forbes & Post, 2006; Purvis et al., 2007). **Adoption, regardless of age, is a traumatic event due to the break in attachment from the primary caregivers.** Children who experience trauma early in life, such as adoption, tend to be reactive and fearful (von der Kolk, 2005) and behave in self-defeating ways in order to protect themselves (West, 1992). For adoptees with insecure attachments, finding safety in the parent-child relationship is challenging, as they desire closeness with their parent but feel threatened by their parents' attempts to comfort and soothe them during times of distress. In addition, adopted children may be hesitant to play (Gil, 2006), because they are tentative and reactive due to their stress responses being activated as they continually search for a way to achieve a felt sense of safety. This emotional searching is commonly manifested in hypervigilance (Perry, 1994). Adopted children tend to experience increased fear, sensory processing issues, difficulty self-regulating, and disorder of memory (Forbes & Post, 2006; Purvis et al., 2007). The child's resulting unpredictable and perplexing behaviors make forming relationships difficult for adoptive parents (Perry & Szalavitz, 2006; Purvis et al., 2007).

Adoptive Parents

Adoptive parents are faced with the challenge of developing a relationship with their adopted child that helps the child discover that relationships can be safe and trusting. Adoptive parents are given the role of mitigating the impact of their children's early relationship experiences; supporting them through recovery, grief, and loss; and facilitating the development of their children's adoptive identities (Brodzinsky, 2013). Providing love, support, and guidance to adopted children throughout their lifetime requires a compassionate environment where adopted children can heal and develop (Hughes, 2006; Perry & Szalavitz, 2006). The journey to healing can be tumultuous due to their children's early trauma. **Children with a history of interpersonal trauma, including disruptions in their attachment relationships, tend to misread and misattune to the cues from their caregivers.** Poor interaction patterns such as hugging the parent one moment followed immediately by aggression, increased parental stress, and parents' own relationship patterns, often connected to early childhood experiences (Purvis et al., 2007), can impact their ability to emotionally respond and attune to their adoptive child (Brodzinsky, 2013).

Rationale for CPRT with Adoptive Families

Children with early relationship trauma struggle in their effort to attune and connect with their caregivers, thus adoptive parents often require attachment- and adoption-specific services to help them form a secure attachment with their adoptee (Purvis, Cross, & Pennings, 2009). According to Barth et al. (2005, p. 264), "It is the parent-child relationship that is the central reason that adoptive parents come to therapy". They encouraged mental health services that focus on attachment-based treatment modalities that are non-coercive and responsive in nature. **The foundational philosophy of CPRT is that the relationship is the vehicle for change, which addresses the core of attachment concerns that many adoptive families experience.** The focus of CPRT is on developing a relationship that provides trust, safety, and understanding to promote healthy, secure parent-child attachments. The four healing messages of I am here, I hear you, I understand, and I care taught in CPRT support the core needs of adoptive families.

Play allows children to communicate their understanding of their world and express their experiences, needs, and feelings through toys, activities, and materials. Play is their natural means of communication and felt safety. For example, adopted children often use the language of play to communicate their own adoption story. Parents of adoptive children frequently share that their empathic understanding of their adoptive child's experience greatly increased as they began to understand how their child utilized play to communicate perceptions, memories, and experience.

CPRT provides adoptive parents the opportunity to learn and implement skills and ways to positively relate and respond to their child that are developmentally responsive and helps parents attune to their adopted child. The focus of CPRT is on training parents in basic Child-Centered Play Therapy (CCPT) skills of reflective listening, recognizing, and responding to children's feelings, therapeutic limit setting, building children's self-esteem, facilitating decision making, and creating an opportunity for children to experience healthy internal control. These skills facilitate and support healing moments for attachment-challenged children and are necessary for building positive parent-child relationships. By helping parents take on a therapeutic role or be an agent of change, **CPRT helps parents learn to understand their adopted child's underlying needs, respond more empathically and effectively to their adopted child's behavioral and emotional difficulties, and facilitate their adopted child's ability to self-regulate.** CPRT is based on the belief that this type of relationship between parent and child promotes a secure attachment and is fundamental for children's healthy development and overall well-being.

Empirical Support

Two studies examined the effectiveness of CPRT with adopted children (Carnes-Holt & Bratton, 2014; Opiola & Bratton, 2018). Carnes-Holt and Bratton (2014) found that adoptive parents who participated in a 10-week CPRT training group reported statistically significant decreases in their children's externalizing and total problems, and that parents demonstrated statistically significant gains in their empathic interactions with their adopted children when compared to the waitlist control group. Carnes-Holt and Bratton concluded that CPRT was responsive to the mental health needs of adoptive families and emphasized the need for replication studies using active control and comparison groups to increase confidence in CPRT's treatment effects.

Opiola and Bratton (2018) investigated the effects of CPRT with adoptive families who reported attachment-related concerns, such as difficulties establishing a mutually satisfying parent-child relationship as well as concerns about the adoptive child's behavior and parental stress. In addition, Opiola and Bratton addressed the need for increased methodological rigor of the Carnes-Holt and Bratton study by adding a "treatment as usual" (TAU) group for comparison. TAU was based on local adoption agency practices, consisting of individual parent phone consultation and focusing on crisis management and behavior modification strategies. Opiola and Bratton found that parents who participated in CPRT, compared to the TAU parents, reported statistically significant improvement in child behavior problems, parent-child relationship stress, and parental empathy, with large treatment effects on all measures.

The combination of the Carnes-Holt and Bratton (2014) and the Opiola and Bratton study provide strong support for CPRT as a responsive intervention for adoptive parents and their children. A recent report issued by the Donaldson Adoption Institute evaluated the empirical support for adoption-related interventions and recognized the Carnes-Holt and Bratton (2014) study in its conclusion that among parent-child interventions, CPRT demonstrated the strongest empirical support for helping adopted children and their parents (Brodzinsky, 2013).

Therapeutic Needs of Adoptive Families

Relationship Stress

Adoptive parents are often stressed by their child's reactive responses, as they are unaware of what triggered the child's behavior. When parents feel discouraged and overwhelmed in their attempts to parent their adopted child, they blame themselves, feel out of control, or doubt their ability to respond and parent effectively. During weekly CPRT group sessions, therapists offer parents alternative perspectives of children's behaviors that highlight the child's best attempts to get his or her needs met. As a result, parents become more accepting of their children and develop a new perception of their children as having possibilities instead of as a problem, thereby positively impacting the parent-child relationship and decreasing relationship stress.

Behavior Problems

Adopted children who experience relationship trauma exhibit signs of developmental delays. Purvis et al. (2007) estimate that adopted children may be delayed at a rate of half their chronological age due to neglect, abuse, and isolation, as well as present with inconsistencies in their displayed behaviors. **Adoption experts propose that adopted children can catch up emotionally, behaviorally, and developmentally when they are in relationships with emotionally attuned and responsive adults** (Brodzinsky, 2013; Purvis et al., 2007; Siegel & Hartzell, 2003; Zilberstein, 2013). **CPRT therapists help parents see past their children's behaviors and identify the underlying cause of their problematic behaviors.**

CPRT therapists help parents focus on the primacy of the parent-child relationship and view themselves as the agent of change in their child's life. Early life experiences for adopted children, especially foster care and international children, are often chaotic, deprived, inconsistent, and/or unpredictable. Such a tumultuous start leaves the adopted child feeling anxious and uncertain when they need to depend on their caregivers (Bowlby, 1980). Adopted children have a strong desire to control their environment for protection, as they cannot trust adults (Hughes, 1999). CPRT therapists teach parents the basic principles, attitudes, and skills of CCPT, in order to foster a more attuned, unconditionally accepting, and consistent relationship with their children (Landreth & Bratton, 2019). Therapists help parents to understand that when adopted children experience this type of safe and secure relationship consistently over time, they begin to feel understood and accepted, experience themselves as lovable and capable, and experience others as safe, dependable, and trustworthy. As a result, children are then free to give up self-defeating behaviors that, for many adopted children, may have been used as a means of self-protection, and choose more self-enhancing and functional behavior (Bratton, Carnes-Holt, & Ceballos, 2011).

It is imperative CPRT therapists understand the social-emotional and behavioral needs of children who experience early trauma in order to help adoptive parents provide a relationship that promotes secure attachment and healing (Perry & Szalavitz, 2006; Purvis et al., 2007). CPRT therapists help parents to observe and respond to their adopted children with empathy and understanding by tuning into the adopted children's underlying needs, often rooted in early experiences.

Attachment and Relational Trauma

Attachment is an important and well-recognized tenet to emotional and social development and is an important construct in CPRT. CPRT therapists need a good understanding of attachment principles and behavioral characteristics of different attachment styles in children and adults. An understanding of these behavioral characteristics helps CPRT therapists understand parent-child relationship challenges and stress. In addition, an understanding of attachment dynamics assists therapists in helping parent's view the children's behaviors as survival skills and as means to create a sense of personal safety and control.

CPRT therapists understanding of attachment and attachment-related characteristics is important in facilitating responsive and attuned verbal communication between parent and child. Typical developmental responses may be inappropriate for an adopted child and lead to further relational breaks. For instance, traditional approaches to discipline often do not work because adopted children feel threatened and fearful (Bowlby, 1980; Cozolino, 2006). Adopted children often have a high need for control, and typical approaches to discipline focus on parents being in control, causing an adopted child to employ a variety of strategies to regain control (Purvis et al., 2007). Instead, **CPRT therapists help parents utilize choice giving. Choices offer children a sense of power in a controlled environment.** Therapists and parents should problem solve in the group a variety of acceptable choices for common behavioral challenges to help parents avoid intense emotional interactions with their children. Adopted parents should also be guided in using choices as consequences sparingly and spend more time focusing on empowering choices for adopted children.

The A-C-T model of therapeutic limit setting (see CPRT Session 4 in the CPRT Treatment Manual, 2nd Edition) can offer alternative discipline models. For adoptive families, it is important that parents acknowledge their children's feelings, wants, and desires by displaying high levels of empathic understanding and acceptance. This is important to help deactivate the child's reactive response. Children who feel heard and understood are more likely to hear the limits parents set and follow through with alternative approaches to getting their needs met. Parents need to be patient and consistent when setting limits with adopted children due to the children's unpredictable early experiences. Adopted children can waver in their level of trust with their parents. Adopted children also have poor self-regulation skills and may repeat the same behavior frequently. Parents who display patience and consistency will help adopted children feel safe, learn, and try out new behaviors.

Another important aspect of facilitating healing of adopted children's insecure attachments is CPRT's focus on helping parents gain awareness of their parenting approaches and emotional reactions to their children. CPRT therapists help parents explore their experiences and feelings associated with their children in weekly meetings. Check-ins, open discussion, normalizing experiences, and weekly supervision of special playtimes allow parents to receive feedback from the CPRT therapists and other parents in the group. A lack of self-awareness on the part of the parents can lead to misunderstandings of adopted children, intense reactions to their children, and the inability to differentiate their needs from their children's needs. Parents' increased self-awareness and ability to differentiate their own emotional response from their child's emotional state enables them to respond to their child with greater empathy, understanding, and acceptance. Parents with good self-regulation skills and self-understanding are more able to remain calm, attentive, and attuned when their child is in a reactive state and provide comfort and support them (Perry & Szalavitz, 2006). Self-awareness and self-understanding are also important because relationships are reciprocal and without awareness, reactive interactions can contribute to stress in the relationship.

Adoption, regardless of age, is a traumatic event due to the break in attachment from the primary caregivers. Attachment and trauma are often integrative factors, particularly in the lives of adopted children. Repeated traumatic events, such as any form of abuse, as well as losses associated with the primary caregivers, significantly disrupt the attachment process. CPRT therapists must have understanding of the interrelationship between trauma and attachment in order to help parents identify and understand their adopted children's underlying needs and behaviors.

Parental Efficacy

Adoptive parents who have participated in CPRT report initially feeling discouraged and challenged in their attempts to connect with and understand their child, causing significant stress in their relationship with their adoptee. Confusion, frustration, and heartache become part of the adoptive parents' daily lives when it appears that their child struggles to connect and displays behaviors that reject or sabotage the relationship (Ginsberg, 1989; Ryan, 2007). CPRT therapists focus on improving parents' confidence and parental locus of control by building parents' relational response skills and helping the parents see more than just their children's behaviors. Parents are taught Child-Centered Play Therapy skills to empower parents to focus on their child's capabilities instead of controlling their child's behavior. CPRT therapists offer adoptive parents alternative perspectives of children's behaviors, one that focuses on the child's best attempts to get his or her needs met. As a result, adoptive parents begin to experience and see their children from a new lens, one of possibilities and acceptance instead of a problem. An adopted parent stated after completing CPRT, "This is not just 10 weeks, this is a lifestyle. I'm a better mom and my spouse is a better dad. I'm so completely grateful. When I screw up I no longer wallow in it. I pick myself up and get back on track." CPRT focuses on encouraging parents and trusting in the parents' ability to utilize new skills to positively impact their child's development.

Adoptive parents can feel isolated, misunderstood, and discounted by others, including family members and parents of biological children, as their adopted children's behaviors may be unique and different from biological children's reactions to similar incidents. Other parents, friends, and family members offer advice that often does not work or lacks understanding of the parent-child relationship struggles. CPRT therapists respond to adoptive parents with empathy, acceptance, and genuineness, and these dimensions help parents feel understood and supported. In the weekly meetings, parents are encouraged to share their feelings and explore experiences they have had with their child. To lessen their feelings of isolation, CPRT therapists help foster a community of support by linking parents' stories, normalizing their struggles, and generalizing their concerns and fears. Parents who are with other parents with similar experiences feel less alone and are validated that their parenting struggles are normal.

CPRT therapists should take time to reflect and explore parents' perceptions and understanding of their children's behaviors. The group's consideration of a variety of reasons adopted children have responded the way they did empowers parents and highlights them as experts on their children's lives. Building parents' confidence helps improve their locus of control and trust in their ability to positively impact their child. In addition to building parents' self-confidence, CPRT therapists focus on parents' observational skills and aid parents' awareness and understanding of their children's behaviors as well as their own.

The process of watching recorded play sessions provides parents an opportunity to see their children and themselves from a new perspective. Viewing their videos also helps parents recognize small, subtle behaviors and interactions that they may have missed in the session. Parents are often not aware of their common behavior patterns, such as the reciprocal cycle of parents being guarded and hypervigilant in the presence of their child in hopes of warding off poor behaviors. Watching their video helps parents develop insight into themselves and offers an opportunity to reflect and process their own personal feelings and reactions as well as highlight their child's response to their behaviors. Throughout this process, CPRT therapists need to be supportive and gently urge parents to further explore their experiences. Only when parents are aware of their reactions and behaviors can they change and approach their child with greater empathy and responsiveness. An adopted mother in CPRT reported,

> I cannot tell you how much this training has meant, how much better I understand myself and my kids and just being accepting of where they are at. Also, this is about the only time I've seen (spouse) move from his views to being able to accept a different perspective on how to help our traumatized kids. We will continue the play sessions, as it's almost as important to my kids as oxygen.

Modifications of Child-Parent Relationship Therapy for Adoptive Families

It is important that CPRT therapists closely follow the Adapting CPRT for Adoptive Families chapter in the CPRT Treatment Manual,

2nd Edition for specific adaptations in content, handouts, and session outlines. There are also some general adjustments that need to be made to meet the unique needs of adoptive families. The original CPRT model is designed for 10 sessions; however, additional sessions are commonly needed with adoptive families. CPRT therapists recognize the hectic lives of adoptive families and work to balance this with CPRT expectations and protocol. The adoption process is commonly associated with intense emotions, struggles, and surprises.

Parents may need an additional session prior to the beginning of the 10-session training to have time to share their family's unique journey of adoption in a supportive and understanding environment. Extending the length of the sessions by 30 to 60 minutes may offer additional time for adoptive parents to share about their current daily struggles. In addition, follow-up sessions are encouraged. The difficult journey of establishing secure attachments in an adoptive family is time consuming, and follow-up sessions may have far-reaching benefits. Parents of adopted children can benefit from ongoing support, resources, and words of encouragement.

The CPRT Treatment Manual, 2nd Edition suggests CPRT therapists use their clinical judgment when deciding how material in each session should be adapted to fit the context of the group and unique needs of parents. For example, in Session 1, the therapist assigns parents the task of noticing one physical characteristic of the child they have not seen before. Therefore, an adaptation of assignments, such as this one, could focus on ways to help parents feel connected in the relationship between parent and child. For the example above, parents could be encouraged to find a physical characteristic or positive behavior that the adopted child has in common with the parents, such as the child and the parent laugh at the same jokes, or they both have a freckle on their right hand.

Due to adopted children's confusing behaviors and misattunement with their parents, CPRT therapists may need to help parents learn how to reflect feelings based on the children's underlying needs and desires rather than typical reflections of obvious behaviors and feelings. For example, a parent may respond with an empathic tone, "*You like being in charge.*" to their child in special playtimes as the child gives frequent directives to the parent. For many adoptive families, parents are unsure of the child's feelings because the child's behavior is confusing and often mismatches his or her current behavior. For example, a parent expressed concern when their adopted child hit the baby doll repeatedly while laughing and smiling. Therapists can highlight and focus on the underlying needs or desires of the adopted child's behaviors. Parents may gain a better understanding of the child's behavior and attune to the child during a period of emotional dysregulation. When parents are able to attune, they can accurately reflect to the child and increase the child's feelings of being understood and worthy.

The dos and don'ts of the play sessions (see Session 3 in the CPRT Treatment Manual, 2nd Edition) need additional discussion during parent training sessions. A discussion of the possible play of adoptive children that may take place during the special playtime needs to be added to Session 3. Children with a history of attachment disruptions and trauma can manifest intense play that may be disturbing and emotionally painful for the parent. For example, the first author of this chapter recalls an emotional session with her adopted child as she intensely used various animal families to play out her experiences of foster care and adoption.

The therapist should normalize the need for personal counseling to deal with unresolved issues regarding the parent's own emotional triggers and traumas. Deeper self-understanding provides parents with the inner resources to increase emotional availability when connecting to their children (Purvis et al., 2007; Siegel & Hartzell, 2003). It may be helpful to have a video demonstration or case example of play therapy with an adopted child to help parents prepare for the first play session.

The location of the first play session may need modification. In the traditional CPRT model, parents perform the first session at their homes. Adoptive parents may benefit from having play sessions directly supervised at the clinic for at least the first few sessions. Filial therapists should use their clinical judgment when offering this option to adoptive parents. This option should be strongly recommended for families in which the child is exhibiting severe behaviors. Direct supervision provides extra support and helps increase parental efficacy and confidence.

Processing of the play sessions is essential in the CPRT model. Additional time and focus that explores the potential intentions of the behaviors from the adopted child's perspective is needed. It is understandable that parents may be quick to judge or get frustrated with their child. With empathy and patience, CPRT therapists help process the parent's reactions and explore multiple ideas (underlying needs or desires) for the child's behavior. Offering parents alternative views of their child's behavior gives parents a greater window of acceptance and increases their problem-solving skills for the more difficult behaviors.

In the majority of sessions, it is suggested in the treatment manual that the therapist present the option to end the group with a motivational poem, story, or Rule of Thumb. Several suggestions are provided in the manual; however, the therapists may want to explore resources that are specifically applicable to adoptive parents. The addition of children's books specifically addressing adoption, ideas for family rituals, calming exercises for the parents, or simple encouraging mantras to repeat during the week could be integrated into the closing portion of the group. It is also helpful to provide parents with a list of book resources that parents can share with their children to focus on a variety of issues that families may face (adoption, foster care, grief and loss, etc.). It is important to suggest books that support the adopted child's culture and country of origin to support the child's self-identity. The CPRT for adoptive families chapter in the CPRT Treatment Manual, 2nd Edition (2019) provides a list of books and suggestions for therapists.

Choice giving is introduced in Session 6. During this session, the therapists should explore specific needs of each child. It may be necessary to recommend that some parents use only basic, positive, and empowering choice-giving skills for a while before progressing to choice giving as a method of discipline. It is essential that the therapist repeatedly reiterate that empathy and patience are the key factors in experiencing success with choice giving. It is common that children will initially make poor choices, exhibit increased opposition, or display angry outbursts. The use of choice giving provides parents empathy for the child's choices without rejecting the child and perpetuating the insecure attachment. In addition, the concept of close proximity instead of time-out as a choice should be discussed. The concept of choice giving, close proximity, and the developmental needs of the child should be woven into the discussion during several sessions.

Adopted children are challenged by daily transitions or major life transitions because of their poor ability to self-regulate when unpredictable events occur. Typically in CPRT, parents are taught to provide their child of focus with alerts before play sessions end.

Adopted children may need more alerts. For instance, children with less developed self-regulation skills may require multiple alerts, such as a 15-, 10-, 5-, and 1-minute alert before the session ends. Adoptive children may also need an advanced notice of when the special playtime will occur and alerts leading up to the sessions to alleviate fear and stress. Setting up a predictable environment helps children to be prepared and to trust their caregivers.

Structured doll play is highly recommended to help parents negotiate stressful and difficult moments for their adopted child. Structured doll play is a method of storytelling for parents to help children who feel anxious or insecure. This skill has numerous benefits for adoptive families, and CPRT therapists may want to introduce the technique earlier in the model. Adoptive parents may or may not have shared with their child that they are adopted or the story behind the creation of their family. Structured doll play can be one way of communicating the family's adoptive journey to the child. (See Companion Website section in the *CPRT Treatment Manual*, (2nd edition) for details about using Structured Doll Play to tell stories.)

> By telling stories about the child's life before he or she came to live with the adoptive family, stories about the family's life before he or she came to live with the adoptive family, and stories about how the parents decided to adopt the child and the process of adoption can build a shared history that will make claiming occur more smoothly.
>
> (Kottman, 1997, p. 348)

Trauma creates a fragmented and disordered memory (Forbes & Post, 2006). Using structured doll play to construct a coherent narrative for the child can have numerous healing benefits: enhanced communication between the parent and child, increased trust of the adopted parent, and increased sense of felt safety in the child's environment. During the group training times, therapists and parents could work together to develop the story and practice this new skill.

References

Barth, R., Crea, T., John, K., Thoburn, J., Quinton, D., & Daniels, F. (2005). Beyond attachment theory and therapy: Towards sensitive and evidenced-based interventions with foster and adoptive families in distress. *Child and Family Social Work, 10*, 257–258. doi:10.1111/j.1365-2206.2005.00380.x

Bowlby, J. (1980). *Attachment and loss*. New York, NY: Basic Books.

Bratton, S. C., Carnes-Holt, K., & Ceballos, P. L. (2011). An integrative humanistic approach to treating adopted children with a history of attachment disruptions. In A. A. Drewes, S. C. Bratton, & C. E. Schaefer (Eds.). *Integrative play therapy* (pp. 341–370). Hoboken, NJ: John Wiley and Sons.

Brodzinsky, D. M. (2013). A need to know: Enhancing adoption competence among mental health professionals. *Policy perspective*. New York, NY: Donaldson Adoption Institute.

Carnes-Holt, K., & Bratton, S. C. (2014). The efficacy of child parent relationship therapy for adopted children with attachment disruptions. *Journal of Counseling & Development, 92*, 328–337.

The Child Welfare Information Gateway Center. (2012). *Adoption disruption and dissolution*. Washington, DC: U.S. Department of Health and Human Services, Children's Bureau. Retrieved from http://www.childwelfare.gov/pubPDFs/s_disrup.pdf.

Cozolino, L. (2006). *The neuroscience of human relationships: Attachment and the developing social brain*. New York, NY: W. W. Norton & Company.

Congressional Coalition on Adoption Institute. (2011). *Facts and statistics*. Retrieved from www.ccainstitute.org/index.php?option=com_content&view=category&layout=blog&id=25&Itemid=43

Forbes, H., & Post, B. (2006). *Beyond consequences logic, and control: A love based approach to helping attachment-challenged children with severe behaviors*. Orlando, FL: Beyond Consequences Institute, LLC.

Gil, E. (2006). *Helping abused and traumatized children: Integrating directive and non-directive approaches*. New York, NY: Guilford Press.

Ginsberg, B. (1989). Training parents as therapeutic agents with foster/adoptive children using the filial approach. In C. E. Schaefer & J. M. Briesmeister (Eds.), *Handbook of parent training: Parents as co-therapists for children's behavior problems* (pp. 442–478). New York, NY: John Wiley & Sons.

Hughes, D. A. (1999). Adopted children with attachment problems. *Child Welfare, 78*(5), 541–561.

Hughes, D. A. (2006). *Building the bonds of attachment: Awakening love in deeply troubled children* (2nd ed). Lanham, MD: Rowman & Littlefield.

Kottman, T. (1997). Building a family: Play therapy with adopted children. In H. G. Kaduson, D. Cangelosi, & C. Schaefer (Eds.), *The playing cure: Individualized play therapy for specific childhood problems* (pp. 337–369). Northvale, NJ: Jason Aronson.

Kreider, R. M., & Lofquist, D. A. (2014). *Adopted children and stepchildren: 2010: Population characteristics*. Washington, DC: U.S. Census Bureau.

Landreth, G., & Bratton, S. (2019). *Child-Parent Relationship Therapy (CPRT): An Evidence-Based 10-session filial therapy model* (2nd ed). New York, NY: Routledge.

Opiola, K. K., & Bratton, S. C. (2018). The efficacy of child-parent relationship therapy for adopted families: A replication study. *Journal of Counseling and Development, 96*(2), 155–166.

Perry, B. D. (1994). Neurobiological sequelae of childhood trauma: Post-traumatic disorders in children. In M. Murburg (Ed.), *Catecholomine function in posttraumatic stress disorder: Emerging concepts* (pp. 253–276). Washington, DC: American Psychiatric Press.

Perry, B. D., & Szalavitz, M. (2006). *The boy who was raised as a dog: and other stories from a child psychiatrist's notebook*. Philadelphia, PA: Basic Books.

Purvis, K., Cross, D., & Pennings, J. (2009). Trust-based relational intervention: Interactive principles for adopted children with special social-emotional needs. *The Journal of Humanistic Counseling Education and Development, 48*(1), 3–22.

Purvis, K., Cross, D., &, Sunshine, L. (2007). *The connected child: Bring hope and healing to your adoptive family*. New York, NY: McGraw-Hill.

Ryan, V. (2007). Filial therapy: Helping children and new carers to form secure attachment relationships. *British Journal of Social Work, 37*(4), 643–657. doi:10.1093/bjsw/bch331

Siegel, D., & Hartzell, M. (2003). *Parenting from the inside-out: How a deeper self-understanding can help you raise children who thrive*. New York, NY: Jeremy P. Tarcher/Putnam.

von der Kolk, B. A. (2005). *Traumatic stress: The effects of overwhelming experience on mind, body, & society*. New York, NY: Guilford Press.

West, J. (1992). *Child centered play therapy* (2nd ed). Croydon, UK: Hodder Education.

Zilberstein, K. (2013). The use and limitations of attachment theory in child psychotherapy. *Psychotherapy*. doi:10.1037/a0030930

CHAPTER 21

ADAPTING CPRT FOR TEACHERS

Mary Morrison Bennett and Wendy Pretz Helker

In the Child-Teacher Relationship Training (CTRT) model, teachers are taught basic Child-Centered Play Therapy skills and relationship-building skills in order to help teachers meet the various emotional and behavioral needs of children ages Pre-K through early elementary school. CTRT is an adaptation of Child-Parent Relationship Therapy (CPRT; Landreth & Bratton, 2019). As in CPRT, "*Teachers* are trained to be therapeutic agents with their *students* through a format of didactic instruction, demonstration play sessions, required laboratory play sessions, and supervision in a supportive atmosphere. *Teachers* are taught basic child-centered play therapy principles and skills including reflective listening, recognizing, and responding to *student's* feelings, therapeutic limit setting, building *student's* self-esteem, and structuring required play sessions with their *students* using a special kit of selected toys." As in CPRT, "*Teachers* learn how to create a nonjudgmental, understanding, and accepting environment that enhances the *teacher-child* relationship thus facilitating personal growth and change for *student* and *teacher*" (Landreth & Bratton, 2019). The purpose of CTRT is to provide opportunities for teachers to gain a better understanding of children's feelings, experiences, and needs; increase teachers' awareness of ways to respond that build children's confidence and self-esteem; and facilitate the development of more positive emotional relationships with children. The CTRT model is also intended as a useful intervention for children experiencing mental health difficulties in early childhood. Initially teachers are trained to have a special playtime with an individual child in a designated playroom or play area. Later in the training, teachers learn to adapt CTRT skills for use with groups of children in the general classroom. Teachers participate in weekly supervision sessions with the CTRT therapist to learn and practice new skills, discuss challenges, ask questions, and gain support and encouragement throughout the training.

Rationale

The catalyst for the development of CTRT was the growing realization that a positive Child-Teacher relationship can have a multitude of benefits for both the young child and for the professional teacher. An increasing body of research indicates the Child-Teacher relationship is an important contributing factor in young children's successful academic, social, and emotional development (Howes et al., 2008). The National Association for the Education of Young Children (NAEYC, 2009) position statement on developmentally appropriate practice for early childhood programs proposes that positive, supportive relationships during the earliest years of life appear to be essential not only for cognitive development but also for healthy emotional development. According to the NAEYC (2009), one of the core values underlying all of NAEYC's work is helping children and adults achieve their full potential in the context of relationships based on trust, respect, and positive regard. These core relationship dimensions are central in CTRT training.

A positive Child-Teacher relationship can impact teachers as well as students. Teachers in positive relationships with children view themselves as competent and successful teachers, according to Guerney and Flumen (1970). Children's mental health needs and behavioral difficulties, and teachers' minimal exposure to skills and training designed to meet children's difficulties, may contribute to a challenging relationship between child and teacher. What is especially challenging to teachers is that the children who tend to cause teachers the most discontent may be the very students who most need a positive, high-quality relationship with the teacher.

When a child is exhibiting challenging behaviors in the classroom, it may be due to a mental health issue or need that is not being addressed. According to the most recent U.S. Surgeon General's report on the status of children's mental health (2000), "growing numbers of children are suffering needlessly, because their emotional, behavioral, and developmental needs are not being met" (p. 3). There are several contributing factors to this increasing problem: a shortage of mental health professionals specially trained to work with children; a lack of accessible services; and perhaps most salient, the need for early intervention specifically involving caregivers in the delivery of services. The President's New Freedom Commission on Mental Health (2003) reiterated the need for early intervention and emphasized a need for mental health services to be offered in accessible, low-stigma settings such as schools. CTRT addresses these issues by focusing on core relationship dimensions as seen in the following comments. **Teachers who participated in CTRT reported that as a result of CTRT, they "knew how to communicate better with their students, knew more helpful ways to respond to students, were better able to acknowledge students' feelings, felt better able to bond with their students, and understood their students better."** After learning the therapeutic skills included in CTRT, teachers also reported feeling more confident in how to work with challenging students. One CTRT participant's powerful comments highlight this idea:

> I believe all teachers should have access to this information. I believe this is especially important in demonstrating how teachers' relationships with their children are so impactful. The limit setting skills and phrases made a tremendous difference in my classroom. Therefore, I truly think I have become a more competent teacher.

Getting Started: Structuring Child-Teacher Relationship Training

CTRT Therapist Qualifications and Responsibilities

The first consideration when planning CTRT is to ensure the CTRT therapist has training and experience with the traditional CPRT model before leading a CTRT group. It is also recommended the CTRT therapist have experience in a school setting working with teachers and an understanding of the structure of a classroom and school culture. The CTRT therapist can be a school-based or outside mental health professional with advanced knowledge and skills in Child-Centered Play Therapy and the CPRT model. These dimensions are crucial since the CTRT therapist is responsible for training and supervising teachers in CTRT skills. This model is possible to execute with one mental health professional. However, if additional qualified professionals are available, dividing up the responsibilities of training, supervision, and general logistics would be helpful.

Planning

The first step in planning for CTRT is to gain administrative collaboration. Presenting administrators with the research supporting CTRT and explaining the philosophy and structure of CTRT can assist with this. Once administrative support is obtained, the CTRT therapist can schedule the CTRT start date and schedule the day and times of initial training and weekly CTRT supervision sessions. Next, begin to create interest in CTRT by talking with teachers about the ways in which participating in CTRT can benefit their work in the classroom and support them in the challenges of working with their students. Both teachers and their teacher aides are encouraged to participate in CTRT at the same time. This allows for consistency and cohesiveness in the classroom. From this point on in the text, teachers and teacher aides will collectively be referred to as teachers.

Staff meetings and teacher in-service days are good opportunities to discuss CTRT with possible participants. The CTRT therapist will need to limit the number of teacher participants based on how many people it is realistic to meet with and supervise each week. A CTRT participant group size of 10 is recommended. Also consider teachers' classroom schedules, space for play sessions, and space for weekly CTRT supervision meetings while planning.

Space and Materials

Ideally, a space in the school building will be allocated for a CTRT playroom. The perfect playroom would be a dedicated space that is warm and inviting and allows for privacy, mess, and noise. For supervision purposes, the room should allow for the capability of video and audio recording of sessions. Because space is highly valuable and often difficult to obtain in a school, creativity in choosing a space may be necessary. A large unused closet or storage space, the corner of an office, an unused classroom, or a section of the school stage are all possible spaces for a play area. Larger spaces can be converted using dividers and shelves to create smaller spaces if necessary.

Categories of toys necessary to furnish a playroom include real-life toys (dolls, dollhouse, puppets, car, truck, boat, cash register), acting out or aggressive toys (toy soldiers, handcuffs, dart gun, something that can be destroyed such as an egg carton, a variety of animals including alligators, dinosaurs, sharks, etc.), and creative release toys (sand, water, blocks, paints).

Given the current conditions of heightened awareness regarding violence in the schools, many schools have a "no tolerance" policy in effect in which items resembling weapons are prohibited on school property. This conflict can typically be resolved when administrators understand that aggressive toys are an essential category to be included in the playroom. Explain to administrators that children use play to express their thoughts, feelings, and needs, and therefore they need an inclusive "vocabulary" to express both pleasant and unpleasant feelings. Aggressive toys are essential for expressing fears, worries, and anger. However, they are also useful for helping the child learn to control his or her own behavior, for developing a sense of mastery and competency, and for understanding limits. It may also help to reassure administrators that the weapons will not leave the playroom. If the weapons are simply not allowed, a foam pool noodle cut in thirds for children to hit things with or an assortment of aggressive animals and puppets (dinosaurs, spiders, snakes, etc.) can be utilized. If you have a dedicated playroom, see Landreth (2012) for a comprehensive list of toys. If you use a temporary space where a small traveling kit is set up for each session, see the Session 2 Toy Checklist in the *CPRT Treatment Manual, 2nd Edition* (Bratton & Landreth, 2019) and descriptions of toys in Chapter 9 of this text. A small storage drawer to hold replacement toys and a map of the arrangement of toys is recommended to allow for consistency in the placement of the toys and materials for the next session in the playroom (Morrison & Helker, 2010).

Participant Training

There are three phases of CTRT. Phase I includes the foundational skills of Child-Teacher Relationship Training and supervision of teachers' individual play sessions with their child of focus. Phase II focuses on instruction and supervision of group play therapy skills used in the classroom. Phase III is an observational/evaluation phase to determine the teacher's ability to generalize the CTRT skills to the classroom after training and weekly supervision has been concluded. Additional detail regarding the training schedule, handouts, and information regarding supervision is included in the Child-Teacher Relationship Training chapter (Helker & Bennett, 2019) in the *CPRT Treatment Manual, 2nd Edition* (Bratton & Landreth, 2019).

Phase I

CTRT is structured to make the most efficient use of the teachers' time. The CTRT model uses 2 days of intensive didactic instruction and practice in CTRT skills, which includes Sessions 1–4 of the CTRT curriculum.

Phase I CTRT Skills Outline

2-Day Intensive CTRT Training (CTRT Sessions 1–4)

- Overview of CTRT Philosophy
- Essential Concepts of Training
- Reflective Responding
- Play Session Dos and Don'ts (see Session 3 Dos & Don'ts in the *CPRT Treatment Manual, 2nd Edition* (Bratton & Landreth, 2019) and in Chapter 10 of this text)
- Play Session Toys and Materials Demonstration
- Limit Setting

CTRT Sessions 5–10 (held during weekly CTRT sessions)

- Supervision of CTRT Playtime Skills
- Choice Giving
- Esteem Building
- Encouragement

Providing intensive training during teacher in-service days at the beginning of the school year and holding the weekly 1-hour CTRT supervision sessions during teachers' planning period has proven to be effective. If an intensive training is not possible, conducting Sessions 1–4 in 1-hour weekly sessions is also an option. In Session 4, teachers select a child of focus and practice the CTRT skills in seven weekly 30-minute play sessions. The child of focus should be a child the teacher struggles with in the classroom or a child the teacher believes to need additional focus. An important component to Phase I is ensuring teachers choose a specific day and 30-minute time block they can commit to on a weekly basis in order to maintain the consistency of the seven play sessions. Keeping in mind several teachers will be using the playroom for play sessions, it is essential for a playroom schedule to be created during this phase.

During the six weekly CTRT sessions in Phase I, therapists provide didactic and experiential practice of skills following the CTRT curriculum. The teachers' play sessions with the child of focus are recorded and then viewed during training/supervision sessions, just as they are in a traditional CPRT group. In CTRT sessions, therapists provide specific feedback regarding teachers' use of skills demonstrated in their recorded play sessions as well as encouragement and support. CTRT therapists help teachers understand children's expression of experiences and feelings during the play sessions.

The following interaction is an example of supervision during Phase I of training. Mr. Orosco struggled with the CTRT philosophy of allowing the child to lead. He reported Jose (4-year-old) stood quietly in the playroom and did not engage with the toys. In the next supervision session, Mr. Orosco reported Jose didn't like the playtime and that he needed to choose another child of focus. After viewing the video in supervision, the therapist was able to help Mr. Orosco notice how unsure and anxious Jose was and suggested that in the next play session he reflect Jose's feelings and allow Jose to lead the playtime, even if he chooses not to play. The therapist engaged Mr. Orosco in role-playing reflection of feeling and then pointed out Mr. Orosco's strengths in the play session, including his efforts to demonstrate the "Be-With" Attitudes. During the next playtime with Jose, Mr. Orosco focused on reflecting Jose's feelings. Soon after, Jose became more comfortable and started playing with the dinosaurs in session, and Mr. Orosco gained a better understanding of Jose's feelings and was able to continue play sessions with Jose.

Consistent with CPRT philosophy, during Phase I teachers are instructed to use the CTRT skills only during play sessions and *not* to practice CTRT skills in the classroom at this time. This is important, as learning these skills for many teachers is like learning a new language. Practicing in the more controlled environment of the playroom sets the stage for more successful integration of these new skills into the classroom. During Phase II, teachers will begin to generalize their newly learned skills into the classroom.

Phase II

The focus of Phase II is to assist teachers in learning how to use relationship-building skills with small groups of children in the classroom setting as well as learning additional skills such as group reflection skills, advanced limit setting, and choice giving. Teachers and therapists continue to meet for 1-hour weekly CTRT sessions.

Phase II CTRT Classroom Skills Outline

Sessions 11–20

- Objectives and Structure of CTRT Time
- Basic and Advanced Group Responding Skills
- Advanced Choice Giving for Teachers
- Advanced Limit Setting, A-C-T for the Classroom
- Anger and Aggression in Children
- Troubleshooting in the Classroom

To facilitate the transition of CTRT skills into the classroom, individual play sessions are discontinued and replaced with Child-Teacher Relationship Training Time (CTRT Time) in the classroom. CTRT therapists and teachers identify a daily time in the classroom in which all students in the classroom are engaged in directing their own play, such as center time, dramatic play, blocks and manipulatives, or arts and crafts. For 15 minutes each day during this child-directed work or playtime, the teacher is asked to respond to a small group of two to four children working or playing together using CTRT skills. The therapist models CTRT skills and assists the teacher as needed. CTRT Time is organized such that if two teachers work in one classroom together, one teacher focuses on practicing the CTRT skills for 15 minutes with a designated small group of children while the other teaching partner focuses on general classroom management. After 15 minutes, teaching partners switch roles to allow for both to have the opportunity to engage in CTRT Time with students. Each teaching partner provides CTRT Time with a different small group of children each day. Ideally, by the end of the week each child in the class will have participated in CTRT Time as part of a small group with the teacher or teacher aide. If there is only one teacher in the classroom, it may be necessary to seek an additional adult helper to assist with classroom management during the 15-minute CTRT Time.

At the beginning of Phase II, teachers learn additional group reflection and group relationship-building skills. Teachers are instructed to limit the use of these new skills to the specifically structured classroom CTRT Time. As teachers become more confident and proficient in using group reflections and group relationship-building skills toward the end of Phase II, it is expected teachers will generalize the use of these skills to their daily interactions with individual and small groups of children.

The following is an example of generalized skills. Mrs. Johnson, a Pre-K teacher, is playing in the block center with Jadon, Miguel, and Andrew. Mrs. Johnson reflects, "*You are all working together. Andrew you are really interested in what Jadon is building.*" Jadon then responds, "I'm making a race car." Andrew then says, "Fast!" Mrs. Johnson then reflects feeling, "*Andrew, you are so excited to build a fast car. You are really focused on what you are building. Jadon, Andrew and Miguel, all three of you know how to build things.*" These reflective responses allow Mrs. Johnson to reflect feeling, build esteem, and build a relationship between the three boys. She is communicating the "Be-With" Attitudes, which strengthens the Child-Teacher relationship and improves student behavior.

At the completion of Phase II, the therapist's role shifts. Weekly CTRT sessions and in-classroom modeling are discontinued but may be offered to teachers on an as-needed basis. At this point, Phase III observation and program evaluation is conducted.

Phase III: Observation and Accountability

The final phase of CTRT includes unscheduled observation of the teachers in the general classroom 3 or 4 weeks after the conclusion of the CTRT training using the CTRT-Skills Checklist (CTRT-SC). The CTRT-Skills Checklist (Helker, 2006) can be found in the Child-Teacher Relationship Training chapter in the *CPRT Treatment*

Manual, 2nd Edition (Bratton & Landreth, 2019). The purpose of the observations is to determine to what degree teachers learned and integrated relationship-building skills in the classroom and as a data collection tool for use in evaluating CTRT.

Based on the results of the observations, a follow-up CTRT supervision meeting can be scheduled to discuss the teacher's strengths and challenges that may be hindering the generalization of skills to the classroom setting. The CTRT-SC can also be used as a pretest-posttest measure to evaluate the effectiveness of CTRT. Detailed information on program evaluation can be found in the Child-Teacher Relationship Training chapter in the *CPRT Treatment Manual, 2nd Edition* (Bratton & Landreth, 2019).

Unique Considerations for Working with Teachers and School Personnel

Each classroom is filled with children who have individual needs that must be met for social, emotional, behavioral, and academic success. Teachers are tasked with the responsibility of trying to identify and meet each of those needs for their students on a daily basis.

The principles of CTRT can be a shift in thinking for teachers who have been taught that their role is to *react* to a child's behavior rather than to *respond* to the underlying needs the child may be communicating with his or her behavior. The following is an example of how the CTRT therapist can respond to this problem. Mr. Gonzales, a teacher, had difficulty understanding the purpose of reflecting feelings. He believed children often behaved in certain ways to get attention, or to be defiant. The therapist explained the difference in responding and reacting to children and that those behaviors may be due to a child not feeling noticed or valued. The therapist explained how reflecting a child's feelings can help a child feel acknowledged and understood, therefore reducing the child's need to use externalizing behaviors to be noticed. The CTRT therapist encouraged Mr. Gonzales to increase reflections of the child's pleasant and unpleasant feelings in his work with children. As teachers adjust to new ways of thinking and understanding children's behaviors, the therapist can be most helpful by being patient and offering understanding and support.

It is also important for the CTRT therapist to consider that the ideas of best practices in the classroom are ever changing. Many teachers have been exposed to a multitude of new ideas, strategies, and techniques, academic or otherwise, and have been required to implement these ideas in their classrooms only to have them replaced with something different the following year. The idea of starting another new program may be met with hesitance and resistance. Case example: Ms. Dean was wary of change in her classroom. Each week when the therapist arrived in her classroom to do CTRT Time, Ms. Dean would moan and say, "Oh, is it time for that again?" The therapist continued to reflect her feeling, providing an opportunity for Ms. Dean to feel heard and understood, "*This is really hard for you. Change is often challenging*." The therapist worked during supervision to continue to reflect Ms. Dean's feelings and offer her support and understanding. Because she felt understood and validated by the therapist, Ms. Dean was willing to try the CTRT Time skills. The therapist was able to help her see how her reflections impacted the children positively, which encouraged her to use the skills more frequently. Eventually, Ms. Dean gained confidence in her use of CTRT Time skills and felt more empowered in her classroom. At the completion of CTRT, Ms. Dean reported she believed one of her students would not be ready for kindergarten the following year if she had not done CTRT with him as a Pre-K student.

An essential goal of CTRT training is that teachers will begin to understand CTRT is a philosophy of working with and understanding children and not simply a collection of tools and strategies. When the philosophy is integrated, teachers' ideas of being with and responding to children is forever changed. Many teacher preparation programs emphasize the teacher's role as one of authority rather than emphasizing the Child-Teacher relationship as one that is mutually respectful. Some teachers may have difficulty adjusting from a more authoritarian role to one that trusts the child with more autonomy. It is important to acknowledge and be understanding of this point of view and patient with teachers as they integrate a potentially new way of thinking and behaving in relationships with their students.

Adaptations for Elementary School Students

CTRT was originally designed and conducted with preschool-aged children and early childhood educators. However, CTRT can be effective with elementary school age children and teachers (through 3rd grade) with some adaptations. Some possibilities for scheduling the seven weekly play sessions include during the teacher's conference period, recess, lunchtime, or before or after school if transportation can be worked out.

If the playtime is scheduled to be held during special area time (music, PE, art, etc.), it is important that the special area teacher understands the child will be missing the special area class once a week for 7 weeks in order to participate in the playtime with the classroom teacher. If recess is selected, it is important to discuss this ahead of time with the child of focus. Recess is one of the only "down" times a child has during the day, and it may be frustrating for the child to miss recess. This could set a negative tone for the play sessions. Recess should only be used as a last resort and only if the teacher and child agree this is an acceptable time for the seven play sessions.

When working with elementary level teachers and students, some adjustments will need to be made in Phase II as well. Due to a differently structured academic focus at the elementary level, there may not be daily opportunities for "free play" in the classroom during which CTRT Time would usually be conducted. It is important to work with the teacher and think creatively to find out what activities are scheduled during the school day that would lend themselves to CTRT Time. Some possibilities include "center time" when students are working in small groups, during interactive hands-on activities, while children are having "Fun Friday" or relaxed classroom time, while children are working on art projects, or during recess time. When planning CTRT Time, consider any classroom activity that has the children working in groups of two to four students, is a child-directed activity (meaning the teacher is not actively instructing the students so is free to respond using CTRT responses), and is a hands-on activity so the teacher can practice interactive responses. Ideally, CTRT Time would occur three times per week, but if this is not possible two times per week can be sufficient.

Assistant teachers or teacher aides are typically not employed on the staff of elementary schools. Depending on the needs of the class, it may therefore be necessary to enlist another adult in the school to assist with classroom management needs while the teacher is engaged in CTRT Time. Discuss whether this is necessary with the classroom teacher before the start of Phase II, so that if an additional teacher is needed those arrangements can be made ahead of time (Helker, Schottelkorb, & Ray, 2007).

What the Research Says: Summaries of CTRT Studies and Results

Morrison and Bratton (2010) examined the effectiveness of training Head Start teachers and their aides in Child-Teacher Relationship Training compared to Conscious Discipline© (Bailey, 2000). A total of 24 Head Start teachers and aides participated in this quasi-experimental design. Teachers identified students (n = 54) with clinical levels of disruptive behaviors to participate in the study. In three points of measure (pre-, mid-, posttest), children whose teachers participated in CTRT had a statistically significant decrease (p = .002) in externalizing behavior problems on the Caregiver-Teacher Report Form (C-TRF, Achenbach & Rescorla, 2000) when compared to children whose teachers participated in the active control group. The large treatment effect ($\eta_p^2 = 0.22$) supports the practical significance of these findings.

Results of the Total Problems Scale indicate CTRT was an effective treatment for these behavioral problems. Compared to the active control group, children in the CTRT group demonstrated a statistically significant (p = .01) decrease in Total Problems, with the magnitude of the effect of the CTRT treatment considered large ($\eta_p^2 = 0.17$). These findings demonstrate the effectiveness of CTRT in reducing children's behavioral problems in the early childhood setting.

Helker and Ray (2009) examined the effectiveness of Child-Teacher Relationship Training (CTRT) when compared to Conscious Discipline© (Bailey, 2000). Head Start teachers and their aides (n = 24) identified students (n = 32) as having clinical levels of disruptive behaviors. Helker and Ray collected data regarding teachers' use of skills and then collected follow-up data regarding behavior change in the children and correlated results to the teachers' use of skills. Helker and Ray found preschool teachers and aides were able to learn and utilize CTRT skills in the general classroom. When compared to an active control group, teachers used CTRT skills more frequently than teachers who had not participated in CTRT. Also, CTRT participants were able to maintain the use of relationship-building skills ($p < .01$) in the general classroom 10 weeks following the completion of CTRT. These results demonstrate that CTRT is an effective means for teaching relationship-building skills to teachers and aides and that CTRT facilitates participants' abilities to generalize the use of relationship-building skills to the general classroom. Authors also found that students whose teachers and aides participated in CTRT demonstrated a statistically significant ($p = .04$) decrease in externalizing problems compared to students whose teachers and aides did not participate in CTRT. An additional noteworthy finding from Helker and Ray's study is that a statistically significant ($p < .05$) relationship was found between teachers' and aides' most frequent use of CTRT relationship-building skills.

Gonzales-Ball and Bratton (2012), replicating Morrison and Bratton (2010), examined the effectiveness of Child-Teacher Relationship Training when compared to Conscious Discipline© (Bailey, 2000). A total of 23 Head Start teachers, aides, and their students ($n = 38$) identified as having clinical levels of disruptive behaviors participated in the study. Results indicated students whose teachers participated in CTRT made a statistically significant decrease ($p < 0.05$) in externalizing behavior problems on the C-TRF (Achenbach & Rescorla, 2000) and a statistically significant decrease in total problems ($p < 0.05$) on the Direct Observation Form (DOF, Achenbach & Rescorla, 2000) when compared to children whose teachers participated in the active control group.

Pronchenko-Jain (2012), replicating Helker and Ray (2009), examined the effectiveness of Child-Teacher Relationship Training when compared to Conscious Discipline© (Bailey, 2000). A total of 23 Head Start teachers, aides, and their students ($n = 38$) identified by teachers as having clinical levels of disruptive behaviors participated in the study. Objective raters utilized the Classroom Assessment Scoring System (CLASS, Pianta, Paro, & Hamre, 2008) and the Child-Teacher Relationship Skills Checklist (CTRT-SC, Helker, 2006) and teacher reports using Index of Teaching Stress (ITS, Abidin, Greene, & Konold, 2004) to determine if teachers could implement the CTRT skills in the classroom. Results indicated a statistically significant interaction effect for the experimental teachers' use of Child-Teacher Relationship Skills (CTRT-SC: $p = .036$), a non-statistically significant interaction effect for the experimental teachers' ability to provide emotional support (CLASS: p = .50), and a non-statistically significant interaction effect on teacher stress (ITS: p = .997). Compared to the active control, teachers in CTRT group demonstrated large treatment effects over time on the CTRT-SC (η_p^2 = .19) and the CLASS (η_p^2 = .16). Study findings provide support for CTRT as an effective intervention for increasing Head Start teachers' ability to provide emotional and relational support to at-risk students.

Coggins (2016) conducted a randomized active control group study examining the effectiveness of CTRT with Head Start teachers when compared to Conscious Discipline© (Bailey, 2000). Teachers (n = 7) identified children (n = 29) exhibiting problem behaviors at pretest participated in the study. Children were measured at pre-, mid-, and posttest using the C-TRF (Achenbach & Rescorla, 2000). Teachers' empathic behaviors were measured at pre- and posttest using the Measurement of Empathy in Adult-Child Interactions (MEACI; Stover, B. Guerney, & O'Connell, 1971). Results of the study indicate child participants in the experimental group demonstrated statistically significant decreases in the total problem behaviors (p = 0.034) when compared to children in the comparison group. Furthermore, teachers who participated in CTRT displayed statistically significant increases in their use of empathic behaviors (p = 0.004) with very large effect sizes.

CTRT provides a viable solution for equipping teachers with therapeutic skills to apply in the classroom under the supervision of a school-based mental health provider. CTRT has strong research to support it as an effective modality in impacting behavior problems of young children. Research also supports teachers' ability to learn and implement the skills. A strong Child-Teacher relationship makes a significant difference in the lives of children, and CTRT provides a structure for teachers to learn the skills they need to facilitate that relationship, impacting children for years to come.

Conclusion

The power of a positive Child-Teacher relationship is well documented both formally through research and anecdotally. When teachers were asked to reflect on their experiences regarding their participation in CTRT, they highlighted positive behavior changes in their students and made statements such as, "His outbursts have become less frequent." "He has greatly improved in his ability to manage frustration. He is no longer as aggressive as he was." "She has completely turned around. She is independent and willing to try new things." "She participates more and is very happy when given responsibilities" (Helker, 2006). Teachers also mentioned positive changes in themselves. "I've learned to stop and listen to what children are trying to say." "I am more patient, taking into consideration the way I see things and the children's view too." "CTRT made me stop and reevaluate some of my ideas about classroom relationships." One teacher said, "This training was invaluable. I believe all teachers should have access to this information."

Child-Teacher Relationship Training utilizes the power of a positive Child-Teacher relationship to make an important and valuable impact on children's and teacher's lives.

References

Abidin, R. R., Greene, R. W., & Konold, T. R. (2004). *Index of teaching stress: Professional manual.* Lutz, FL: Psychological Assessment Resources, Inc.

Achenbach, T. M., & Rescorla, L. A. (2000). *Manual for the ASEBA preschool forms & profiles.* Burlington: University of Vermont, Research Center for Children, Youth, & Families.

Bailey, B. A. (2000). *Conscious discipline.* Oviedo, FL: Loving Guidance.

Bratton, S. C., & Landreth, G. L. (2019). *Child-Parent relationship therapy training manual: An Evidence-Based 10-session filial therapy model* (2nd ed). New York, NY: Routledge.

Coggins, K. (2016). *The efficacy of Child-Teacher relationship training as an early childhood mental health intervention in head start centers* (Order No. 10113687). Available from ProQuest Dissertations & Theses Global. (1801725449). Retrieved from http://libproxy.txstate.edu/login?url=http://search.proquest.com/docview/1801725449? =5683

Gonzales-Ball, T.L., & Bratton, S.C. (2019). Child-Teacher relationship training as a Head Start early mental health intervention for children exhibiting disruptive behavior. *International Journal of Play Therapy, 28*(1), 44–56.

Guerney, B. G., Jr., & Flumen, A. B. (1970). Teachers as psychotherapeutic agents for withdrawn children. *Journal of School Psychology, 8*, 107–113.

Helker, W. P. (2006). *The impact of child teacher relationship training on teachers' and aides use of relationship-building skills and the effect on student classroom behavior* (Order No. 3254192). Available from ProQuest Dissertations & Theses Global. (305295221). Retrieved from http://libproxy.txstate.edu/login?url=http://search.proquest.com/docview/305295221?accountid=5683

Helker, W., & Bennett, M. (2019). Child-Teacher relationship training manual. In G. Landreth & S. Bratton, (Eds.), *Child-parent relationship therapy training manual* (pp. 119–123). New York, NY: Routledge.

Helker, W. P., & Ray, D. C. (2009). Impact of child teacher relationship training on teachers' and aides' use of relationship-building skills and the effects on student classroom behavior. *International Journal of Play Therapy, 18*(4), 70–83.

Helker, W. P., Schottelkorb, A. A., & Ray, D. C. (2007). Helping students and teachers connect: An intervention model for school counselors. *Journal of Professional Counseling: Practice, Theory, and Research, 35*(2), 31–45.

Howes, C., Burchinal, M., Pianta, R., Bryant, D., Early, D., Clifford, R., & Barbarin, O. (2008). Ready to learn? Children's pre-academic achievement in pre-kindergarten programs. *Early Childhood Research Quarterly, 23*(1), 27–50.

Landreth, G. L. (2012). *Play therapy: The art of the relationship* (3rd ed). New York, NY: Routledge.

Landreth, G. L., & Bratton, S. C. (2019). *Child-parent relationship therapy: An Evidence-Based 10-session filial therapy model* (2nd ed). New York, NY: Routledge.

Morrison, M. O., & Bratton, S. C. (2010). Preliminary investigation of an early mental health intervention for head start programs: Effects of child teacher relationship training (CTRT) on children's behavior problems. *Psychology in the Schools, 47*(10), 1003–1017. doi:10.1002/pits

Morrison, M. O., & Helker, W. P. (2010). Child-Teacher relationship training: Using the power of the Child-Teacher relationship as a school-based mental health intervention. In A. Drews & C. Schaefer (Eds.), *School-based play therapy* (2nd ed) (pp. 181–195). Hoboken, NJ: John Wiley & Sons.

National Association for the Education of Young Children. (2009). *Developmentally Appropriate Practice in Early Childhood Programs Serving Children from Birth through Age 8*. Retrieved from www.naeyc.org/files/naeyc/file/positions/PSDAP.pdf

New Freedom Commission on Mental Health. (2003). *Achieving the promise: Transforming mental health care in America*. Final report (DHHS Publication No. SMA-03-3832). Rockville, MD: U.S. Department of Health and Human Services.

Pianta, R, C., La Paro, K. M., & Hamre, B. K. (2008). *Classroom assessment scoring system*. Baltimore, MD: Paul H Brookes Publishing.

Pronchenko-Jain, Y. (2012). *Child Teacher Relationship Training (CTRT) with children exhibiting disruptive behavior: Effects on teachers' ability to provide emotional and relational support to students and on student-teachers relationship stress* (Order No. 3538127). Available from ProQuest Dissertations & Theses Global. (1335545982). Retrieved from http://libproxy.txstate.edu/login?url=http://search.proquest.com/docview/1335545982?accountid=5683

Stover, L., Guerney, B., & O'Connell, M. (1971). Measurements of acceptance, allowing self-direction, involvement, and empathy in adult-child interaction. *Journal of Psychology*, 77, 261–69. doi: 10.1080/00223980.19719916879

United States Public Health Service. (2000). *Report of the surgeon general's conference on children's mental health: A national agenda*. Washington, DC: United States Public Health Service.

CHAPTER 22

CULTURALLY RESPONSIVE CPRT

Angela I. Sheely-Moore, Peggy L. Ceballos, Yung-Wei Dennis Lin, and Yumiko Ogawa

Many countries in the world, including the United States, represent large racially and ethnically diverse populations. Within the U.S., these diverse populations have consistently grown in the past two decades, with persons of color projected to become the numerical majority by the year 2045 (U.S. Census Bureau, 2015).

In the U.S., individuals and families of color are more likely to live in poverty and lack health insurance coverage (Denavas-Walt & Proctor, 2015). Approximately 13% of the Asian American population lives below the poverty line compared to the national average of 12% (National Commission on Asian American and Pacific Islander Research in Education, 2008).

Furthermore, culturally diverse children in the U.S. are more likely to develop behavioral and emotional concerns. Results of the 2007 National Survey of Children's Health indicated that almost half of all Latino and African American children under the age of 5 developed physical, behavioral, or social concerns (Data Resource Center for Child and Adolescent Health, DRCCAH, 2007). Approximately 12% of children of color between the ages of 6 and 17 consistently demonstrate problematic social behaviors, compared to 7.5% of their white counterparts (DRCCAH, 2007).

Despite the increasing attention to multiculturalism in the mental health profession, ethnically diverse children and families are still likely to remain underserved (Kataoka, Zhang, & Wells, 2002). With the rapidly growing numbers and the prevalent mental health needs of children and families in these ethnic minority groups, the play therapy mental health community has become increasingly aware of the need to address the application of play-based interventions with children and families of diverse cultures.

Play as the Universal Language

Across disciplines and cultures, there is agreement that play is the universal language for children and is critical to children's cognitive, socio-emotional, and motor skills development (Landreth, 2012; Remorini & Renda, 2014). Children use play to express their emotions and thoughts. Remorini and Renda (2014) reported that "play . . . allows [for] the expression of their creativity and autonomy, and contributes with the construction of their identity, the command of their mobility and the progressive knowledge of their own body and environment" (p. 241). While play behaviors are largely influenced by the child's cultural group (Remorini & Renda, 2014), developmentally all children use play as a natural form of expression (Landreth, 2012). In fact, it is through play that children *process* cultural values, including internalization of familial and peer socialization rules (Paradise & de Haan, 2009).

Children from all cultures engage in play spontaneously and find it to be enjoyable. Similarly, play is symbolic; it represents children's perceptions, feelings, and attempts to make sense of their experiences (Landreth, 2012). Given the universal qualities of play, Child-Parent Relationship Therapy (CPRT), which uses play as the vehicle to strengthen the parent-child relationship, demonstrates responsiveness and sensitivity to racially and ethnically minority children and their families.

CPRT focuses on helping parents understand the internal world of their children by becoming attuned to children's needs and responding to those needs in ways that promote optimal child development. During special playtimes, children communicate through their natural language, play, while parents respond with understanding within their cultural framework. Communication through play allows for the integration of the family culture within CPRT. Hence, the parent-child dyad communication within the context of CPRT demonstrates respect and honor to their cultural background. Glover (2001) declared that the nondirective, empathetic, and accepting relationship one provides with Child-Centered Play Therapy is the ideal treatment for all children. Similarly, communication through play allows for parents to better understand their children's developmental needs and respond accordingly. In addition to the use of a universal language, CPRT empowers parents to be the agent of change in their children's lives.

In many minority communities, seeking mental health services is not commonly accepted. Such feelings and perceptions can be augmented when therapists assume the role of "expert" as treatment providers for the child, and thus minimize contributions parents can make in this context. CPRT allows for the empowerment of parents by having *them* apply the necessary therapeutic skills during scheduled playtimes with their own children. **With the strong Child-Parent bond found in some minority families, parent involvement within the CPRT training would seem most fitting.**

Many minority cultures have a more collective orientation rather than an individualistic orientation to life and view one's sacrifice for the family unit as pivotal (Drewes, 2006). CPRT honors these cultural values by intervening at the family level and focusing on the parent-child dyad. The group modality of CPRT also serves to honor the collective orientation racial and ethnic minority families share. Conducting the intervention in a group setting provides parents additional support systems and promotes a feeling of community membership.

Understanding Children and Families through Their Unique, Cultural Lens

It behooves mental health professionals to anticipate possible resistance to counseling services based upon the lived experiences of marginalization and institutional oppression for minority groups. Experiences of mistrust within therapeutic services is affirmed with the underutilization of mental health services for racial/ethnic minorities when compared to whites (Ojeda & Bergstresser, 2008).

In order to provide culturally responsive therapeutic services, it is critical for play therapists to understand that play is *culturally contextualized* while acknowledging a global orientation of play as a catalyst of children's expression and development across cultures. For example, myriad cultural differences, values, and practices exist among and within all racial and ethnic groups: common parenting practices, family values, educational systems, connotation of "play," and expected age for developmental milestones, to name a few (Bornstein, 2013). It is recommended that play therapists engage in an *ongoing, active* role in understanding the world of their clients. This commitment begins with an exploration into one's own intersecting cultural identities.

Unwrapping one's own ethnic and racial identity based upon historical, psychological, and socio-political viewpoints would help play therapists to respect the myriad parenting approaches shared during the CPRT experience. The likelihood of ascribing a different parenting experience from one's own upbringing as "wrong" can be minimized with a strong grounding in one's own cultural framework and an openness to other parenting styles from a culturally different background. In order to understand the cultural complexity of ethnic and racially diverse clients, CPRT facilitators should already possess an understanding of their own cultural grounding.

CPRT therapists will also need to be sensitive to differences *between* members of the same minority group and to acknowledge parents' cultural identity. For example, familiarity with various racial identity models may enhance CPRT therapists' understanding of each minority parent's acculturation level. Asking parents how they self-identify themselves ethnically and racially communicates acceptance on behalf of the CPRT facilitator (Glover, 2001). This question can then lead to a robust discussion of parents educating the CPRT facilitator in the ways of family customs, traditions, rituals, and celebrations. Considering the intergenerational dimension within a parent-child dyad may provide clues for CPRT therapists to conceptualize the parent's struggle in understanding the child's internal frame of reference. Helping parents become aware of the difference in cultural identity between themselves and their child may advance their understanding of their children's unique world.

Modifications to CPRT Protocol When Working with Ethnic and Racially Diverse Families

In order to maximize the benefits of CPRT, the following recommendations are provided to group facilitators of CPRT when organizing a CPRT group comprising a specific ethnic-racial minority group.

Increasing "Buy In"

Deconstructing the CPRT process to parents is key. To increase "buy in" of the CPRT approach, parents of racial/ethnic minority groups who have successfully completed CPRT training can be invited to share their experiences by handing out flyers within their respective communities and the use of "word of mouth" to increase turnout rates for upcoming CPRT groups. The CPRT facilitator can accompany volunteer parents into their communities: residential neighborhoods, hair salons, recreation centers, churches, grocery stores, and school settings. Having face-to-face interactions with community members can provide an opportunity for prospective CPRT parents to view the group facilitator as an ally and additional source of support.

Cultural values specific to the ethnic representation of the local community can be added to flyers advertising upcoming CPRT groups. If possible, these flyers should be in the native language of the targeted group and can include phrases highlighting key ethnic values such as "CPRT provides parents skills to instill *respeto* in children" for Spanish-speaking populations. The cultural value of *respeto* is important for parents within Latino communities, and this value can be stressed when teaching parents the purpose of therapeutic limit setting. Such encounters with parent prospects allow CPRT group facilitators to start building trust with parents. These personal interactions honor, for example, the Latino value of *personalismo*, which refers to the valuing of personal relationships over status. For CPRT treatment providers, honoring this value means being able to convey that they genuinely care for parents and by avoiding a business-like approach.

Some minority groups often conduct "Saturday school" in communities where ethnic minorities learn their language and culture, as well as study the standard curriculum (e.g., math, science, language arts) in their primary, non-English language. It is a rarity for mental health professionals to be assigned to work in Saturday schools; however, children's behavioral and emotional issues, as well as family and parenting issues, can be observed in this setting. For example, a creative CPRT facilitator collaborated with a Japanese Saturday School, established a relationship with the principal, teachers, and volunteer parent members, and eventually conducted CPRT at the site.

Establishing rapport and gaining the trust of parents serves to mitigate the possible stigma related to mental health services. It is essential that group facilitators of CPRT remain patient during marketing efforts for CPRT training. Providing face-to-face contact and an open Q&A forum featuring parents who are CPRT graduates facilitates trust, veracity, and openness with CPRT group facilitators.

Emphasizing the impact of CPRT special play sessions in mitigating potential cognitive and behavioral problems later in life is a message that resonates with minority caregivers and encourages them to try on new behaviors. This "sales pitch" is one that many parent CPRT graduates often openly share during the grassroots recruitment strategy.

Addressing Confidentiality

To promote safety and group cohesion, it is important that parents be educated about confidentiality and obtain their commitment to keep what is shared within the CPRT group meetings. This is especially crucial for parents who know one another as a result of living in a small, racially and ethnically dense community. Requesting verbal and/or written consent to maintain confidentiality may communicate to members the seriousness of this matter. At the same time, it is also important to highlight that in some ethnic minority communities, extended families are an important part of child rearing, and there is a tendency for parents to include these family members in the CPRT process. For example, two CPRT facilitators reported that Latino and African American parents brought extended family members (e.g., child's godparents, grandparents, aunts) to some of the group sessions from time to time. In these instances, the facilitators consulted with parent group members and found that they felt open and welcoming of having additional family members come and go throughout the CPRT training sessions. Hence, for some parents of diverse ethnic-racial background, the value of an open group is greater than the value of confidentiality.

Option to Provide Individual CPRT Sessions

Although benefits of the group format and process of CPRT are well documented (Bratton, Landreth, & Lin, 2010), conducting individual CPRT can be a viable option when confidentiality becomes an issue. For example, one CPRT facilitator conducted individual CPRT training with a Sudanese community leader. The rationale behind the decision to conduct individual CPRT was to promote the willingness for the parent to share his struggles without fear of losing respect in his role as a community leader. In CPRT, parents are encouraged to provide an environment where their children experience unconditional acceptance. This way of being is also translated to working with parents.

CPRT leaders need to be open to conduct make-up individual sessions to reduce the pressure of parents attending for every group meeting. Transportation issues and inflexible work schedules can prevent parents from attending on a regular basis. Remaining flexible with one's schedule by offering make-up individual sessions or conducting individual CPRT sessions communicates to parents the therapist's acceptance of their life roles and willingness to meet them where they are.

Structuring CPRT Training Sessions with Flexibility and Inclusivity

The composition of the contemporary family varies. Honoring the myriad presentations of family structure through language and in the general format for CPRT meetings is a modification CPRT facilitators have reported to be important to the CPRT training experiences with ethnic and racial minority families. Specifically, the following adjustments have been included to demonstrate cultural responsiveness and sensitivity: (1) fluidity of the start time for group meetings; (2) inclusion of a brief "check-in"; (3) reaffirmation of the importance of the family unit by including meal times as part of the training experience; and (4) adjustment of homework assignments via culturally specific play/activity.

The concept of time can be viewed within a cultural lens. According to Katz's (1985) seminal work, the counseling discipline itself has been described as the exemplification of white culture. In the practice of CPRT with minority groups, punctuality is not deemed as critical for some cultures as compared to others. For example, Latinos are present-oriented; thus, they focus more on the immediacy of the moment rather than on future appointments. This emphasis results in Latino parents being less concerned about punctuality and more concerned about the quality of interactions they have with others. What is key for CPRT therapists is unconditional acceptance of CPRT participants. A delayed arrival to group sessions should not have an impact on the group facilitator's way of being with the tardy parent.

The inclusion of a "check in" time at the start of each training session is especially helpful in providing an outlet for parents who encounter economic, social, political, and environmental stressors on a daily basis. Providing this platform of group sharing can promote group cohesiveness, trust, and support. The importance of a collectivist perspective can also be demonstrated in sharing a meal before the start of each CPRT session. This is a time for all family members (including children) to convene and interact. For Latino families, this sharing time exemplifies the value of *personalismo* by having members spend time engaging in informal conversations, which strengthens the group connection.

Homework assignments in CPRT are provided to reinforce teaching points shared during sessions. Some assignments, especially ones that include physical interaction between parent and child (e.g., Sandwich Hug and Sandwich Kiss assignments for Session 5, play-wrestle homework in Session 9), may not reflect typical parent-child interaction in particular cultures. Such homework assignments can be replaced with traditional play or activities from a specific culture, which facilitate positive parent-child interaction and communicate a "Be-With" Attitude.

Toy Selections for Ethnic and Culturally Diverse Families

As toys serve the role of children's words, it is paramount to provide an extensive "vocabulary" through the inclusion of toys and play materials for the special playtime kit that reflect the child's cultural world: dolls representing family composition, appropriate skin tones, clothing attire, plastic foods germane to the country of origin, music instruments, to name a few. Another area to consider is transportation: scooters, motorcycles, or trains are common forms of transportation in some Asian countries. The absence of such culturally responsive toys may inhibit children's full range of expression.

One CPRT facilitator of a Japanese group added traditional Japanese toys to the portable play kit: kamifusen (paper balloon), denden daiko (one-handed, small drum), *otedama* (juggling balls), and be-dama (marbles). The parents reported that seeing traditional toys tapped into their own playfulness. On the other hand, the CPRT facilitator observed some parents fighting the urge to teach their children how to play with those toys as their children who were born and raised in the U.S. had never encountered these toys before. This struggle the parents experienced was utilized as a teachable moment about not labeling toys as a way to respect children's imagination and creativity. A variety of culturally sensitive toys provide children the opportunity to work through issues that are significant to them. See the *Toy Checklist for Play Sessions* in Session 2 in the CPRT Treatment Manual, 2nd Edition.

Use of Language

When parents choose to conduct special playtimes in their native language other than English, it behooves CPRT facilitators to make sure the intent of parents' therapeutic responses is not lost in translation while simultaneously keeping the selected words, used in the parents' primary language, natural and culturally sensitive. For example, Lillard (2015) pointed out that Japanese mothers are prone to speak to their infant's affect using onomatopoeia. A CPRT facilitator reported that this strategy of Japanese parents using onomatopoeia to be effective during special playtime, particularly when parents reflected a child's feelings (e.g., "waku waku" to express excitement, "doki doki" for nervousness). Another CPRT facilitator found it difficult to identify an appropriate Chinese feeling word for proud, as the literal translation connotes bragging. Thus, a more appropriate Chinese translation for the English CPRT phrase "*You are proud of yourself*" would be "*You feel good about yourself.*"

Another strategy involves translating acronyms used in the CPRT English materials to help parents remember skills via the use of acronyms germane to their first language. For example, the acronym A-C-T for limit setting was translated to *S-E-D* for Latino parents. This acronym, which means thirst, gives Latino parents the opportunity to easily memorize the steps. Modifying English phrases used within CPRT therapeutic responses and training material into another language requires CPRT therapists to have a thorough understanding of the philosophy behind CPRT, intentionality of each therapeutic response, and the cultural aspect of the parents' native language.

Empirical Research Supporting Use of CPRT with Ethnic and Racially Diverse Families

Researchers have confirmed the benefits of involving parents or caregivers in the treatment process of children's psychotherapy (Bratton, Ray, Rhine, & Jones, 2005; Lin & Bratton, 2015). CPRT is the most empirically researched, play-based child psychotherapy approach with full parent involvement, with more than 40 empirical studies investigating the effectiveness of CPRT. Several of these studies targeted specific racial and/or ethnic populations: Latinos, African Americans, Native Americans, Asians/Asian Americans (Bratton et al., 2010). Empirical findings from these studies supported the effectiveness of CPRT with children's behavior problems and parent–child relationship stress in Latino families (Ceballos & Bratton, 2010; Villarreal, 2008); in African American families (Sheely-Moore & Bratton, 2010); as well as in Asian or immigrant Asian families (Chau & Landreth, 1997; Jang, 2000; Kidron & Landreth, 2010; Lee & Landreth, 2003; Yuen, Landreth, & Baggerly, 2002). Research findings also confirmed CPRT's positive effect on increasing the empathy levels of Native American parents (Glover & Landreth, 2000) and Asian or immigrant Asian parents (Chau & Landreth, 1997; Jang, 2000; Kidron & Landreth, 2010; Lee & Landreth, 2003; Yuen et al., 2002).

Conclusion

Given the mental health needs of children and families of racially and ethnically diverse groups, play therapy researchers have begun to establish research evidence for culturally responsive interventions and modalities. Lin and Bratton's (2015) meta-analysis involving 52 empirical studies that used a Child-Centered Play Therapy modality, which includes CPRT, included 15 studies of primarily non-Caucasian participants (e.g., African American,

Latino/Hispanic, Asian/Asian American), with an additional 15 studies that recruited mainly Caucasian participants. The results of this meta-analysis revealed an average effect size of 0.76 for Child-Centered Play Therapy studies, which included CPRT, with non-Caucasian participants. This effect size was statistically significantly larger than the average effect size of 0.33 produced by the studies with Caucasian participants. The findings of this meta-analysis and other previously mentioned empirical studies strongly support the effectiveness of CPRT with culturally diverse children and families. For ethnic and racially minority parents, who may have encountered disempowerment within social, political, economic, and environmental contexts, CPRT can serve as a means to help parents become change agents in their children's lives while honoring their cultural framework—a clear demonstration of a culturally responsive play-based intervention.

References

Bornstein, M. (2013). Parenting and child mental health: A cross-cultural perspective. *World Psychiatry, 12*, 258–265.

Bratton, S., Landreth, G., & Lin, Y. (2010). Child parent relationship therapy: A review of controlled-outcome research. In J. N. Baggerly, D. C. Ray, & S. C. Bratton (Eds.), *Child-centered play therapy research: The evidence base for effective practice* (pp. 267–293). Hoboken, NJ: John Wiley & Sons.

Bratton, S., Ray, D., Rhine, T., & Jones, L. (2005). The efficacy of play therapy with children: A meta-analytic review of treatment outcomes. *Professional Psychology: Research and Practice, 36*(4), 367–390. doi:10.1037/0735-7028.36.4.376

Ceballos, P., & Bratton, S. (2010). Empowering Latino families: Effects of a culturally responsive intervention for low-income immigrant Latino parents on children's behaviors and parental stress. *Psychology in the Schools, 47*(8), 761–775.

Chau, I., & Landreth, G. (1997). Filial therapy with Chinese parents: Effects on parental empathic interactions, parental acceptance of child and parental stress. *International Journal of Play Therapy, 6*(2), 75–92. doi:10.1037/h0089409

Data Resource Center for Child and Adolescent Health. (2007). *2007 national survey of children's health*. Retrieved from www.childhealthdata.org/browse/survey?q=236&r=1

Denavas-Walt, C., & Proctor, B. D. (2015). *Income and poverty in the United States: 2014.* Retrieved from www.census.gov/content/dam/Census/library/publications/2015/demo/p60-252.pdf

Drewes, A. A. (2006). Suggestions and research on multicultural play therapy. In E. Gil & A. A. Drewes (Eds.), *Cultural issues in play therapy* (pp. 72–95). New York, NY: Guilford Press.

Glover, G. (2001). Cultural considerations in play therapy. In G. Landreth (Ed.), *Innovations in play therapy: Issues, process, and special populations* (pp. 31–41). Philadelphia, PA: Routledge.

Glover, G., & Landreth, G. (2000). Filial therapy with Native Americans on the Flathead Reservation. *International Journal of Play Therapy, 9*(2), 57–80. doi:10.1037/h0089436

Jang, M. (2000). Effectiveness of filial therapy for Korean parents. *International Journal of Play Therapy, 9*(2), 39–56. doi:10.1037/h0089435

Kataoka, S. H., Zhang, L., & Wells, K. B. (2002). Unmet need for mental health care among US children: Variation by ethnicity and insurance status. *The American Journal of Psychiatry, 159*(9), 1548–1555.

Katz, J. (1985). The sociopolitical nature of counseling. *The Counseling Psychologist, 13*, 615–624.

Kidron, M., & Landreth, G. (2010). Intensive child parent relationship therapy with Israeli parents in Israel. *International Journal of Play Therapy, 19*(2), 64–78. doi:10.1037/a0017516

Landreth, G. L. (2012). *Play therapy: The art of the relationship* (3rd ed). New York, NY: Routledge.

Lee, M., & Landreth, G. (2003). Filial therapy with immigrant Korean parents in the United States. *International Journal of Play Therapy, 12*(2), 67–85. doi:10.1037/h0088879

Lillard, A. S. (2015). The development of play. In L. S. Liben, U. Muller, & R. M. Lerner (Eds.), *Handbook of child psychology and developmental science, Volume 2, cognitive process* (7th ed) (pp. 425–468). Hoboken, NJ: John Wiley & Sons.

Lin, Y., & Bratton, S. (2015). A meta-analytic review of child-centered play therapy approaches. *Journal of Counseling and Development, 93*(1), 45–58. doi:10.1002/j.1556-6676.2015.00180.x

National Commission on Asian American and Pacific Islander Research in Education. (2008). *CARE reports: Asian Americans and pacific islanders: Fact not fiction: Setting the record straight: The Steinhardt Institute for Higher Education Policy at New York University.* Retrieved from http://care.gseis.ucla.edu/care-reports

Ojeda, V. D., & Bergstresser, S. M. (2008). Gender, race-ethnicity, and psychosocial barriers to mental health care: An examination of perceptions and attitudes among adults reporting unmet need. *Journal of Health and Social Behavior, 49*, 317–334.

Paradise R., & de Haan, M. (2009). Responsibility and reciprocity: Social organization of Mazahua learning practices. *Anthropology and Education Quarterly, 40*(2), 187–204.

Remorini, C., & Renda, M. (2014). Play and child development: Considerations from a comparative ethnographic research in two rural Argentinian communities. *The Oriental Anthropologist, 14*(2), 241–266.

Sheely-Moore, A., & Bratton, S. (2010). A strengths-based parenting intervention with low- income African American families. *Professional School Counseling, 13*(3), 175–183.

U.S. Census Bureau. (2015). *National population projections*. Retrieved from www.census.gov/population/projections/data/national/

Villarreal, C. E. (2008). School-based Child Parent Relationship Therapy (CPRT) with Hispanic parents. *Dissertation Abstracts International: Section A. Humanities and Social Sciences, 69*(2).

Yuen, T., Landreth, G., & Baggerly, J. (2002). Filial therapy with immigrant Chinese families. *International Journal of Play Therapy, 11*(2), 63–90. doi:10.1037/h0088865

CHAPTER 23

DEBBIE'S JOURNEY THROUGH CPRT TRAINING: A 1-WEEK, 4-YEAR, AND 13-YEAR FOLLOW-UP

In previous chapters, we have followed Debbie's journey through 10 sessions of CPRT as she struggled with her own feelings of inadequacy and her relationship with her daughter. At this point, it might be helpful to revisit some of Debbie's reasons for wanting CPRT training. Debbie had been married for 5 years and had two children, Rachel, who was 4 years old, and Josh, who was 3 months. She was a stay-at-home mother and struggled with feelings of isolation from her husband, depression, and anger, and she was overwhelmed by the requirements of parenting.

Her relationship with her husband was characterized by a lack of communication and an inability to connect with each other on most matters of importance. Debbie felt as though she was parenting by herself with no support from her husband in efforts to parent: "I do all the parenting by myself. He undermines me. I put Rachel to bed at night, later she wakes up, he decides she is hungry and feeds her. Then she's wide awake and tearing around the house, and I'm supposed to take care of her." (Several years later, Debbie described this time as "the darkest period of my marriage.")

Debbie felt out of control and felt everything in the home was out of control. Many little factors seemed to create an explosive situation. Debbie felt powerless to create the kind of home and to be the kind of parent she would like to be because "I don't know what a home and family is supposed to look like. I don't know what is normal for a family. I have no role model." She wanted a sense of peace and calm in her home but didn't know how to make that happen. "I have no building blocks to create a home. I have no routine in my life." Debbie didn't have a sense of home; she didn't know how to stay home and create order and routine. "When Rachel was a tiny baby, I would put her in a car seat and be gone all day long. I would come home just before my husband came home from work. The house was always a disaster area." Debbie didn't know how to build routine into her life, her home, and her children. Yet, she wanted this desperately. "I want to figure things out, to make my home better, to be a better parent. I need skills so I won't feel so overwhelmed and angry toward my children. I need to know what I am supposed to do. I'm hungry for information."

As was evident in her interactions in the first few sessions, she questioned, challenged, and struggled with some of the basic concepts, but was still open to the process of attempting the new behaviors required in the special play sessions. Her questioning and challenging was not motivated by resistance, but was a function of her natural tendency to want details and facts and her long-standing history of doubting herself and feeling inadequate. Some of her interactions revealed remarkable insight, and her experience in filial therapy was a time of tremendous personal growth as she incorporated, practiced, and internalized the Child-Centered Play Therapy philosophy, skills, and attitudes taught in the 10 sessions.

Parent Reactions to CPRT: A 1-Week Follow-Up

Three parents in the CPRT group we followed in earlier chapters through their 10 sessions of training were randomly selected and interviewed 1 week following the tenth session for their responses to the following questions. Debbie was one of the parents interviewed.

What did you like best about the training setting?

Debbie: I liked the fact that the training was done in a group. I now know that I am not the only one out there who has problems with her child. I don't feel as isolated. I enjoyed the shared experience and the bonding that took place between parents.

Kathy: I liked the fact that the group was small enough so we could have discussions. I also enjoyed learning about other parents' experiences and hearing their opinions.

Kim: I enjoyed the group setting, and I liked hearing the other mothers' opinions and feedback.

What was the most effective skill that you learned?

Debbie: I really like the choice-giving skill. It has definitely helped me the most, especially when I am trying to get my daughter to stay in her bed. The choice giving has cut down on her getting out of bed at night by at least 50 percent.

Kathy: The choice giving; it really helps my son make decisions, and it gives him power and responsibility for his actions.

Kim: The reflective listening and the reflection of feelings. I think my child perceives me as being more understanding towards him now. I also liked the choice giving, and making him more responsible for his actions.

What was the most difficult skill to master?

Debbie: I have problems reflecting my daughter's feelings. I still feel very awkward when I do this, and it seems very unnatural to me.

Kathy: The limit setting. I have problems following through with the alternatives.

Kim: The tracking and reflecting what I see. I feel like I sound like Mr. Rogers.

Is there something new that you learned about yourself?

Debbie: I have learned that I can control my anger, and that it is OK to be angry with my daughter. I now have new alternatives to spanking and yelling, and I am not feeling as frustrated as I did before. I am feeling more like a parent now.

Kathy: I have learned that I don't have to be perfect, and that I am more capable than I once thought. I have learned that it's OK if I get angry, and it's OK if I am frustrated. I feel more in control.

Is there something new that you learned about your child?

Debbie: I learned that Rachel is especially bright and very perceptive. She has caught on to the choice giving very quickly, and she now has limits and boundaries. I also discovered that I like her. I have always loved her, but now I like her, too. It's a great feeling.

Kathy: I have learned that Cody is more capable than I thought. He can control himself if he wants to, especially when he has choices.

Kim: I have noticed Toby more in general. I notice that he needs attention, and I also noticed that he is very bright.

How has your child responded to the special playtimes and the skills you are using?

Debbie: Rachel really enjoys the time that I am spending with her. She seems to appreciate that I understand her more now, and that I don't spank her as much. She seems to respect me more, and I think she senses that I am being a better parent.

Kathy: Cody usually enjoys the play sessions. However, he sometimes wants to end them early. I think we get along better after the play sessions.

Kim: Toby loves the playtimes and looks forward to them every week. He is not getting into trouble as he used to. Now he has a place where he knows he will get one-on-one attention.

How is your child different as a result of the filial therapy training?

Debbie: She now has more freedom to be herself, and she seems to feel more secure now that she has limits and boundaries. She seems to be more free.

Kathy: Cody seems to have slowed down a lot. He seems happier and more in control of himself.

Kim: Toby seems to have more self-confidence. He is more secure, and he seems happier because he knows I am "there."

Have you taught your spouse any of the skills?

Debbie: Yes, I have taught my husband choice giving and limit setting, but I would like for us both to go to a filial group together. I think he would benefit more from that setting, rather than me trying to teach him.

Kathy: (Single parent, so she did not respond.)

Kim: Yes, he is now a better listener to Toby.

Was the video-recording beneficial to you?

Debbie: Yes, I video-recorded every play session. I watched each one over and over with Rachel, and I corrected myself with her watching. If I forgot to give a self-esteem-building response, I would interject one while we were watching together. She loves it.

Kathy: I liked the video-recording, but I was very embarrassed for you all to see how Cody acts. He is far worse than any of the other children, and I was embarrassed about my video.

Kim: Yes, I still watch the first play session I recorded.

Was the supervision feedback you received beneficial?

Debbie: Yes, it was excellent. I learned something new about myself that I might not have ever known had it not been pointed out to me.

Kathy: Yes, it was. However, next time I would like for Dr. Landreth to have a play session with my child, so that I could see how someone else handles him.

Kim: Yes, it's just not possible to learn some things about yourself until someone points them out to you.

4-Year Follow-Up

As a part of the activities of the graduate level filial therapy class I was teaching one semester at the University of North Texas, I arranged for the class to observe the following interview with three parents from the CPRT therapy group whose transcribed sessions are provided as a part of the descriptions for the 10-session training model described in earlier chapters. This interview served as a 4-year follow-up to that training. Debbie was one of the parents interviewed.

Dr. L.: Well, I'm glad you all are here, Laura, Debbie, and Kim. I know the group appreciates you being here and sharing your experiences with us about what the filial therapy training was like for you 4 years ago. That's a long time in a person's life, and a long time in a child's life. I think we would all be interested in knowing what you remember most about the filial training.

Laura: With Dawson, in the beginning I remember the tracking and the play sessions. At that time, the kids' faces would just light up when they were being tracked, even in play. I could feel some of the joy seeing their faces light up. And choice giving, letting them know they could make choices was a big help.

Dr. L.: So the playtimes and the choice giving made a difference. Kim or Debbie, what do you remember most about the filial training?

Kim: Choices, and I've told a million people the Oreo® Cookie Theory! That changed not only what I do with my kids, it has changed how I deal with other adults in my life by giving them choices. I don't know how I would have parented or made it through the last 4 years without the choice-giving approach, especially with my son. I mainly took the course for my son, and he has come such a long way. I can't imagine life without the discipline techniques that you taught me.

Dr. L.: Kim, I remember 4 years ago, one of the things you were concerned about was your son's poor self-esteem.

Kim: He has ADD and I wanted to take more of an active role in his development instead of just letting the school district do it. The choice giving has made a big difference in his learning self-control. And allowing him to make decisions by saying, "*It's whatever you want it to be, Toby*," empowered him.

Dr. L.: You have been able to give some of the responsibility back to him instead of being the answer source.

Kim: Yes, and I had a 6-month-old when I first took the course. The difference in her discipline compared to the 8-year-old is dramatic, because she never knew any other way. The minute I say, "*You can choose*," she stops what she is doing and says, "OK Mom, I don't even want to hear it. I know what to do."

Dr. L.: Debbie, what do you remember?

Debbie: I can't say one specific thing, because everything in the training has changed my entire outlook on being a parent. When I began the training, I had a feeling that I wasn't really a parent. Somebody else was controlling things. I didn't feel like I was the grown-up. I acted just like my 4-year-old daughter did, short of throwing myself on the floor. During the training and seeing her responses in the special playtimes, I realized I was a parent. I felt like a parent inside of myself. And that is what I wanted. That awareness of being the parent has carried over to my son. He was only a couple of months old when we started the filial training. Now he is the age that my daughter was, 4½. I feel like an adult with him, I feel like the parent and that is a good feeling.

Dr. L.: I remember one of the things you said in reference to Rachel, who was 4 years old at the time, was that you were wishy-washy with her. You weren't really sure about yourself in that relationship and that you found yourself sometimes rejecting her.

Debbie: Yes, I felt like her playmate, because when she wanted cookies and milk, we had cookies and milk because she decided we would have cookies and milk. I didn't know anything better. Nobody told me, "It's 9:00 in the morning, you don't have that." In the filial training, I had a sense of growing up. I had a sense of taking my role, my position as a parent.

Dr. L.: So, what is it like now for you?

Debbie: I'm older inside. I'm in my place and I know who's in charge, so to speak. Not that I am in control, because you taught us that children can have control and choices. It's a relief to know I can be in control. I'm not caught up in a major struggle for position and for power. It's an automatic, it's a given now. I'm the parent.

Dr. L.: Laura, I saw you shaking your head in reference to that. What were you reacting to?

Laura: About being in charge and giving children choices when there are choices. And letting them know it's not negotiable.

Dr. L.: Standing firm.

Laura: Standing firm on the choices given.

Debbie: And knowing the difference.

Dr. L.: Kim, is taking a firm stand any different for you?

Kim: My kids get excellent reviews at school because they do what they are told immediately. All three of them go to different schools and I think their behavior at school has to do with what we do at home now.

Dr. L.: So you not only see a difference in your own home, but the differences carry over into your children's school activities.

Kim: They always get excellent reviews, not always in math, but always in behavior. When someone is older or in charge, like the babysitter tells them what to do, they do it because they know they choose to lose Nintendo or whatever if they don't. But they still test us.

Dr. L.: Sure. There are some things that don't change; children still try to do some of the things they have always done, but I hear you all saying you are different in the way you respond to what your children are doing. How have you changed personally as a result of the filial therapy training? Have you seen any differences in yourself?

Kim: I would say I have taken a more active role. You gave us the tools to express feelings. I didn't have the words to express myself, and you gave us the words. I really agreed with what you taught about how to discipline without spanking. All of a sudden, that came home to me in one of our classes. You wouldn't hit your coworker if she did something you didn't like. So you are giving more respect to your coworker than your own children. I expressed that to my husband, and it was hard to get him to see things my way. I would take home my stuff every day and show him what we are doing. I would say, "This is what we are going to implement." (Laughter.)

Dr. L.: So you were training him.

Kim: Yeah, I would come home and tell him, "Look, this is the deal." Every once in a while, I will tell him to count to 10 because I could tell he was going to spank. I would tell him, "Would you treat your boss this way?" No, so give the children the same respect. I guess it was the words. I needed the words and I got the words from you just telling me what I am feeling.

Dr. L.: So you are different in that you respond differently and have some tools to teach self-discipline.

Kim: Yeah, I can verbalize what I want, and I can describe the skills we learned. A lot of people I work with are a lot younger than I am and they will come to me and ask me questions about child rearing. Now I can actually put into words my theory of how I parent my children. I can even explain why physical punishment or spanking isn't right.

Dr. L.: So one of the additional changes is you have some reasons now for doing what you do. How about you, Debbie or Laura, have you changed in any way? Are you any different than you were 4 years ago because of the training?

Debbie: I think I'm stronger inside. I think I know what I believe. You encouraged me to trust that I had some correct answers and to believe in myself. Now, when my daughter is pushing me in the wrong direction, I can say, "This isn't right," and I don't have to do it just because she wants it done. I think that helped me to internalize what I was doing.

Dr. L.: So, one of the ways you are stronger is to stand up to your children now—not just give in to them.

Dr. L.: Laura, are you any different?

Laura: When I was in the filial group, I was a single parent and parenting was a real struggle. Trying to do things differently than the way I was raised was really hard. I had lost a lot of the joy of being with my children. That changed while I was in the filial group. I became aware of the consequences of having so much anger and strong feelings inside myself. I learned to be more objective about acknowledging my child's feelings.

Dr. L.: So, you have become more aware of your own feelings. Speaking of feelings, Debbie, I remember one of the things you shared with us was there were times when you didn't like your child.

Debbie: No. No I didn't.

Dr. L.: Can you get back in touch with what that was like and how it changed for you?

Debbie: She was and still is very strong inside herself about what she wants to do and how it should be done. If she wanted to bake a cake, she wouldn't do it the way I asked her to do it. Any kind of interaction with her became a major struggle. I rejected not only what she wanted us to do, but her. And so she was taking in all those feelings. I hated her because she controlled me. It really helped me to learn how to separate her actions from her as a person. Learning how to give her choices and letting her suffer the consequences of her choices was a real turning point for me. I was able to see a little girl, a different little girl emerge.

Kim: We still have the 30-minute playtimes, even though on some Saturdays I just don't want to do it. I do it anyway, because I know the end result will be worth it.

Dr. L.: So, 4 years later you're still having the special playtimes with Toby. You sound really committed to the playtimes.

Kim: Yes, because it is very important. I also have special playtimes with my other two children. My playtimes with Toby are really special and he likes it. You can tell he waits for it. And he knows it will come every Saturday. On vacation, I don't have a playtime, but I take him on a walk for 30 minutes, just the two of us.

Dr. L.: That sounds very satisfying. Laura and Debbie, would you bring us up to date on whether you are still having special playtimes or doing any of the things that you applied during the special playtime?

Laura: We bike ride together or walk together, and we spend time together reading. Dawson needs a lot more of my time than the other two children.

Dr. L.: What's it like for you, Debbie?

Debbie: I still have the 30-minute playtime with Rachel. I incorporate story time with Mark and a quiet time where we have time together. We still do the Sandwich Hug. They like that. I do wish that I was still doing the playtimes, because it does something different than just your reading time and together time. It accomplishes something different.

Dr. L.: Have your children changed?

Kim: Well, it's hard to tell with my littlest one, because the filial approach is all she's ever had, but Toby has definitely changed. Before, he was such a handful, I would throw my hands up in exasperation and not deal with him. Now I deal with him immediately. I drop everything and deal with him because I have found out that it only gets worse. Ignoring bad behavior doesn't work. When I'm in the grocery store and my children start getting disruptive, they know we will walk out and go home. They know I'm serious. They know I'm serious about what I do now.

Dr. L.: So now you will follow through with what you say you are going to do, and they know it.

Kim: If I say we aren't going to do something because of their behavior, they know they are not going to get it. Before, I would have given in. If we had planned to go to the park and they did something they weren't supposed to do, I would still take them to the park because I wanted to go, too. I also learned not to give a choice about things I can't control. If it's not a realistic choice, then they know you won't enforce it. I have learned to limit that so they know whatever I say is definitely going to be done.

Dr. L.: Kim, you sound firm and committed. Laura, 4 years ago you were concerned because Dawson was so demanding. Is that any different?

Laura: Yes. At that time he used to just leave home. He and the dog would just stray off. The doors on our house had deadbolts, but Dawson would go out the window. He would hide underneath the other mobile homes. He could disappear in a minute. I would bolt the doors and he would find another way out. Now, he definitely knows the boundaries. When I call his name, he responds to me and answers me. Before, he wouldn't even answer me.

That has definitely improved. He was very demanding and things had to be his way. If he asks for more time, and doesn't get it, he's no longer destructive. He is much more content now.

Dr. L.: It sounds as though he is calmer. Debbie, 4 years ago, one of the things you were concerned about was Rachel's temper tantrums. She was also very demanding. Is she any different in those areas?

Debbie: Yes. She has changed. She is calmer now. She might cry, but she doesn't throw herself on the floor and try to use guilt trips on me. Even at 4, she was real big on guilt trips. My son is now 4 and he is able to say, "I'm berry, berry, berry angry with you." He doesn't throw a tantrum.

Dr. L.: So, you have seen your children use your skills in identifying feelings.

Debbie: Oh yeah. It's interesting to hear them say it.

Dr. L.: Kim, I saw you shaking your head.

Kim: Yes, my middle child thinks she is the mother of the house. She disciplines her little sister the way I discipline by giving choices. I think it's funny.

Laura: All of my children are more in tune with their feelings and communicate more openly.

Dr. L.: Debbie and Kim, have you seen any differences in your relationships with your husbands because of the training? Are you aware of responding in that relationship any differently?

Debbie: I do. I felt like I grew up during the training. I felt like I took a role and I wasn't a kid anymore. I wasn't throwing tantrums anymore myself. I was able to respond to my husband differently because I was responding to the children differently. Four years ago, I felt like I was fighting with siblings all day long and when my husband came home at night, he was just another sibling to fight with. Everything in our relationship has shifted.

Kim: Some people say money is a sore spot in people's marriages, but I think our problems came from the children. The parenting techniques I learned in the filial training gave me a solid goal for what I wanted. The training also gave me something to back me up on what I wanted. "Excuse me, Dr. Garry Landreth taught me this." (Laughter.)

Kim: I used to say that all the time. When we do the Sandwich Hugs, my husband becomes more emotional, giving kisses and actually showing his love and telling his love. He doesn't do the play sessions, but he sets aside a block of time for each child. I think that helps our relationship, because it makes me so proud to see him being an excellent father. I take pride in the fact that I taught it to him. I think those things have helped our relationship.

Debbie: The filial training has changed my entire life. There are only a handful of things that you can really pinpoint that have significantly changed your life, and the filial training is one of those for me. The 30-minute playtimes gave my daughter confidence and provided a place to work on all the things that I was able to work with her on. The training changed me inside. I keep saying that, but it's important to say that. Once you change in your heart, it spills onto your children. It's not a technique. It's not something you're teaching your children; they are not monkeys. They are not going to perform; change has to begin in their heart.

Dr. L.: It is obvious from listening to you all that parts of the training have become a part of you. And you and your children are different in some ways because of that. I'm sure some of the students in my class would like to ask you all some questions.

Student: It's been 4 years since the three of you had the filial training, and it has made a big impact on you that went from a level of learning a skill to a level that entered your heart. What was it about taking the filial training that made it different for you? How is it different than any other parenting class you may have taken 4 years ago? After the filial training, you all are able to identify tracking, reflecting feelings, and limit-setting skills that you remember 4 years later. I'm not sure you could be that specific about other parenting classes. What makes the difference? Why are you able to recall things from the filial training?

Debbie: Giving choices is probably a good example of what happens and why we can remember. When I began choice giving in the playtimes, choice giving was pretty much surface stuff and superficial, not really life issues as occurs outside the playtimes. Then when I transferred the choice giving to other times outside the playtimes, I began to realize there was a deeper meaning, because the choice giving put the responsibility back on the child and the child learned decision-making skills and morals at 4 years of age, something most of us didn't learn until we were adults. I began to realize I'm making choices and that what I was learning in the class also applied to me.

Dr. L.: So the choice giving had some real-life application immediately.

Debbie: Exactly.

Dr. L.: Kim and Laura, did either of you react to the question?

Kim: Yes, I work at night and don't put the kids to bed four nights a week. I realized that I needed to make a choice about which is more important, me working or putting my kids to bed. They're only going to be in the house another 10 years, so I chose to give up a night of work so I would be at home to put them to bed another night. I made the choice that my children were more important. The filial training infiltrates your mind and everything you do. I think the reason I learned the skills and this new approach to parenting so quickly, and took it on and kept it for 4 years, is because of the simplicity that Dr. Landreth adds to the training. It's easy to say give your children a Sandwich Hug, but just hugging isn't what is important. It's the whole idea of what's behind the hugging. Dr. Landreth just made it so easy by calling it a Sandwich Hug. It sinks into your life.

Dr. L.: Laura, you were reacting.

Laura: We were really active in participating in the training, too. We did the play sessions; we wrote notes to our children; we discussed our playtimes in class—so we were able to apply what we were learning to our lives where we were then. Two years ago I remarried, and I have used the rule of thumb, The most important thing may not be what you do but what you do after what you have done, in my relationship with my husband when I get angry and say things I shouldn't have said. Another thing I use a lot is the 5-minute warning. When we are out somewhere, that helps my children to get ready to leave.

Kim: That is so funny, because I had forgotten that Dr. Landreth taught us that rule of thumb. I just thought that was something I had come up with. (Group laughter.) I was thinking about that principle the other day. So many of the things I use, I have forgotten the source, like the 5-minute warning you mentioned.

Debbie: And the 30-second burst of attention was fabulous.

Dr. L.: So these skills have become a part of you. You don't even think about where you got them. Other questions?

Student: What did you all look forward to each time you were preparing to go to class?

Debbie: The sharing. We would have this big huge problem and Dr. Landreth would say, "Here, try this." He was so soft and calm. The next week we would run back to class and say, "That worked!" The sharing was the greatest for me.

Kim: For me, it was empowerment. The more classes I went to, I got more and more power as a parent.

Dr. L.: We need to stop for today. I want to thank you for sharing so personally with us today.

The personal sharing of Debbie and the other parents makes it quite clear that the filial therapy training helped them gain a sense of personal adequacy and empowerment not only as a parent, but also in other relationships in their lives.

13-Year Follow-Up with Debbie

In July 2004, I conducted a CPRT workshop in the Center for Play Therapy Summer Play Therapy Institute on the University of North Texas campus and invited Debbie to share her experience with the workshop participants. As a part of the training experience, I had shown video segments of Debbie's filial therapy group (with their permission) so the participants already had a limited acquaintance with Debbie.

Dr. L.: Group, this is Debbie, 13 years later. Debbie, I'm sure everyone is eager to hear what you remember about the filial therapy training and what impact it had on you.

Debbie: First of all, I would like to say thank you to Dr. Landreth because he empowered me as a parent to do what I needed to do with my child. Prior to the filial therapy lessons, I had a 4-year-old daughter who was pretty much running the household, and she would tell me what to do. To give you an example, we would be in my van driving, and I would start to sing a song. She would say, "No! We're not singing that song!" So I would say, "Ok, what song are we going to sing?" My thought was if Rachel was happy, I was happy. And she would say, "We are going to sing 'Jesus Loves Me.'" So I would start singing. Then she would tell me what part of the song I was going to sing, how long I was to sing, and when I was supposed to stop singing it.

This is what I lived with day in and day out, a child telling me what to do. I didn't know any better, so I would do what she told me to do. I was under the assumption that if she was happy, everything was OK. But I felt inside myself major frustration and anger. I can still remember the comment I made in the filial group saying the anger came out of frustration. My rejection of Rachel came from not knowing what to do with her. She was a bundle of energy and she was in control. At 18 months, she was telling me what she was going to wear. Her being in control started very young. I had no parent training. Most parents don't. I didn't have anywhere to go for the basic tools of child communication, so I pushed her away. I was so angry with her and tired of her. I put her in day care because I didn't know how to deal with her.

I don't know how I found out about Dr. Landreth's class, I was just told about it. I came to his class, and he began to teach us how to relate to our children. As you saw in the videos, I was really involved in the training because I was so eager to learn how to be a parent. I started the training with the idea of learning how to control my child. How can I make my child do what I want to do? How do I make her sing the songs I want to sing? I discovered in the training that as Dr. Landreth began to give me tools to use, I wanted to know more. I didn't miss any of the sessions. I was in his face every session asking him all my questions about parenting. He wrote my questions down saying, "We will work on that later." I was probably one of the parents he wanted to go to and say, "Will you please leave my group." (Laughter.) "The other people need to talk."

Rachel was a very precious little girl, but she controlled our lives. She was very strong-willed and determined. I didn't see those as good personality traits, which she still exhibits today. But back then, she ruled the house. Logically, I could not understand going into a 30-minute play session and allowing her to control it. It didn't make any sense because she was already controlling my life. In the filial training, I realized the change needed to be in me, not in my daughter.

In the special playtimes, I could relax because most of what Rachel did there was OK. Actually, she learned very quickly where the boundaries were. I didn't have to explain the rules to her ahead of time. Those special playtimes began to change me and the way I viewed my daughter. I began to see her in a more positive way, that she wasn't really trying to make my life miserable all the time. The skills I learned to use in the special playtimes worked; they were wonderful and I began using them outside the playtimes. I sensed a change in Rachel. It was as though she knew there was a change in the atmosphere of our relationship. She had more freedom in her choices and she became less demanding of me.

The infant you all saw in the video of one of our filial therapy training sessions is my son. I saw things that came out in our play sessions that helped me to understand what Rachel was feeling about the new baby. Even though I had to set limits and boundaries on her behavior, our new relationship was so freeing to me that all my anger began to evaporate. Today, we have a wonderful sharing relationship, and Rachel wanted to come with me today to hear what I have to say to you all.

Dr. L.: Rachel, stand up so the group can see you. (Applause.)

Debbie: Rachel remembers our special playtimes and the different things we did together. The important thing about Rachel is that she is extremely self-sufficient today. She is very strong-willed but that is tempered with sensitivity to other people. She has a lot of confidence in herself. She tackles problems and goes after a lot of things I wouldn't dream of doing. And she is very successful doing the things she has chosen to do.

If I had not had the filial therapy training and learned the skills and tools I was taught, there's no telling what Rachel's personality traits would have become and what would have been manifested in them. There is just no doubt when I say that the filial therapy and the tools I received changed my life. It changed my home, it changed my family, it changed everything.

Dr. L.: Thank you Debbie. Would you all like to ask Debbie a question?

(Question asked by audience member.)

Dr. L.: The question is, Debbie, did you continue to do the play sessions after the training ended?

Debbie: Yes, I continued them for a little while. Then, as my son got older, it became a little more difficult to do. As

Rachel got older, we changed the structure of the playtimes to doing special things together, like going shopping and allowing her to make decisions about where to shop and what we would do, but she didn't decide how much money to spend.

Rachel is now 17, my middle child is 13, and I have a 10-year-old. Instead of a playtime, I give each of them 20 dollars, and they decide what we are going to do for our special time together. It is a time where I let go. It's an internal letting go and the focus of the time is on them. Even though it isn't a playtime with toys, it is still basically the same thing because each child has all of my attention and none of my control during our special date time.

Dr. L.: Is there another question or two you would like to ask?

(Question asked by audience member.)

Dr. L.: Debbie, the question is what specific changes did you make after the training?

Debbie: Everything. The way I approached Rachel, the way I dealt with her, the way I even saw her. One of the first assignments Dr. Landreth gave us was to notice a physical characteristic about our child that we had not noticed before. I had to go home and look at Rachel in a wondering way and for a few minutes in that process I saw her differently. Another change was that, in the special playtimes, I stopped emotionally pushing her away from me. Before the training, I rejected her because I didn't know how to deal with her.

I recognized Rachel wasn't very happy having all of the control I allowed her to have. With that awareness, my attitude about myself began to change. It was amazing what happened when I began taking control of myself and began giving Rachel choices. I started using choices, setting boundaries, and setting limits in my interactions with Rachel. It was just amazing what wonderful things happened in our relationship. I think we both began to like each other better.

Dr. L.: Thank you so much for sharing with us, Debbie. I appreciate you being here. (Applause.)

Debbie was eager to share her experiences in these interviews and continues to be a strong advocate for filial therapy training. Perhaps I should point out that I had no contact with Debbie after the conclusion of the filial therapy training until I contacted her just prior to the 4-year follow-up interview. After that interview, I lost contact with her until 1 year prior to the 13-year follow-up session, when she happened to learn that I was teaching a family-focused training class and joined the group.

CHAPTER 24

SOLUTIONS TO COMMON PROBLEMS AND QUESTIONS PARENTS AND CHILDREN ASK

Therapists who plan to use filial therapy need to be prepared to answer questions parents may ask about filial therapy training. Anticipating many of these questions and responding to them in the intake interview or during the first filial therapy training session can help alleviate parents' confusion and anxiety, thus helping parents to relax, feel more secure about the training, make a commitment to the process, and more readily engage in the process of learning new skills.

Questions Parents Ask About CPRT

Question: **How will having playtimes with my child correct his behavior problems? He already plays with toys a lot.**

Response: That does seem unlikely, doesn't it, that a special playtime could help change behavior problems? Yes, most children play with toys a lot. However, they usually are not playing with a parent in the kind of relationship I am going to teach you to build with your child. The special playtime you will have with your child is a different kind of playtime, a time when you will work on building a different kind of relationship with your child. We have found that when children experience a play relationship in which they feel accepted, understood, and cared for, they play out many of their problems. They feel better about themselves, they develop self-control, and they assume greater self-responsibility. How children feel about themselves is what makes a significant difference in their behavior. In these special playtimes where parents learn to focus on the child rather than the problem, children learn to correct their own behavior because how children behave, how they think, and how they perform in school is directly related to how they feel about themselves. When children's needs are met in the special playtimes, their behavior problems diminish. When children feel better about themselves, they behave in more self-enhancing ways rather than self-defeating ways.

Question: **How do I explain to my child why we are having these special playtimes?**

Response: Tell your child, "I like to be with you, and I want to spend more time with you, so I am taking a special class to learn how to play with you." This helps to make the playtime really special. Your child can brag to his friends that his parent is taking a special class to learn how to play with him. How many other children can say that? That makes it a big deal. Your child doesn't need a lengthy explanation and facts are not necessary. Yes, you are experiencing some problems with your child, but the reason you are having the playtimes is to build a better relationship with your child, not to fix the problem.

Question: **We live in a really small apartment. There's just no place for a special playtime.**

Response: The special playtime should be scheduled for a time when other family members are out and could take place in your kitchen. Another possibility is to fold a blanket, place it on the floor in one of your rooms, and designate the blanket as the special place for the playtime each week. The borders of the blanket become the boundaries for the playtime. If you can only have the special playtime when other family members are home, you can use the bathroom as your private place. Although not ideal, this space can work quite well. It is important that your child have a private time and place where other family members will not watch or interrupt.

Question: I am a single mom with three kids, and I just can't keep the other two, ages 4 and 8, out of my special playtimes with my 6-year-old.

Response: Their behavior is normal and may indicate they want to have their own special playtime with you. You could ask a friend or relative to take the 4- and 8-year-old for a special time at the park or to get a treat. You might be able to swap some time with another single parent. Be sure to explain to your children that you will be having a playtime with them in 5 weeks or 8 weeks (identify the number of play sessions left in the first child's sequence of 10 sessions). In the meantime, each child can choose to do something special each week with you: read a story, bake cookies together, go get an ice cream cone, or some other special time. You might swap babysitting with a friend or neighbor who could babysit your 4- and 8-year-old while you have your playtime. You could give the 8-year-old babysitting responsibility for the 4-year-old during the 30 minutes of the playtime and pay her to play with the 4-year-old and keep him out of your playtime. You might try having the playtime in the evening after the 4-year-old has gone to bed and elicit the 8-year-old's cooperation. If that doesn't work, you could use choice giving with the 8-year-old: "If you choose to stay out of the room while I am having a playtime, you choose to get to watch TV that day. If you choose to interrupt the playtime, you choose not to get to watch TV that day."

Question: **My son is 10 years old and probably isn't going to be interested in most of the toys on this list. How do I get him to play?**

Response: This is your child's time to decide what to do for 30 minutes. Whether or not he plays with the toys is his decision. He might decide to talk for 30 minutes. There is no requirement that your child play. However, our experience is that even 10-year-old children find very creative things to do with the toys on this list. Some of the things your child does with the toys may surprise you, or you may have difficulty accepting some of the ways your child chooses to play, such as ignoring you and playing silently for 30 minutes, or sucking on the baby bottle. One of the parents in our filial therapy training reported that her 9-year-old daughter chose to sit in the middle of the bed and talk for 30 minutes during her first play session. In succeeding play sessions, she played actively with the toys. Let's find out how your child reacts to the toys. If he chooses not to play with any of the toys, we will talk about adding some different toys.

Question: **What's wrong with asking questions if I am interested in my child's play?**

Response: Tracking statements that describe what you see and statements that reflect the content and feeling of what you hear convey your interest in a more positive and encouraging way. Questions imply you don't understand. Questions also put you in the lead in the relationship and can interfere with your child's creativity and decision making during the playtime. It is important that your child be allowed to stay in the lead and discover how it feels to make his own decisions for 30 minutes.

Question: **I don't see anything significant in my child's play. What can I do to help her begin to work on her problem during our playtime?**

Response: The relationship you are building with your child during the special playtimes is more important than whether or not your child is working on a problem. As your relationship with your child is strengthened, your child's problem will diminish. Your child may be working on issues through her play that you are not aware of. Remember the lesson of the Band-Aid (see transcript of CPRT Session 2 in Chapter 9). What you are doing in the playtimes is working even when you don't see any change. Children can change as a result of what they do in play sessions with parents or play therapists even though we are not aware of what they are working on. Your job during the special playtimes is to follow your child's lead and to be nonjudgmental, understanding, and accepting of your child. Your empathic responses will help your child to focus on the issues that are important to her.

Question: **My child really likes to play with these toys, and keeping them out of his hands is a major problem. Why can't I let him play with them at other times?**

Response: Allowing your child to play with these toys only during the 30-minute playtimes helps to convey the message that this is a special time, a time just for the two of you, a fun time. Setting the toys apart makes the playtime unique and more desirable. Another reason is that this time with your child is an emotional relationship time and the toys become a part of that emotional relationship during which your child expresses and explores emotional messages through the toys because of the kinds of empathic responses you make. This same kind of emotional exploration cannot occur during other playtimes because you are not there to communicate understanding of your child's play. Additionally, being allowed to play with these toys only during the special playtimes helps your child learn to delay his need for gratification. If you are having trouble keeping your child from playing with the special toy kit, try storing it out of sight on the top shelf of your closet. If that doesn't work, lock it in the trunk of your car.

Question: **I always thought it was good to praise my child. What's wrong with praising for doing a good job?**

Response: Praise is evaluative, judgmental, and leading. "Oh, that's such a beautiful picture you painted" communicates an evaluation of the picture and reinforces the child to paint similar pictures to obtain similar praise, thus stifling the child's creativity and self-direction. A person who makes such praise statements also has the power to evaluate the picture to be ugly, and that is what a child fears. A statement such as, "*You worked hard on that picture*," or "*You put a lot of colors in that picture*," recognizes the child's effort or prizes what the child has done. How your child feels about herself is always more important than what your child does. Praising what a child does results in children becoming externally motivated to seek praise for what they produce by pleasing. Recognizing a child's effort results in children becoming internally motivated. Such children are more creative, have better self-concepts, and are self-motivated. **Rule of Thumb: Recognize the child's effort rather than praising the product.**

If your child is persistent about seeking praise—"Do you like my picture?"—and you have already responded with "*You put lots of colors on your picture*," "*You're proud of your picture*," "*You worked hard on your picture*," etc., you can say, "*I know you want me to decide if I like your picture, but during our special playtime, the important thing is whether or not you like your picture.*"

Question: **I'm having trouble finding some of the items on the toy list. Is it really important that I have all of this stuff?**

Response: The toys are like words for your child, and play is your child's language, so it would be helpful for you to try to find as many of the items as possible. All of the items are on the list because we have found they help children act out a wide range of experiences and express a wide range of feelings about those experiences. You should go ahead and have your play sessions and add the missing items as soon as possible. Let's take a few minutes and find out what toys everyone had trouble finding and share information about where some of you found the toys that other parents are having trouble locating. The toys don't have to be new or best quality. Check out garage sales, dollar stores, and grocery store toy aisles.

Question: **I'm bored. What's the value of this if my child just plays with the same toy over and over? Am I doing something wrong?**

Response: Playing with the same toy or playing out the same theme repetitively is not unusual for some children and may indicate they are trying to master a new skill, solve a problem, or work through an intense emotion or something significant in their life. Play that is repeated within a session or across several sessions may be the result of a child trying to process and integrate a new experience or previous event into his life, or it may be the child's way of expressing a particular need in his life. The important consideration is whether or not the child seems interested and involved in the play. If the child is interested, then the play has meaning for the child and something important is happening. It is not necessary that you figure out the meaning.

Being bored in a playtime is not an unusual happening because parents have busy schedules, are on the go a lot, and are not used to sitting and interacting quietly for 30 minutes. You can increase your interest level and involvement in your child's play by responding to what you see in your child's face, asking yourself questions such as, "What is he feeling?" "What is he trying to say in his play?" "What does he need from me?" "What is so interesting to him about the toy or the play?" and by making more tracking responses and reflective responses. The most important thing you can do is continue to be patient with the process of the play sessions. (Being bored may be an indication that the parent has not acquired the necessary skills or is not putting enough effort into using the new skills. In either case, additional training in the form of modeling and role-playing the skills of tracking and empathic responding is needed.)

Question: **My child asks lots of questions and gets mad when I don't answer all of them. What am I supposed to do?**

Response: We always begin by reflecting the child's feelings. "*You're angry at me.*" Sometimes a child feels insecure when a parent changes typical ways of responding and is angry because he doesn't know how to react. Your child may feel insecure and be trying to get your attention the way he has done in the past. Your objective is to encourage your child's self-reliance and self-acceptance. "*In our special playtime, the answer can be anything you want it to be.*" Your child asks, "What should I draw?" You want your child to know he's in charge of his drawing during the special playtime, so you respond, "*You've decided to draw, and in this special playtime, you can draw whatever you decide.*" Our objective is to empower the child, to enable the child to discover his own strengths.

Question: **What do I do when my child wants my help?**

Response: This is a playtime, this is not a time to sit and observe your child. You are to be involved in and a part of your child's play as you might at other times, with one major difference—you are to get instructions from your child. You are not to assume you know what your child wants or how your child wants something done. Remember, for 30 minutes, you are dumb. Therefore, you will need to get instruction and direction from your child. "*Show me where you want me to line up the soldiers.*" "*Tell me what you want me to cook for breakfast.*" "*We can go to the kitchen, and you can show me what you want in the baby bottle.*" "*You can show me what kind of cat you want me to draw.*" Your objective is to keep your child in the lead so your child experiences making decisions and doing things for himself.

Question: **My child wanted to leave after 10–15 minutes. What am I supposed to do?**

Response: You always want to communicate your understanding, so you could say, "*You would like to go do something else, but we have 15 more minutes in our special playtime. I would like to be with you longer. When could we have our whole playtime?*" Another possible approach would be to reflect your child's desire to leave and add, "*We have 15 more minutes in our special playtime. I will tell you when you have 10 more minutes, and then you can decide to stop or play for the last 10 minutes.*" This is a time to negotiate. Forcing your child to stay another 15 minutes might interfere with the reason for having the special playtime. On the other hand, the relationship can't be worked on if the child is not present. Patient understanding is needed. The important thing is that the special playtime occur this week sometime. That is more important than adhering to the scheduled time.

Question: **When it was time for our special playtime, my child didn't want to participate at all. What can I do?**

Response: Communicating understanding is always important. "*You don't want to have the special playtime. You would rather do something else. Let's have the special playtime for 10 minutes, then you can decide if* *you want to have the rest of the special playtime or do something else.*" This response helps your child to feel understood and to feel in control. A child in that position in a relationship is much more likely to compromise. In most cases, a child will get started playing and will decide to have the rest of the playtime.

Question: **Why can't I have a special playtime with each of my children each week or rotate each week so each child gets a playtime with me?**

Response: You have three children, so that would mean three playtimes each week. My experience is that parents are very busy and being consistent in having just one playtime each week can often become a problem. I wish you had the time to have two or three playtimes each week with each of your children. It is crucial, though, that you be absolutely consistent in having the playtime each week so you and the playtime become predictable. This communicates a powerful message to your child that he is important, so important that nothing will interfere with your special playtime with him. Let's begin with a playtime each week with just one child and see how that works out with your schedule. We'll consider adding playtimes with the other children later.

You can learn best how to build this new kind of relationship by having the playtimes with the same child each week for 8 or 10 weeks. All of your children do not always need you equally at the same time in their lives. Which of your children needs you most at this time in their life, or which child are you having the most difficulty with now? That is the child who needs the special playtimes most right now. If all three of your children climb a tree in the back yard, and one child fall out of the tree and breaks a leg, which child will you take to the emergency room at the hospital? Yes, the one with the broken leg. Why not take all three children to the emergency room? Because two of them don't have a broken leg, so they don't need you as much at that time as does the child with the broken leg. In 8 or 10 weeks, we will talk about you adding playtimes with the other children or rotating playtimes so each child gets a playtime with you.

Questions Children Ask and Comments They Make about the Play Sessions

One of the most common concerns of parents in the early stages of CPRT training is how to respond to children's questions and unexpected comments. Parents frequently feel unprepared for the barrage of questions children have during the initial play sessions and the surprising comments they make. Therefore, the therapist will need to help parents anticipate some of the questions and comments children may spontaneously present and formulate short, standard responses parents will be able to readily call to mind when needed. This preparation will do a lot to ease parents' anxieties and help them to feel more in control in the new experience of a nondirected play relationship.

A common practice of children is to ask the parent a multitude of questions, which may be their way of making contact with the parent in this new playtime relationship. However, the parent should consider that children already know the answer to many of the questions they ask. Examined from this perspective, responding to children's questions becomes a matter of trying to understand the motivation behind the question rather than attempting to provide an answer. Providing answers to questions can inhibit children's use of items by binding children to the parents' world of reality. When 5-year-old Hershel holds up the handcuffs and asks, "What are these?" and his parent answers, "Handcuffs," they can no longer be the special new kind of spaceship he was thinking about. The parent could facilitate the coming forth of Hershel's creativity and imagination by responding, "*That can be whatever you want it to be.*" Hershel is then free to proceed with what he already had in mind but had not verbalized. When Judy asks, "*What happens if something gets broken in here?*" a sensitive parent would respond, "*Sometimes accidents happen in here.*" Judy then knows this is not a place of punishment, or a place where you must be careful. She then feels freer to express herself more spontaneously and completely.

RULE OF THUMB:

Don't answer questions that haven't been asked.

Answers to obvious questions can result in lengthy question-and-answer routines that increase children's dependency. When children ask questions during special playtimes, the parent would do well to consider what the underlying meanings are before responding to what seems to be the objective of their questions. Trying to anticipate what children are saying in their questions, rather than attempting to answer the questions, is usually much more facilitative of expression and exploration. What the parent senses at the moment would determine the kind of response to be made.

Question: **What do you want me to do?**

Response: "*In this special playtime, you can decide what you want to do.*" (This response clarifies the special nature of the playtime and returns responsibility to the child. We do not worry about the possibility that this response may result in the child deciding to do something that would not be allowed. The need to set a limit is not considered until the moment a limit is needed. The parent does not suggest any activities or offer any solutions for the duration of the 30-minute playtime.)

Question: **Can I play with my computer game?**

Response: "*It would be fun to play with your computer game, but these are the toys for playing with during our special playtime. You can play with your computer game later today if there's time.*" (The alternative should be truly an alternative. Don't say something you can't follow through on. Items that are not similar to the filial therapy items are not allowed in the special playtime because they are too structured, do not facilitate playing out personal experiences by the child, and do not allow the child to express a wide range of emotions. (The response recognizes the child's desire, gently sets a limit, and grants fulfillment at a later time, thus communicating understanding and conveying to the child that he will get to do what he wants. This elicits the child's cooperation and avoids an adversarial position. The words "later today" are deliberately chosen instead of "after our playtime is over" because computer games are so highly attractive to many children that saying, "after our playtime is over" might result in the child then insisting on ending the playtime.)

Question: **Can we go play outside?**

Response: "*You would like to play outside, but our special playtime is for this room. You can choose to play outside when our special playtime is over.*" (Reflects the child's desire and communicates that the child will get to go outside later. There are too many distractions outside and too many opportunities for unexpected happenings for the inexperienced parent to handle. The confined area inside the house helps promote the desired relationship. After the sixth or seventh play session, it would probably be OK to allow the playtime outside, but with all the playtime structure and requirements intact.)

Question: **Why can't we play longer?**

Response: "*You're really having fun and would like to play a lot longer, but our special playtime is over for today. We will have another special playtime next Tuesday.*" (Even though parent and child are having lots of fun, the time limit is adhered to because this promotes consistency, affords the parent an opportunity to be firm, and provides the child with an opportunity to bring himself under control and end a very desirable playtime. If your child persists, you could say, "Joey, I wish we had more time, too, but our 30 minutes are up for today. We'll get to have another playtime next Tuesday.")

Question: **Why do you keep saying what I say?**

Response: "*Sounds like what I am saying bothers you. I just want to let you know I understand what you are saying and what you are playing, so you will know I am interested.*" (There is the possibility the parent is reflecting word-for-word exactly what the child says too often, or the parent sounds too stilted and unnatural, and it is irritating to the child.)

Question: **You sound weird. Why are you talking like that?**

Response: "*I sound different to you. That's my way of letting you know I heard what you said. Remember, I'm going to that special class to learn how to play with you.*" (The child may be saying he notices the parent is different; having a surprise reaction to the verbal attention; annoyed by too much reflection of words; or saying he notices the difference in the parent's reflective-type responses. The child may also be saying he doesn't want the parent to change because that will mean he must then change and adjust to the parent's new way of responding.)

Comment: **Guess what I am going to do next.**

Response: "*You have something in mind you are going to do. You can tell me.*" (A variation might be "*Sounds like you have something planned. You can tell me.*" This shows understanding and frees the child to continue to be in the lead. Guessing what the child will do next places the parent in the lead and is structuring because the child may then feel obligated to do what the parent guesses. Trying to guess what a child will do next could go on indefinitely. If the child is unusually insistent or demanding, as some older children might be, you might want to consider going along with the child's insistence and making a guess.)

Question: **Do you know what I am going to do next?**

Response: "*You have something planned. You can tell me.*" (This response says, "I heard your underlying message," and keeps the child in the lead. The child is really making a statement rather than asking a question. A response should be directed to what the child is saying rather than respond to the obvious question.)

Question: **What is this?**

Response: "*That can be whatever you want it to be.*" (This response keeps the child in the lead, returns responsibility to the child, and frees the child to label the item whatever the child wants it to be. There are several subtle possibilities in this child's question: She might be unfamiliar with the toy and unsure of how it is supposed to be used, trying to decide what she would like to do with the toy, testing the permissiveness of the special playtime, trying to engage the parent, seeking direction or approval from the parent, or wanting to use the item for something other than the apparent use. Labeling the item would prevent any of these possibilities from being expressed.)

Comment: **I'm bored.**

Response: "*You're not having any fun. This is a time when you can decide what you want us to do. You can decide to play with the toys, or talk, or create something.*" (This response shows understanding and returns responsibility to the child to decide how she wants to spend the time together. Such a comment by a child is often disconcerting to a parent, resulting in the parent feeling responsible to make the child happy, a behavior usually typical of the relationship outside the playtime. The parent is not responsible for the child's happiness in the special playtime. Conveying this principle to parents prior to their special playtimes can help prevent some of their anxiety.)

Problems and Solutions in CPRT Training

The unique dimensions of CPRT in training parents to be therapeutic agents in their children's lives creates a number of problems for the filial therapist that must be dealt with prior to initiating filial therapy training and during the process of training. A few of those potential problems and possible solutions are presented here to help the filial therapist anticipate and prepare for their occurrence.

Problem: Making the transition from being a therapist to being a teacher/trainer.

Solution: Mental health professionals who pursue training in filial therapy typically have had little or no training or experience as a teacher, educator, or supervisor. This issue is explored again in this section because many of the skills required of a filial therapist go counter to much of what a therapist does with clients. Since most mental health professionals do not have a background of training or experience as a teacher or educator, they may lack the basic skills required to involve individuals in a learning process. They have graduated from graduate programs that have emphasized broad philosophical and theoretical issues and conceptual skills. Many graduate classes in these programs encourage a learning-on-your-own approach. These approaches to learning, while appropriate for graduate students, are not effective in training parents to be therapeutic agents in their children's lives. The filial therapist must make the transition from therapist to the task of teaching specific skills, and these skills must be taught in small incremental steps—no exploration of broad conceptual issues here. In filial therapy, the focus is on developing specific skills and accepting attitudes.

Becoming a filial therapist requires a significant shift in the mental health professional's emphasis in a number of significant dimensions: the identified client, focus on what is deemed important, identified objectives in the therapist–client relationship, methodology utilized in working toward a solution of the problem, skills employed in facilitating behavioral change, and personal need fulfillment. Parents generally seek out filial therapy because they are having "problems" with their children, but in filial therapy, the therapist does not work directly with the identified children.

The relationship between parents and children occupies the central focus of the filial therapist, yet the therapist is dependent on the parent to develop a therapeutic relationship with the child that will facilitate change.

Unlike counseling relationships, wherein the identified objective is the emotional growth of the clients, in filial therapy, the objective is facilitation of the acquisition of therapeutic skills by parents. The methodology utilized in working toward a solution of the problem is teaching and training, a procedure foreign to most mental health professionals because they do not have experiential backgrounds in teaching and training. Although some mental health professionals have natural teaching skills, most have not been attracted to teaching methodology because it does not meet their needs for close interpersonal relationships, or planning and organization have a low priority in their need fulfillment. Supervised experience in leading a filial therapy group is key to the beginning filial therapist in learning what the teaching process is like. This discovery is described in the self-critique of a graduate student:

> The most important thing that I learned in this session is that I know more information than I give myself credit for. I was really worried about teaching parents what I know about play therapy, but I found out that I could do it! I learned that I can teach this material! I thought that since I did not have teaching experience, I would not be able to teach parents very well. It is my interest and passion for working with children in play therapy that inspires me to teach everything that I know to parents. I believe that it is this love for what I am doing that helps make me a better teacher.

The skills employed by parents in interactions with their children in the special playtimes to facilitate behavioral change are basic Child-Centered Play Therapy skills, and the filial therapist must be able to train parents in how to incorporate those skills into their interactions with their children. Therefore, filial therapists must first be competent and experienced child-centered play therapists. Second, they must be able to skillfully train parents in the appropriate use of Child-Centered Play Therapy principles and skills, and in that process they must be able to draw on their own play therapy experiences to add sparkle to the learning process.

The solution to this problem can only be thorough training and experience in play therapy, and then in-depth filial therapy training and experience that have a strong component focused on how to be an effective trainer and supervisor. Just as parents do not automatically know how to parent effectively simply because they become parents, mental health professionals do not automatically know how to be effective trainers just because they decide to become filial therapists.

Problem: Covering all of the specified material for each filial therapy training session.

Solution: One of the problems that plagues inexperienced filial therapists and filial therapists who do not have a background of teaching experience is staying on track each session and covering the designated material for that session. Organizational experience, a sense of timing, and group facilitation skills are needed to keep the group moving toward the learning objectives for each session. Each session should begin on time. This may mean interrupting social conversations that are generated as parents wait for the session to begin. Beginning on time models for the parents what is expected of them in their play sessions and communicates to the parents that they are expected to be on time for the training sessions.

The therapist must be able to keep the group from getting bogged down in relating personal stories, child behaviors that are problematic, or issues that sidetrack the discussion from the learning topic at hand. The key is organization, organization, organization. The therapist should be well prepared prior to each session with the agenda well thought out, handouts ready, homework assignments prepared, and toys for role-playing and video equipment ready prior to the parents arrival. The prescribed material must be covered or parents won't be prepared to conduct play sessions, nor will they be successful in doing so.

The therapist may find it helpful to make an agenda outline for each training session showing topics to be covered and activities, such as viewing a video or role-playing, to be utilized, and assign specific clock times to each topic and activity. The therapist will then know, for example, that at 3:10 parent role-playing should begin. A brief time outline for CPRT training Session 2 might be:

2:00	Review homework
2:15	Empathic responding, demonstrate with a parent playing role of her child
2:45	View video of therapist playtime
2:55	Explain basic principles and guidelines of 30-minute play sessions
3:10	Parents role-play in pairs
3:20	List of toys to be used in special playtimes; show toys and demonstrate responding
3:50	Select a time and place for special playtimes and assign empathic response sheet
4:00	Adjourn

At times it may be necessary to cut off discussion and say, "We need to move on to the next activity for today." Such structuring, although difficult for therapists because they are accustomed to following the client's lead and facilitating exploration, is essential because 2 hours with an active group of parents can zip by in a hurry. In early training sessions especially, parents often bring up problematic issues, such as bedtime problems, that are unrelated to the training at hand. These concerns are responded to respectfully, and the therapist tells the parent, "I am making a note about your concern" (writes note to self), "and we will come back to the bedtime problem in later sessions. Right now, we need to work on . . ." Writing a reminder note gives the parent a sense that she was heard and reassures the parent that the therapist recognizes the importance of the problem to the parent and that the problem is being dealt with. Many of these concerns are not an issue in filial therapy training for a couple or one parent.

Problem: Parents who do not complete homework assignments or have persistent difficulty applying the skills.

Solution: Not all parents enter CPRT with an equal commitment to developing a new approach to relating to their children. Some parents enter filial therapy training to get their children "fixed" by the therapist and may be reluctant to enter fully into the training regimen because they want a quick fix for their children's behavioral problems. Many parents in filial therapy training are stressed by the problems they experience with their children and may feel helpless. Given such circumstances, it is understandable that some parents may not think homework assignments are important. After all, it has been years since a teacher gave them a homework assignment, so they show up with nothing to report. As exasperating as this may be for the therapist, patience and an encouraging attitude from the therapist are the rules of the day. It may be necessary to clarify for parents that the problems they are concerned about will be worked on in their special play sessions as they utilize their skills as therapeutic agents in their children's lives. Helping parents understand how the homework assignments relate to their roles in the play sessions and their relationships with their children will be encouragement enough for most parents. The key to working with the reluctant parent is persistent encouragement and an attitude of expectancy.

Sitting down privately with the reluctant parent for tutoring on the homework and exploring the difficulty with the homework often will elicit cooperation. The therapist may discover during this one-on-one time that the content of the homework assignment reminded the parent of an unresolved emotional issue that resulted in the parent avoiding the homework assignment. Exploring such issues can be very releasing to the parent and free the parent to become more directly involved in the training.

Some of the skills taught in CPRT training may touch on a parent's difficulty in his or her life or relationships and may result in the parent persistently having unusual difficulty in applying some of the skills. Sometimes these issues can be worked through quickly in the group, as in the case of a mother who had difficulty applying limits effectively in her play sessions. As she struggled with the dynamics of trying to set limits, she fairly quickly gained insight into her own long-standing struggle with boundary issues. In the course of the training session discussions, she shared the following insight into her difficulty:

> I was the youngest and was spoiled rotten. I never had any limits. Setting limits has been the hardest thing for me. I wanted my children to like me so much, to be their friend. I wanted my children to know that they were

> loved all the time, and it was hard to discipline them. But I've learned that disciplining them is loving them. Now I'm not afraid to go to restaurants. Now, my children are so much more in control of their behavior.

Asking a parent who is having persistent difficulty in applying certain skills to make a video of her play session, and critiquing the video with the parent, will often produce quick insight on the part of the parent. This approach must be undertaken with much patience and sensitivity to the threatening nature of the experience. When a point of difficulty is observed in the video, it is sometimes helpful to stop the video and ask the parent if she is aware of what is needed at that point or how her response needs to be changed. The therapist will need to avoid providing a quick answer or solution. It is more important that the parent make the discovery and, in the process, achieve insight. If the parent is unaware of what needs to be done, replay the segment a couple of times if needed. When the parent is able to provide an acceptable response, the therapist can then offer a self-esteem-building response to the parent: "There, you figured it out," or "You knew how to respond all along. It just didn't come out." This could then be a good time to explore what was blocking the response. The therapist should role-play various scenarios of the situation several times with the parent to help the parent feel comfortable with the new "language."

Do not assume that the parent's difficulty is a result of a crisis the parent is experiencing. Although this may be a factor, our experiences with incarcerated parents, single parents, nonoffending parents of sexually abused children, and many other parents in crisis situations have shown that these parents can quickly learn the skills taught in CPRT training. Parents, as is true of children, are quite resilient and, given an understanding, supportive, encouraging, and safe environment, can and will learn, change, and draw upon their inner coping mechanisms.

Problem: Parents who are noncompliant or inconsistent in having parent-child play sessions at home.

Solution: A good starting place to process this problem is to ask the parent, "What do you think you need to do differently to solve the problem?" Any confrontation with parents who are having difficulty must always be done gently. The therapist is always attempting to understand the parent's viewpoint. Parents who are not compliant in having playtimes at home may have serious doubts about their ability to use the skills that have been taught even though they may have adequately demonstrated use of the skills in role-playing experiences with toys in training sessions. Patient encouragement, although highly recommended, seldom results in these parents changing their behavior because they are convinced they will "mess up." A personal interview with the parent may be necessary to clarify the underlying causes for the noncompliance. If the therapist determines that self-doubt is the central factor, one solution is to schedule the parent to bring his child of focus to the agency or therapist's office at a time other than the CPRT training time for supervision and video-recording of their play session. In the supervision feedback time, the therapist is especially sensitive and responsive to the parent's feelings of anxiety and apprehension and responds with encouragement and support by pointing out specific positive responses and skills the parent exhibited. A part of the video can then be shown in the next CPRT training session. The other parents are usually sensitive to the noncompliant parent's reluctance and are generous in their praise and support, thus breaking down defensive barriers.

If a deeper emotional issue of rejection or resentment of the child by the parent emerges in the personal interview as the basis for the noncompliant behavior, exploration of the issue can proceed rapidly because the filial therapist has already established a therapeutic relationship with the parent. This initial therapy session can be such a powerful insight-producing experience that the parent will decide to go home and have her first parent-child play session. If nothing seems to work with the noncompliant parent, the therapist may need to have a private session with the parent and suggest that in light of the difficulty the parent is having in following through with the special playtimes, this may not be a good time for the parent to be in filial therapy training.

Problem: Resistant parents.

Solution: When parents are resistant to the training, look for underlying causes. Some parents are threatened by the possibility of changing their typical reactions to their children because changing may mean having to accept the fact that what they have been doing has not worked. Other parents are resistant because they came to filial therapy with the expectation that the therapist would change their children, and then they discover there are some attitudes and behaviors they are expected to change.

Dealing with a resistant parent can be frustrating to the beginning filial therapist, as revealed in this self-critique:

> An area for improvement involves my discomfort in redirecting or keeping a parent on task. During the first part of this third training session, I divided the group into dyads to practice reflection. Mr. Smith was very hesitant to practice his reflection skills. He asked numerous questions which I believe he already knew the answers to and often changed the subject. It was quite clear to me that he was using these tactics to avoid practicing reflection. I knew he understood the skill, so his delay tactics were those of resistance to practicing them. I am really uncomfortable dealing with his resistance. It was very difficult for me to get him back on task. Since I often hate to be put on the spot when I am unsure about something, I found it too easy to let him "off the hook" when he strayed off task. I realize that it is important for me to help parents practice all the skills and not just the ones that are comfortable. Practice is the only thing that will increase Mr. Smith's comfort. Yet, I found myself going along with his resistance so I wouldn't offend him or make him uncomfortable. This issue isn't going to go away! I must become more skilled at dealing with parent resistance.

In the case of Mr. Smith, there are no techniques that will solve this problem, and trying to figure out just how to break through Mr. Smith's resistance is not the solution. The issue is not making Mr. Smith uncomfortable; the issue is the therapist's discomfort. The therapist feels intimidated and lacks confidence. The problem lies with the therapist, and this issue was dealt with in supervision. One helpful thing the therapist could do would be to share his concern with Mr. Smith about wanting to be helpful to him but feeling apprehensive about keeping him on track or correcting him because he might feel hurt in the process.

RULE OF THUMB:

The therapist should model what she teaches.
In CPRT, we hope parents will share their
feelings and reactions with us.

Problem: A parent who dominates the training time.

Solution: A highly verbal parent who dominates the discussion time can be a deadly element in a filial therapy group. Other parents may roll their eyes, look knowingly at each other, stare at the floor, and begin to "tune out" when the domineering parent begins talking. Domineering individuals are typically insensitive to other people's reactions and continue to plow ahead. The experience can be so frustrating to parents that some may decide to drop out of the training. A general principle of group work is that no member should be allowed to destroy a group.

There are several methods of intervention to be considered in dealing with a domineering parent. After listening empathically to several minutes of the domineering parent's story, gently inserting (interrupting if necessary) a response summarizing the parent's story, and then asking "Anyone else in the group ever have that kind of problem?" can take the domineering parent out of the lead. Another way to intervene at this point is to relate the domineering parent's point to a teaching point and push ahead with the training plan:

> Jan, sounds as though you are really frustrated with your husband's parents. Group, there may be times when you are frustrated with your child during a special playtime. At such moments, you will need to work hard to get back in touch with your child. Look through your child's eyes. Ask yourself, "What is my child feeling?" "What does my child need right now?" "What is my child trying to communicate?" and try to make an empathic response as quickly as possible. Getting frustrated with your child is

natural, and we will talk about your frustration and other feelings here in our training sessions.

The filial therapist should always be sensitive to a parent's emotional needs and may determine that it is necessary to have a special counseling session with the parent. Sometimes, a one-on-one counseling session with the domineering parent will meet enough of the domineering parent's needs and result in less verbal activity in the filial therapy training sessions. If a counseling session does not seem necessary, another possibility would be to have a private session with the offending parent, explaining that other parents are having a difficult time entering into the discussion and eliciting the cooperation of the domineering parent to help other parents to participate.

Problem: The therapist is not a parent and is apprehensive about having anything of value to offer parents.

Solution: Being an effective filial therapist is not dependent on having experienced parenthood, although the experience can have some positive benefits for the filial therapist in helping parents feel they are understood and in helping the therapist to be sensitive to some parenting issues and struggles. The Child-Centered Play Therapy principles and skills the filial therapist has acquired from training and experience and can teach to parents are more important than the experience of being a parent. Feelings of inadequacy related to not being a parent are often related to other generalized feelings of inadequacy resulting from lack of experience. Supervision can be a significant help in this area. A part of the solution to feelings of doubt related to the absence of parenting is supervised experience as a filial therapist to discover that inexperience in parenting is not a deterrent to effectiveness as a filial therapist.

Many inexperienced filial therapists who are not parents feel inadequate about trying to teach parents how to relate to their children. These feelings of inadequacy and how they were worked through can be seen in the self-critiques of the following filial therapists who were enrolled in a graduate course in filial therapy that had a supervised practicum experience.

Judy: During the first two or three filial therapy sessions I led, I was extremely nervous because I thought I did not know enough because I have never been a parent. I now realize that just because I have never been a parent does not make me unknowledgeable about children.

Geri: I felt awkward during the first few training sessions because I do not have children. I questioned why these parents would listen to me. After our last filial therapy training session, one of the moms approached me and told me that at the beginning of the training group, she questioned how I would be able to understand or to help her, since I had told the parents that I had no children. She said that she had been skeptical of my ability and competency, but she had changed her mind over the past 10 weeks. She said that she now felt my responses to parents facilitated their thought and growth. I am now confident in my skills despite not having children of my own. I now realize I only need to be myself and to convey to parents the information I do know about children, play therapy, and filial therapy.

Megan: I was nervous at first because I am not a mother. I felt that the parents would question my experience and knowledge because I have never dealt with a child on a day-to-day basis like a mother does. I now realize that being a mother does not matter. In fact, not being a mother may even strengthen what I have to say. A mother will see things that I cannot even if I was a parent, and I will see things that a mother does not see. So if we work together, we get to see the whole picture, and this will benefit the child. I found that I was able to use examples from my own life, and the parents related to them.

Alisha: I felt uncertain about my ability to teach parents, since I have no parenting experience. I was surprised that the parents seemed to trust and respect me as a leader, without questioning my expertise or experience. Throughout the filial therapy training sessions, I began to feel more comfortable with the parents and more confident in my ability to instruct and guide them, despite our differences in parenting experience.

CHAPTER 25

VARIATIONS OF THE 10-SESSION CPRT MODEL

The model of once-a-week training sessions is considered ideal; however, the emotional needs, availability, or schedule of parents or children may necessitate consideration of other sequences of training sessions. The traditional concept of scheduling once-a-week sessions does not always match the dynamic needs of a family. A week between sessions can be a terribly long time in the life of a family in the midst of trauma or crisis. We have achieved positive results in adapting the 10-session CPRT model to meet the emotional and situational needs of families.

Although the frequency of CPRT training sessions may vary as suggested in this chapter, the content and structure of the training sessions remain virtually the same. The content of the 10-session model of training is considered to be the minimal amount of training needed to equip parents with the skills necessary to enable them to become therapeutic agents in their children's lives. A reduction in the content is likely to result in a corresponding reduction in effectiveness of the training. Although we do not have research findings to verify this assumption, our experience with a multitude of parent and child populations in a variety of settings supports this conclusion at this time. Research findings in the future may prove our assumptions to be incorrect, since the capacity of the human organism to assimilate experiences and adjust is not fully known or understood. We do have scientific studies that verify the effectiveness of condensing the time between training sessions while maintaining the content of the 10 sessions of training in the Landreth CPRT filial therapy model.

Once-a-Week Filial Therapy Schedule

Since the once-a-week CPRT model has already been thoroughly described, additional information is not needed here. The once-a-week CPRT model is mentioned here simply to provide a complete listing of the possible variations in scheduling the 10-session model of CPRT. The once-a-week structure does provide an opportunity for parents to take a more leisurely approach to scheduling the parent-child play sessions. When the time between training sessions is condensed, play sessions need to be scheduled more frequently during the week for supervision purposes. The parent should have a play session to report on in each training session after the first three training sessions. The parent-child play sessions are considered to be a key part of the 10-session model.

Twice-a-Week CPRT Schedule

The scheduling of once-a-week counseling or filial therapy sessions is generally done to meet the needs of the therapist—but what about the needs of clients? Could it be that clients are capable of assimilating and integrating experiences more rapidly and do not need a week between therapy sessions? This is an especially key consideration when families have been torn apart and their lives shattered by traumatic experiences that leave them feeling helpless with no relief in sight. These families may need short-term intensive CPRT training sessions twice a week for 5 weeks to help them get through the crisis more quickly.

Another consideration is parents who are not able to sustain continued focus for long periods of time. We found this to be the case in working with a group of teenage mothers. They seemed to lose interest and focus after about 50 minutes, so the format was changed from once-a-week 2-hour sessions to meeting twice weekly for 45 minutes. This shorter time frame seemed to be a much better learning experience. Some of the material also had to be adapted in very concrete ways to help this group learn. A lot of role-playing was added to the format, and initially the therapist had to assume the role of the child because the young mothers were uncomfortable playing the role of a child. These teenage mothers were dealing with huge personal issues that, if unaddressed, would hinder their ability to learn. Therefore, it was necessary to devote a larger amount of time to the process dimensions of the model and to be especially sensitive in determining when the group was ready to move on.

What is to be done for families who are not available for 10 weeks of therapy? This was the case for incarcerated mothers we wanted to involve in CPRT training before they were sent to another correctional facility. They were awaiting trial and/or sentencing or had been sentenced and were remanded to the county jail before being sent to a regional correctional facility in another part of the state. Since the majority of incarcerated female inmates are single mothers of dependent children, these children are usually placed with extended family members. Incarceration of the mother can be a terrifying experience for young children who can visit their mother only at designated times and in the frightening setting of a jail.

Arrangements were made with the county sheriff's department to provide 2-hour CPRT training sessions twice a week for 5 weeks for four groups of mothers. Almost 75% of these mothers had not completed high school and almost half of them had annual incomes of less than $5,000. Fifty percent of the mothers were Caucasian and 41% were African American. The CPRT training sessions were conducted in a small room in the county jail. After the third training session, parent-child play sessions were scheduled between each training session in a small space that could be supervised. CPRT toy kits were provided for the parents to use, and each play session was video-recorded for supervision and research purposes.

We found that the mothers in the CPRT training groups significantly increased their empathic interactions with their children, significantly increased their attitude of acceptance of their children, and reported a significant reduction in the number of behavior problems with their children (Harris & Landreth, 1997). These are encouraging results, and they demonstrate the power of the

10-session CPRT training model as well as the efficacy of the intensive training. The results of this study are truly remarkable given the extreme conditions and stressful circumstances of a county jail setting and the restricted backgrounds of the mothers. We anticipate similar results using a twice-a-week format with other parent populations.

Every Day CPRT Schedule

Some families may be experiencing such intense situational circumstances and/or emotional and physical trauma that CPRT training sessions every day are warranted.

Mothers and children who reside in a domestic violence shelter or homeless shelter are often there for only 2 or 3 weeks and then are relocated to a halfway house, return to their homes, or find some other place of residence. Even twice-a-week CPRT training sessions would not be sufficient under these circumstances. Therefore, CPRT training sessions every day are necessary in such a setting. Smith and Landreth (2003) modified the structure of the 10-session filial therapy model to provided intensive CPRT training (12 sessions in 14 days) for mothers and children in a domestic violence shelter and a homeless shelter. In order to accommodate the mothers' hectic and stressful work schedules, shelter-assigned chores, and shelter training schedules, the training segment of the model and the parent-child play sessions were merged into 1½-hour training sessions 5 nights a week and during the day on weekends.

Smith and Landreth found that children in the CPRT group demonstrated a significant increase in self-concept; a significant decrease in overall behavior problems; a significant decrease in internalizing and externalizing behavior problems; and a significant decrease in aggression, anxiety, and depression, compared to children in a control group. Mothers who received CPRT training demonstrated a significant increase in empathic interactions with their children, based on analysis of pre and post video-recordings of mother-child play sessions. These results are extraordinary considering the high levels of stress, anxiety, depression, and fatigue these mothers were experiencing on a daily basis. The results are also significant in view of the fact that children's relationships to their mothers have been identified as a key factor in how children are affected by witnessing domestic violence.

A comparative analysis of the results of this study with the Kot, Landreth, and Giordano (1998) intensive, short-term, child-centered individual play therapy study (12 sessions in 14 days) in the same domestic violence shelter and the Tyndall-Lind, Landreth, and Giordano (2001) intensive, short-term, child-centered, sibling group play therapy study (12 sessions in 14 days) in the same domestic violence shelter showed no significant differences on the dimensions identified above between the intensive CPRT training, the intensive short-term individual play therapy, and the intensive short-term sibling group play therapy groups. Intensive CPRT training was found to be as effective as intensive individual play therapy and intensive sibling group play therapy conducted by professional play therapists.

The significant results of scientific studies on the effect of collapsing the time between sessions attest to the robustness of the 10-session CPRT model.

Multiple Weekend CPRT Schedule

The weekday schedule for some families is so hectic and stressful that they have difficulty making a commitment to 10 weeks of training. For these parents, it may be necessary to lengthen training sessions and significantly reduce the number of training sessions. To assess the impact of collapsing the time between CPRT training sessions and reducing the number of sessions, parents were given the opportunity to enroll in CPRT training for four consecutive Saturdays or the traditional model of 10 weekly sessions. The parents in each group lived in a large city, and their children were displaying a wide spectrum of behavioral problems. Since there were fewer opportunities for parents in the four-session Saturday group to have home play sessions with their children and receive supervision from the therapist, parent-child play sessions were added to the training schedule, and child care was provided on-site for the children. An advantage of this arrangement was that the therapist always had a child available for demonstration of the skills being taught, as well as providing an opportunity for parents to immediately practice those skills.

Test results showed that parents in the four-session Saturday training group were initially much more stressed than parents in the 10-week training group. After training, no significant differences were found between the two training groups on parental stress, parental empathy, parental acceptance, and child behavior problems. Parents in the 10-week filial therapy training group demonstrated greater skill development in empathic responding. Parents in the four-session Saturday group seemed to become a more cohesive group than parents in the 10-session group. This may have been a function of a smaller number of parents in the four-session Saturday groups (Ferrell, 2003).

Weekend CPRT Schedule

A couple called me about concerns for their 6-year-old son, James, whom they described as bossy, manipulative, angry all the time, "wants to sleep in our bed every night," and a severe discipline problem. "We can't do anything with him. Spanking doesn't work anymore. Nothing works." I recommended play therapy, but the only play therapist I could locate in their rural area of west Texas was a 3-hour drive away. I called them back and described CPRT training to them. They were eager, excited, and said, "That sounds like just what we need!" Since they lived several hundred miles away, arrangements were made for them to come to the Center for Play Therapy for a weekend of filial therapy training.

I condensed the 10 sessions of CPRT training into 2 hours of training on Friday evening and 7 hours on Saturday. In the Friday evening session, I focused on parts of the first three sessions of the 10-session model: active listening, reflecting feelings, returning responsibility, and tracking. My primary objective was to help both parents acquire a few of the basic skills needed for a first 10-minute mini-play session with their son that evening. This decision was based on their high level of commitment, the intensity of the setting, and my thoughts that a mini-play session that evening would help reduce their anxiety about the experience. The schedule for the second hour was:

- 10 minutes — Demonstration play session with James, which the parents observed through a two-way mirror.

- 15 minutes — Critique of the play session focused on what they saw (nonverbal behaviors: sat down quickly, smiled, nodded head, tracked James with my whole body), what they heard (verbal responses: reflected content, reflected feelings, returned responsibility, made tracking responses), and answers to their questions.
- 10 minutes — Mother-child play session. As we observed, I pointed out to the father the positive responses the mother made.
- 5 minutes — Feedback to the mother.
- 10 minutes — Father-child play session. As we observed, I pointed out to the mother the positive responses the father made.
- 10 minutes — Feedback to the father and outline of what to expect the next day.

A babysitter was hired to take care of James when he was not in the playroom Friday evening and all day Saturday.

Saturday content schedule was determined by the immediate needs of the parents but was still content within the framework of the 10-session model (flexibility was the rule of the day):

- 1 hour — Therapeutic limit setting training, role-played in the playroom.
- 1 hour — Supervision; 15-minute parent-child play session with 15-minute feedback for each parent.
- 1 hour — Training, role-playing, viewing of video segments of my play sessions.
- 1 hour — Lunch.
- 1 hour — Supervision of parent play sessions.
- 1 hour — Training, role-playing, viewing segments of one parent play session.
- 1 hour — Supervision of parent play sessions.
- 1 hour — Training, viewing segments of one parent play session, wrap-up, and planning for at-home play sessions by both parents and telephone follow-up supervision.

At the 1-month and 2-month follow-up, both parents enthusiastically reported feeling empowered and described significant behavioral changes for James. By the end of the second week, he was sleeping in his own bed. By the end of the first month, the angry outbursts had disappeared and there were no discipline problems. They reported the Oreo® Cookie Theory of choice giving was the most helpful tool they acquired.

Long-Distance CPRT Training

The number of mental health professionals and agencies that provide filial therapy training is minimal because the majority of existing play therapists have not been trained in filial therapy. Therefore, this highly effective procedure for improving the mental health of families is not readily available to the majority of parents. Entire regions of the United States and other countries do not have the services of a filial therapist. Indeed, some entire nations may not have a single filial therapist. One temporary solution to this dilemma is the provision of filial therapy training via the telephone. We have had several successful experiences using the telephone to provide long-distance CPRT training for parents. The following cases describe what happened in two families when CPRT training was conducted via the telephone.

A Traumatized Child in Israel

Nine-year-old Rachel, an Israeli, was riding in a bus that was attacked by three terrorists who shot and killed 11 of the adults and children aboard. Rachel was not physically injured, but after witnessing the brutal attack, she withdrew into herself and became very subdued and quiet although she had formerly been a playful, talkative child. She also developed severe mouth ulcers that were so painful she had to be placed on a liquid diet. She was taken to several physicians, but the ulcers seemed immune to medication.

Seven months after the attack, Rachel's mother was desperate for help and called her cousin, Suzi Kagan, one of my doctoral students in the play therapy program at the University of North Texas at that time. Suzi, who had completed filial therapy training and supervision, was faced with the dilemma of responding to the mother's concerns on the phone, hoping to help her find a mental health worker nearby in Israel or wait to provide help in person when she returned to Israel two months later. The mother was so distressed that Suzi concluded that immediate support was crucial to the family.

In the span of about 20 minutes, the significance of a special playtime was quickly explained, and examples of tracking and empathic listening were described. A few toys were recommended, and the mother was encouraged to sit on the floor and allow Rachel to decide how to spend the time together, playing or just sitting quietly in mom's lap if Rachel chose to do so. Suzi also suggested that the mother tell Rachel, "I know how scared you are and how hard it is to talk about what you saw on the bus."

Suzi made a commitment to call her cousin in a week. However, 24 hours later, Rachel's mother called again to report the play session had produced some immediate and startling results. Excitedly, she described the experience for Rachel as being like a huge, bulging ball of anxiety, pain, and fear that had finally been burst. Rachel, who had attempted to avoid crying since the terrorist attack, cried throughout the whole day after the playtime and into the night. She talked about how frightened she was and that every day she believed another terrorist attack would occur. That night Rachel slept through the whole night without waking up frightened, something she had not done since the attack.

Encouraged by the dramatic impact of the first play session, Suzi continued CPRT training once a week via the telephone for 10 weeks. During that time, she mailed the mother handout material typically used in the Landreth 10-session CPRT training. In the second telephone training session, the mother reported Rachel's mouth ulcers had begun to heal and Rachel had started eating solid food. As the play sessions progressed, she became more expressive and vocal in the special play sessions and in her daily life. By the tenth week, she had returned to her normal level of functioning and displayed no major trauma symptoms. The mother also described significant positive changes in her own relationship with her daughter and with other family members, as well as improvement in the overall atmosphere of the home. She was also able to generalize the new skills comfortably in her relationships outside the special play sessions.

An Isolated Family in a Rural Area

The parents and three children, ages 5, 3, and 4 months, lived in an isolated rural area of Minnesota, a 3-hour drive to the nearest airport. The mother was not employed outside the home, was taking graduate level correspondence courses, and often felt overwhelmed by the amount of time required to care for three small children, especially in the winter when they were confined to the house much of the time due to extreme cold and heavy snows.

David, the 5-year-old child of concern, was described as unmanageable, strong-willed, manipulative, exhibiting infantile behavior at times, with an extremely low threshold for frustration, and a physical threat to his 3-year-old brother. His kindergarten teacher reported no behavioral problems. The parents, who had not heard of play therapy or filial therapy, learned about these approaches to helping children from a relative who lived 1,000 miles away. Arrangements were made for a graduate student at the University of North Texas to provide long-distance CPRT training for the mother once a week under the close supervision of Dr. Garry L. Landreth.

The format of the 10-session training model was followed, information and homework assignments were faxed, and the mother was encouraged to e-mail pressing questions that occurred between the weekly phone sessions. Since the mother was so stressed, a part of the early training sessions was spent responding empathically to her feelings. Since she had not seen a demonstration play session, she seemed to have a great deal of difficulty in the early training sessions grasping the concept of empathic listening and acknowledging feelings, and had a hard time keeping evaluative and problem-solving statements out of her reflections, so the video *Child-Centered Play Therapy* by Garry L. Landreth was mailed to her. Viewing this video seemed to crystallize for the mother many of the concepts and skills she had difficulty understanding.

A major benefit of the CPRT training was that the mother gained insight into how she normally responded to David and did not allow him enough responsibility in his play. She was able to incorporate her new skills into her interactions outside the play sessions. David became less rigid, demanding, and aggressive, and his acting-out behavior diminished. His mother reported he had fewer serious "blow-ups." At conclusion of the 10 sessions of training, arrangements were made for the mother to continue to e-mail her questions to the graduate student and to video-record a play session once a month for more specific supervision.

Problematic Areas in Long-Distance Training

It is difficult to teach and practice reflective listening skills over the phone. For every emotion reflected, there must first be a verbal statement to communicate the emotion. The subtleties of facial expression and mood conveyed through the body are lost in this format. Scenarios that communicate particular emotions without using the feeling words themselves must be developed. The use of computers equipped with webcast (video cameras) would alleviate some of this problem.

The use of toys to demonstrate a child's behavior in a play session and corresponding recommended responses is not possible via the telephone, nor can tracking skills be demonstrated. The absence of these concrete examples is a significant hindrance to training. Therefore, it is imperative that arrangements be made early in the training to send the parent a video demonstrating a play session with a child. It is essential that the parent be able to see what a play session is supposed to look like. Filial play sessions are so foreign to how parents typically react that it is almost impossible for parents to visualize the nature of the play sessions. Scheduling the viewing of a specified section of the video by the trainer and the parent at the same time during a CPRT training phone session enables the trainer to have the parent stop the video so the trainer can explain what is happening in the play session or call attention to specific responses. This procedure greatly enhances the learning experience for the parent. If the trainer does not have a video that can be mailed to the parent, we recommend the video *Child-Centered Play Therapy* by Garry L. Landreth. Again, the use of webcast-equipped computers can alleviate some of these problems because the more technically advanced cameras, also more expensive, can be set to focus on a table containing toys for demonstration purposes.

The potential benefits of supervision are significantly diminished when the trainer is not able to observe a parent-child play session. Parents are simply not skilled enough to be aware of the subtle happenings in play sessions that make a huge difference in the impact of the sessions and then describe those happening to the trainer in a supervision session. Parents' interpretation of events in play sessions often do not match what is seen on videos. The graduate student's critique of one of her training sessions with the mother in the second case described above highlights this difficulty.

Some of the essential problems with the long-distance format were revealed in full force during this session. Audio messages without a visual component are less-than-reliable messages, and so communication by phone makes it more difficult to give and receive accurate information about feelings or to communicate genuine support. The mother's report of the first play session had been encouraging. Based on what the mother said, it sounded like she had a good grasp of how to conduct the sessions. However, after viewing the video of her second play session, I was no longer sure that what she reported fully reflected what was really happening. She reported that the second session had also gone well, but the tension in her voice and happenings I saw on the video told another story. For example, the mother described a scene in which David was so frustrated with not being able to untie a knot in the rope that she decided to take the rope out of his hands and undo it for him. What I saw on the video was David picked up the rope, mentioned there was a knot in it, and then his mother immediately took the rope out of his hands to undo the knot.

This problem can be largely overcome by requiring the parent to video-record play sessions, make copies for herself, and mail the videos to the trainer for supervision. Skills the parent has difficulty utilizing can be focused on in the following training session through role-playing and modeling by the trainer. Segments of the videos can also be viewed at the same time by the trainer and parent during training sessions to reinforce positive parent behaviors and highlight areas that need to be improved. This simulcast or long-distance viewing of a video-recorded session at the same time by the trainer and the parent facilitates a supervision process similar to face-to-face supervision when a video is being watched.

Based on our experiences, we encourage the limited use of CPRT training via the telephone with parents who live in areas where filial therapy training is not available. A caution: The filial therapist must have had extensive training and supervision in play therapy and filial therapy. One or two workshop experiences in filial therapy training are not sufficient.

Individual Parents and Couples

Having both parents attend CPRT training and learn the skills required for conducting special play sessions is highly desirable since these principles and skills will be generalized outside the play sessions. An important principle in child rearing is that both parents "be on the same page" in utilizing general child rearing principles, especially in areas such as discipline. When parents do not use a similar approach in child rearing, children become confused, feel insecure, and may compensate by acting out or becoming manipulative. Therefore, the therapist makes every effort possible to encourage and accommodate a reluctant spouse's schedule to make it possible for both parents to attend, even if the reluctant parent can only attend every other session or once a month. The therapist can also offer to schedule a special training session at the reluctant parent's convenience: an hour before reporting to work, during lunch, on the way home from work, a night session, etc. After obtaining permission from the child, a parent in training can invite their reluctant spouse to sit in on the at-home special playtimes to observe. This can be highly effective in helping to lower defensive barriers. When a parent is invited to sit in on the special playtime, a caution is in order: The invited parent is to sit on the floor and observe, and the parent in training will do all the talking for both parents. This requirement is necessary to prevent the nontrained parent from taking over the playtime, offering inappropriate suggestions to the child, asking leading questions, etc.

Our experience has been, however, that attendance at CPRT training sessions by both parents is not the norm. Fathers are notorious for being "too busy." In many cases, mothers have reported that they have taught fathers many of the skills they learned. One particularly "take charge," forceful mother said, "I just told my husband to listen up, this is the way we are going to start responding to our son." Many parents have reported teaching the skills they have learned to the absent parent and have been rewarded when they later observed the absent parent responding empathically or giving choices. Parents often jokingly relate stories about using the skills with the absent parent and how effective the skills were. A multitude of research studies have reported significant positive results in correcting children's behavioral problems even though only one parent received CPRT training. This is understandable since the parent is the child's therapeutic agent and is therefore somewhat similar to a play therapist in the child's life. In play therapy, significant positive results are often achieved even though the parents are not involved in therapy. This fact is demonstrated daily in elementary schools where elementary school counselors utilize play therapy and seldom have direct contact with the children's parents.

The 2-hour training format is usually not needed when working with one parent or a couple. One hour of training each week should be sufficient because so much more material can be covered. Skill development is speeded up because of the one-on-one mentoring, making it possible for the parent or couple to begin at-home play sessions the first week of training.

When training one parent or a couple, arrangements can be made for the child of focus to be brought to each CPRT training session for therapist demonstration play sessions and parent practice play sessions. A typical format for the first training session might be:

- 25 minutes — Basic information, skill development, and role-play; the therapist points out what the parent is to look for in a demonstration play session.
- 10 minutes — The therapist demonstrates a play session with the child as the parent observes through a two-way mirror. Alternatively, a video camera could be set up in a corner of the playroom and the parent could watch on a TV monitor from another room. Less desirable, but workable, the parent could sit in the hall and observe through the partially open door or sit in the playroom and observe but not interact.
- 5 minutes — Critique; therapist directs parent's attention to what she did, explains the purpose of responses to the child, and answers parent questions.
- 10 minutes — Parent-child play session; therapist observes and makes notes.
- 10 minutes — Feedback to parent; therapist takes the role of the child to help the parent practice needed response changes.

The one potential problematic factor with this format is arranging for someone to babysit the child while the therapist is training the parent or couple. If a secretary is not available, an older sibling could fill the role of babysitter. Another possibility is to provide the child with toys to play with in the hall outside the office or playroom door, if the hall dead-ends on one side of the door and there are no office or exit doors in that part of the hall. The therapist can position her chair so she can see the child if the child walks past the open door of the playroom or therapist's office. This same arrangement could be utilized if the playroom or office door opens into a waiting room, and toys can be placed on one side of the waiting room with the open door of the playroom or therapist's office between the toys and the entrance door to the waiting room so the child would not be able to leave the area without being seen.

The format of the first filial therapy training session is recommended for the second and third training sessions. The format for the remaining filial therapy training sessions might be:

- 30 minutes — Reviewing homework assignments, supervising at-home parent-child play sessions, and training.
- 15 minutes — Parent-child play session.
- 15 minutes — Therapist feedback and training.

This training format could be revised to meet the needs of a parent or couple, as in the case of a parent who is having difficulty in her play sessions and needs to observe the therapist more.

References

Ferrell, L. (2003). *A comparison of an intensive 4-week format of the Landreth 10-week filial therapy training model with the traditional Landreth 10-week model of filial therapy.* Unpublished doctoral dissertation, University of North Texas, Denton.

Harris, Z., & Landreth, G. (1997). Filial therapy with incarcerated mothers: A five-week model. *International Journal of Play Therapy, 6*(2), 53–73.

Kot, S., Landreth, G., & Giordano, M. (1998). Intensive child-centered play therapy with child witnesses of domestic violence. *International Journal of Play Therapy, 7*(2), 17–36.

Smith, N., & Landreth, G. (2003). Intensive filial therapy with child witnesses of domestic violence: A comparison with individual and sibling group play therapy. *International Journal of Play Therapy, 12*(1), 67–88.

Tyndall-Lind, A., Landreth, G., & Giordano, M. (2001). Intensive group play therapy with child witnesses of domestic violence. *International Journal of Play Therapy, 10*(1), 53–83.

CHAPTER 26

RESEARCH EVIDENCE FOR CPRT

Sue Bratton and Alyssa M. Swan

CPRT is one of the more well-researched treatment protocols in the field of play therapy and in the broader area of child therapy practices. The considerable body of CPRT research rests firmly on the empirical foundation laid by the Guerneys and their colleagues in the 1960s and 70s (Guerney & Ryan, 2013). Although early filial therapy studies lacked the methodological rigor of contemporary studies, the encouraging findings from the Guerneys' groundbreaking research (Guerney, 1975; Guerney & Stover, 1971; Oxman, 1972; Stover & Guerney, 1967) provided the catalyst for the significant production of CPRT research over the past two decades (Bratton et al. 2015). There are more than 50 studies investigating CPRT's process and outcomes (cpt.unt.edu); however, for the purpose of this chapter we include only research findings from published controlled outcome research. Controlled outcome studies prove the effectiveness of an intervention when compared to a control or comparison group and contribute to recognition of a treatment as an evidence-based practice. Since the publication of the first edition of this text, recognition of the empirical support for CPRT has grown substantially. Important happenings include the national recognition of CPRT as an evidence-based practice by the National Registry of Evidence-based Programs and Practices (NREPP, www.nrepp.samhsa.gov) and by the California Evidence-Based Clearinghouse (CEBC) for Child Welfare (www.cebc4cw.org). Specific to mental health treatments for adoptive families, the Donaldson Adoption Institute released a report in 2013 in which CPRT was evaluated as the parent-child intervention that demonstrated the most robust research support for this population of parents and children (Brodzinsky, 2013). An outgrowth of CPRT's designation as an evidence-based practice has been the development of certification to insure that practitioners who use CPRT in their practice are adhering to the CPRT protocol. Information on the certification process and requirements is found at www.cpt.unt/Child-Parent-therapy-certification.

Individual Outcome Studies

Since Bratton and Landreth published the first CPRT outcome study in 1995, the evidentiary base for CPRT has grown as studies' methodological rigor increased. An impressive 22 are published peer-reviewed studies, and of those 22 studies, 17 employ random assignment to groups considered the "gold standard with regards to questions of treatment efficacy" (Nezu & Nezu, 2008, p. vii). The remaining studies used quasi-experimental designs primarily due to challenges in conducting research in community settings that interfered with random assignment. As an indicator of the high level of treatment fidelity in CPRT research, the 22 published studies were conducted by investigators that were directly trained and supervised in the CPRT protocol The preponderance of studies showed statistically significant results and moderate to large treatment effects for CPRT over control groups using standardized measurements to assess improvements in the areas of child behavior problems and parent-child relationship stress. Sixteen of the 22 studies used objective raters blinded to participant group assignment to examine the effects of CPRT training on parents' and other paraprofessionals' empathic behavior with the children of focus. Although the majority of outcome studies focused on the effects of training and supervising parents as therapeutic agents, the benefit of CPRT delivered by teachers and student mentors was the focus of investigation in five of these studies. Table 26.1 presents a concise summary of the 22 CPRT studies that met the following criteria: (a) published in refereed journal; (b) CPRT was compared to a no-treatment, active-control, or comparison group; and (c) treatment integrity ensured through use of a protocol by CPRT-trained therapists. Readers are directed to evidencebasedchildtherapy.com (Bratton et al., 2015) to review detailed summaries of the study characteristics and findings for the studies included in Table 26.1, as well as to review additional studies that failed to meet the stated criteria.

Several conclusions can be drawn from reviewing the findings from the body of research included in Table 26.1 Overall results indicate CPRT is effective on reducing children's behavior problems, decreasing stress in the parent-child relationship, and increasing parental empathy. That both children and parents demonstrated beneficial outcomes indicates the robustness of this approach. Specifically, studies show CPRT's efficacy across multiple populations and issues, including adopted/fostered children with attachment difficulties, children whose mothers or fathers were incarcerated, children who were sexually abused, children living in domestic violence shelters, children living with chronic illness, at-risk children of single parents, and children diagnosed with learning differences, speech problems, adjustment difficulties, and various behavior problems. The strongest CPRT finding is its effectiveness with adoptive families. Two well-designed, randomized controlled trials involving 110 parents and children demonstrated large treatment effects and statistically significant improvements in child behavior problems, parent-child relationship stress, and parental empathy (Carnes-Holt & Bratton, 2014; Opiola & Bratton, 2018). CPRT's transportability is demonstrated by its successful use in a variety of real-world settings, including community agencies, churches, public and private schools, Head Start programs, shelters, prisons/county jails, and hospitals.

The effectiveness of CPRT with diverse populations is a strength of the treatment model. Multiple studies show CPRT's efficacy across ethnic, socioeconomic, and cultural groups, including African American, Native American, Israeli, Korean, immigrant Latino, immigrant Korean, and immigrant Chinese populations. In addition, study participants ranged in age from 2 to 11 years, indicating CPRT's responsiveness to a range of developmental needs. With a participant mean age of 5 years, CPRT appears particularly sensitive to the treatment needs of young children and, as such,

Table 26.1 Child-Parent Relationship Therapy (CPRT) Published Controlled Outcome Research—1995 to Present

Study	**Intervention Model/** Control Group Type • Randomization • # Sessions • Frequency; Length • Setting *Treatment provider	**Sample** • Age • Ethnicity • Sex	**Child Outcome Variable/Target Problem**	**Findings**
Baggerly, J., & Landreth, G. L. (2001). Training children to help children: A new dimension in play therapy. *Peer Facilitator Quarterly*, *18*(1), 6–14.	**Modified CPRT/**WC • Non-randomized • 10 play sessions • 1/wk; 20 min • School *CPRT-trained 5th-grade mentors	*N* = 29 Behaviorally at-risk students • Age: 5–6; M = 5.7 • 76% Cauc, 14% AfAm, 10% Lat • 58% male	Internalized behavioral problems; Self-esteem	Compared to the WC, parents of experimental group children reported a statistically significant reduction in their kindergarteners' internalizing behavior problems over time. Although not statistically significant, teachers and parents reported a greater reduction in overall behavior problems of children receiving CPRT and an increase in self-esteem following 10 supervised play mentoring sessions with their 5th grade mentors, compared to control group.
Bratton, S. C., & Landreth, G. L. (1995). Filial therapy with single parents: Effects on parental acceptance, empathy, and stress. *International Journal of Play Therapy*, *4*(1), 61–80.	**CPRT**/WC • Randomized • 7 play sessions • 1/wk; 30 min • Community agency *CPRT-trained parents	*N* = 43 behaviorally at-risk children of single parents • Age: 3–7; M = 4.7 • 90% Cauc, 5% Lat, 5% other • 56% male	Behavioral problems; Parent-child relationship stress	Between-group differences over time revealed that parents in the CPRT group demonstrated a statistically significant increase in empathic interactions with their children as directly observed by independent raters. CPRT parents also reported a statistically significant gain in parental acceptance, as well as statistically significant reductions in parent-child relationship stress and in their children's behavior problems, compared to the control group over time.

Note: Control group type denoted by WC = waitlist control/delayed start, AC = active control, COMP = comparison treatment; AfAm = African American; Asian = of Asian descent living in U.S.; Cauc = Caucasian/European American; Lat = Latino/Hispanic.

Carnes-Holt, K., & Bratton, S.C. (2014). The efficacy of Child-Parent Relationship Therapy for adopted children with attachment disruptions. *Journal for Counseling and Development*, *92*, 328–337.	**CPRT**/WC • Randomized • 7 play sessions • 1/wk; 30 min • Community agency *CPRT-trained parents	*N* = 61 Adoptees • Age: 2.5–10; M = 5.7 • 47% Cauc, 15% Lat, 9% AfAm, 18% other • 55% male	Attachment difficulties; Clinical comorbid behavior problems	Statistically significant findings and large treatment effects on all measures indicated the effectiveness of CPRT over the WC on (1) reducing adopted children's externalized behaviors and global behavior problems, and (2) increasing parental empathy as measured by objective raters blinded to the study.
Ceballos, P., & Bratton, S. (2010). Empowering Latino families: A culturally responsive, school-based intervention with low-income immigrant Latin parents and their children identified with academic and behavioral concerns. *Psychology in the Schools*, *47*(8), 761–7.	**CPRT**/WC • Randomized • 7 play sessions • 1/wk; 30 min • Head Start school *CPRT-trained parents	*N* = 48 At-risk, low-income PreK students • Age: 3–4; M = 4.3 • 100% Lat • 56% male	Clinical comorbid behavior problems	Statistically significant findings and large treatment effects on all measures indicated the effectiveness of culturally adapted CPRT over the WC on (1) reducing children's externalized and internalized behavior problems, and (2) decreasing parent-child relationship stress. 85% of children in the CPRT group moved from clinical levels of concern to more normative functioning. Cultural considerations discussed.

(*Continued*)

Table 26.1 (Continued)

Chau, I., & Landreth, G. L. (1997). Filial therapy with Chinese parents: Effects on parental empathic interactions, parental acceptance of child and parental stress. *International Journal of Play Therapy*, *6*(2), 75–92.	**CPRT**/WC • Randomized • 7 play sessions • 1/wk; 30 min • Community agency *CPRT-trained parents	*N* = 34 children • Age: 2–10; M = 5.1 • 100% Chinese • 50% male	Parent-child relationship stress	Compared to the control group over time, parents in the CPRT group demonstrated a statistically significant increase in empathic interactions with their children as directly observed in play sessions by independent raters. From pre to post, parents in the CPRT group also reported a statistically significant increase in parental acceptance and a statistically significant decrease in parent-child relationship stress, compared to the control group.
Costas & Landreth (1999). Filial therapy with nonoffending parents of children who have been sexually abused. *International Journal of Play Therapy*, *8*(1), 43–66.	**CPRT**/WC • Randomized • 7 play sessions • 1/wk; 30 min • Community agency *CPRT-trained, non-offending parents	*N* = 22 children who had experienced sexual abuse • Age: 5–9; M = 7.2 • 8% Lat, 92% Cauc • 32% male	Behavioral problems; Parent-child relationship stress	Between-group differences over time revealed that parents receiving CPRT demonstrated statistically significant gains in (1) empathic interactions with their children as rated by objective raters, (2) acceptance of their children, and (3) improvement in parent-child relationship stress. Although not statistically significant, CPRT-trained parents reported a marked improvement in their children's behavior problems, anxiety, emotional adjustment, and self-concept.

Glover, G., & Landreth, G. L. (2000). Filial therapy with Native Americans on the Flathead reservation. *International Journal of Play Therapy*, *9*(2), 57–80.	**CPRT**/WC • Non-randomized • 7 play sessions • 1/wk; 30 min • Native American reservation	*N* = 21 children living on a reservation in western U.S. • Age: 3–10; M = 5.4 • 100% Native American • 48% male	Behavioral problems; Parent-child relationship stress	Compared to the control group over time, parents in CPRT group demonstrated a statistically significant increase in their empathic interactions with their children as directly observed in play sessions by independent raters, and their children also demonstrated a statistically significant increase in desirable play behaviors with their parents (independent raters). CPRT-trained parents also reported an increase in parental acceptance and a decrease in parent-child relationship, and their children reported increased self-concept, although these results were not statistically significant.
Harris, Z. L., & Landreth, G. L. (1997). Filial therapy with incarcerated mothers: A five-week model. *International Journal of Play Therapy*, *6*(2), 53–73.	**CPRT**/WC • Randomized • 7 play sessions • 2/wk; 30 min • Jail *CPRT-trained, incarcerated mothers	*N* = 22 children with incarcerated mothers • Age: 3–10; M = 5 • 5% Native American, 5% Lat, 41% AfAm, 50% Cauc • 53% male	Behavioral problems; Adjustment difficulties	Compared to the control group over time, mothers in the CPRT group demonstrated a statistically significant increase in their empathic interaction with their children as directly observed by independent raters, and reported statistically significant gains in their parental acceptance and a statistically significant decrease in their children's behavior problems.

(*Continued*)

Table 26.1 (Continued)

Helker, W. P., & Ray, D. (2009). The impact of child-teacher relationship training on teachers' and aides' use of relationship-building skills and the effect on student classroom behavior. *International Journal of Play Therapy*, *18*(2), 70–83.	**CTRT**/AC • Randomized • 24 play sessions • 3/wk; 15 min • Head Start school *CPRT-trained Head Start teachers	*N* = 32 behaviorally at-risk preschool children • Age: 3–4; M = 3.5 • 53% Lat, 19% AfAm, 28% Cauc • 56% male	Comorbid behavioral problems	Between-group differences over time revealed: (1) CTRT-trained teachers/aides demonstrated a statistically significant greater use of relationship-building skills in the classroom; (2) a statistically significant relationship between CTRT-trained teachers/aides' higher use of relationship-building skills in the classroom and students' decrease in externalizing behaviors. Experimental group children demonstrated a statistically significant decrease in externalizing problems from pre to mid to post when compared to the children in the active control group.
Jones, L., Rhine, T., & Bratton, S. (2002). High school students as therapeutic agents with young children experiencing school adjustment difficulties: The effectiveness of filial therapy training model. *International Journal for Play Therapy*, *11*(2), 43–62.	**Modified CPRT**/COMP • Randomized • 20 play sessions • 1/wk; 20 min • School *11th–12th grade CPRT-trained mentors	*N* = 26 behaviorally at-risk PreK to K children • Age: 4–6; M = 5.4 • 96% Cauc • 57% male	Comorbid behavioral problems	Parents who were blinded to children's treatment group reported CPRT group children demonstrated a statistically significant decrease in internalizing and total behavior problems, compared to the COMP group, PALS®, which used a manualized curriculum. According to blinded raters' direct observation, CPRT mentors demonstrated a statistically significant improvement in empathic interactions with their child of focus compared to PALS® mentors.

Kale, A. L., & Landreth, G. L. (1999). Filial therapy with parents of children experiencing learning difficulties. *International Journal of Play Therapy*, *8*(2), 35–56.	**CPRT**/WC • Randomized • 7 play sessions • 1/wk; 30 min • School *CPRT-trained parents	*N* = 22 children identified with learning difficulties • Age: 5–10 • 5% Native American, 23% biracial, 73% Cauc	Comorbid behavioral problems; Parent-child relationship stress	Results indicated statistically significant improvement in parental acceptance and reduction in parent-child relationship stress from pre- to post-testing for the CPRT-trained group compared to the no treatment control. While not statistically significant, parents trained in CPRT reported greater improvement in child behavior problems compared to the control group.
Kidron, M., & Landreth, G. L. (2010). Intensive Child-Parent Relationship Therapy with Israeli parents in Israel. *International Journal of Play Therapy*, *19*(2), 64–78.	**CPRT**/WC • Non-randomized • 7 play sessions • 1/wk; 30 min • Community agency *CPRT-trained parents	*N* = 27 children • Ages: 5–10, M = 6 • 100% Israeli • 44% male	Parent-child relationship stress	Compared to control parents, the CPRT group demonstrated a statistically significant increase pre to post in empathic interactions with their children as rated by observers blind to study, and reported a statistically significant reduction in parent-child relationship stress. Compared to the control group over time, CPRT parents also reported a statistically significant reduction in their children's externalized behavior problems.

(Continued)

Table 26.1 (Continued)

Landreth, G. L., & Lobaugh, A. (1998). Filial therapy with incarcerated fathers: Effects on parental acceptance of child, parental stress, and child adjustment. *Journal of Counseling & Development*, *76*, 157–165.	**CPRT**/WC • Randomized • 8–10 play sessions • 1/wk; 30 min • Jail *CPRT-trained, incarcerated fathers	*N* = 32 children with incarcerated fathers • Age: 4–9; M = 6.5 • 30% Lat, 18% AfAm, 52% Cauc • 41% male	Adjustment difficulties; parent-child relationship stress	Compared to the control group over time, fathers in the CPRT group reported a statistically significant increase in their parental acceptance towards their children, and a statistically significant reduction in parent-child relationship stress. In addition, children whose fathers were in the CPRT group reported a statistically significant increase in their self-esteem from pre- to post-testing.
Lee, M., & Landreth G. L. (2003). Filial therapy with immigrant Korean parents in the United States. *International Journal of Play Therapy*, *12*(2), 67–85.	**CPRT**/WC • Randomized • 7 play sessions • 1/wk; 30 min • Community settings *CPRT-trained parents	*N* = 32 Korean children • Age: 2–10; M = 7.3 • 100% Korean • 53% male	Comorbid behavioral problems; Parent-child relationship stress	Between-group differences over time revealed that parents in the CPRT group (1) demonstrated a statistically significant increase in their empathic interactions with their children as directly observed by independent raters, and (2) reported a statistically significant increase in their parental acceptance toward their children as well as a statistically significant reduction in parent-child relationship stress.

Morrison, M., & Bratton, S. (2010). Preliminary investigation of an early mental health intervention for Head Start programs: Effects of Child Teacher Relationship Therapy (CTRT) on children's behavior problems. *Psychology in the Schools*, *47*(10), 1003–1017.	**CTRT/**AC • Randomized • 16 wks • Daily center time play • Head Start school *CPRT-trained teachers	*N* = 52 At-risk, low-income PreK students • Age: 3–4; M = 3.9 • 56% Lat, 31% AfAm, 13% Cauc • 58% male	Clinical comorbid behavioral problems	Compared to the AC (Conscious Discipline®) across three points of measure, teacher-adapted CPRT (CTRT) demonstrated statistically significant improvements and large treatment effect on children's externalizing behavior problems and moderate effect on internalizing problems; 84% of CTRT group children moved from clinical to normal functioning.
Morrison, M., & Bratton, S. (2011). The effects of child-teacher relationship training on the children of focus: A pilot study. *International Journal of Play Therapy*, *20*(4), 193–207.	**CTRT/**AC • Randomized • 16 wks • Daily center time play • Head Start school *CPRT-trained teachers	*N* = 22 At-risk, low-income PreK students • Age: 3–4; M = 3.8 • 59% Lat, 18% AfAm, 23% Cauc • 59% male	Clinical comorbid behavioral problems	Compared to the AC (Conscious Discipline®) across three points of measure, teacher-adapted CPRT (CTRT) demonstrated statistically significant benefits and large treatment effect on children's externalizing behavior problems. CTRT demonstrated a large treatment effect on reducing children's internalizing behavior problems, although no between group differences were found. 84% of CTRT group children moved from clinical to normal functioning.

(*Continued*)

Table 26.1 (Continued)

Opiola, K., & Bratton, S. (2018). The efficacy of Child-Parent Relationship Therapy for adopted children with attachment disruptions. *Journal for Counseling and Development,96* (4), 155–166.	**CPRT**/AC • Randomized • 7 play sessions • 1/wk; 30 min • Community agency *CPRT-trained parents	*N* = 49 Adoptees • Age: 2.5–8; M = 5 • 40% Cauc, 19% Lat, 19% AfAm, 22% other • 50% male	Attachment difficulties; Clinical comorbid behavioral problems	Statistically significant findings and large treatment effects on all measures indicated the effectiveness of CPRT over the AC on (1) reducing adopted children's global behavior problems, (2) decreasing parental stress, and (3) increasing parental empathy as measured by objective raters blind to the study.
Sheely, A., & Bratton, S. (2010). A strengths-based parenting intervention with low-income African American families. *Professional School Counseling, 13*(3), 175–183.	**CPRT**/WC • Randomized • 7 play sessions • 1/wk; 30 min • Head Start school *CPRT-trained parents	*N* = 23 At-risk, low-income Pre-K students • Age: 3–5; M = 4.2 • 100% AfrAm • 62% male	Clinical behavioral problems	Statistically significant findings and large treatment effects on all measures indicated the effectiveness of culturally adapted CPRT over the WC on (1) reducing children's global behavior problems and (2) decreasing parent-child relationship stress. Cultural considerations discussed.
Smith, D. M., & Landreth, G. L. (2004). Filial therapy with teachers of deaf and hard of hearing preschool children. *International Journal of Play Therapy, 13*(1), 13–33.	**CTRT**/WC • Randomized • 7 play sessions • 1/wk; 30 min • Preschool for Deaf *CPRT-trained teachers	*N* = 24 Deaf & hard of hearing Pre-K children • Age: 2–6; M = 4.1 • 33% Cauc; 42% Lat; 25% AfAm • 54% male	Behavioral problems; Social-emotional functioning	Compared to the WC, (1) children whose teachers participated in teacher-adapted CPRT (CTRT) made statistically significant improvement in behavior problems and social-emotional functioning, and (2) CTRT-trained teachers demonstrated statistically significant gains in their empathic interactions with students according to direct observation by independent raters.

Smith, N., & Landreth, G. L. (2003). Intensive filial therapy with child witnesses of domestic violence: A comparison with individual and sibling group play therapy. *International Journal for Play Therapy*, *12*(1), 67–88.	**CPRT**/COMP • Non-randomized • 7 play sessions • 1–2/wk; 30 min • Community agency *CPRT-trained parents	*N* = 44 children who had witnessed domestic violence • Age: 4–10; M = 6.2 • 17% Lat, 40% AfAm, 2% Arabic, 40% Cauc • 45% male	Comorbid behavioral problems	Compared to no treatment control over time: (1) CPRT-trained parents reported statistically significant decreases in their children's behavior problems, and (2) children in CPRT group reported a statistically significant increase in self-esteem. Additionally, CPRT parents demonstrated a statistically significant increase from pre to post in their empathic interactions with their children (direct observation by blinded raters). Results across treatment groups revealed no statistically significant differences between interventions.
Tew, K., Landreth, G. L., Joiner, K. D., & Solt, M. D. (2002). Filial therapy with parents of chronically ill children. *International Journal of Play Therapy*, *11*(1), 79–100.	**CPRT/**WC • Non-randomized • 7 play sessions • 1/wk; 30 min • Children's medical center *CPRT-trained parents	*N* = 23 hospitalized, chronically ill children • Age: 3–10 • 13% Lat, 87% Cauc	Adjustment difficulties	Compared to control group, CPRT-trained parents reported a statistically significant reduction in parent-child relationship stress and in their children's behavior problems. CPRT parents also reported a statistically significant increase in parental acceptance, compared to control parents over time.

(Continued)

Table 26.1 (Continued)

Yuen, T. C., Landreth, G. L., & Baggerly, J. (2002). Filial therapy with immigrant Chinese parents in Canada. *International Journal for Play Therapy*, *11*(2), 63–90.	**CPRT/**WC • Randomized • 7 play sessions • 1/wk; 30 min • Community agency *CPRT-trained parents	*N* = 35 Behaviorally at-risk immigrants • Age: 3–10; M = 6.4 • 100% Chinese Canadians • 54% male	Comorbid behavioral problems; Self-concept	Compared to the WC, the CPRT group demonstrated statistically significant improvements in (1) child behavior problems, parent-child relationship stress, and parental acceptance according to parent report, and (2) parental empathy according to raters blinded to treatment groups. CPRT group children also reported greater gains in perceived competence and social acceptance

Also see evidencebasedchildtherapy.com for detailed summaries of these and other CPRT/filial therapy outcome studies as well as play therapy outcome studies.

responds to the dearth of evidence-based treatments for young children (Chorpita et al., 2011; Weisz & Kazdin, 2010; www.effectivechildtherapy.com).

Meta-Analyses

Meta-analyses (Bratton, Ray, Rhine, & Jones, 2005; LeBlanc & Ritchie, 2001; Lin & Bratton, 2015), as well as comprehensive systematic reviews (Bratton, Landreth, & Lin, 2010; Lindo, Bratton, & Landreth, 2015) conducted in this millennium, support and strengthen the findings from individual CPRT studies. Bratton et al., LeBlanc and Ritchie, and Lin and Bratton conducted meta-analyses on play therapy outcome studies including CPRT/filial therapy and found stronger outcomes for studies in which caregivers were trained and supervised in CPRT/filial therapy methodology to use with their children than play therapy studies in which professional play therapists provided treatment (Bratton et al., 2015). Readers can access and download detailed summaries of the Bratton et al. (2005), Lin and Bratton (2015), and LeBlanc and Ritchie (2001) meta-analyses at evidencebasedchildtherapy.com. Landreth & Bratton (2006) used the meta-analytic data from Bratton et al. (2005) to analyze only those studies using the CPRT model and calculated an overall effect size. CPRT demonstrated a large treatment effect size of 1.25 (Cohen, 1988). These results indicate the average child-caregiver dyad receiving CPRT performed one and a quarter standard deviations better on outcome measures compared to the average child/caregiver dyad not receiving the treatment.

Strengths and Limitations

The evidence base for CPRT firmly establishes the model as an effective child therapy intervention. CPRT research has increased in methodological rigor over its relatively short history by (a) investigating clearly defined populations and target behaviors, (b) employing randomized controlled designs, (c) recruiting sample sizes determined by a priori power analysis, (d) following a manualized protocol with treatment fidelity checks, and (e) using objective raters blinded to group assignment. As noted previously in this chapter, CPRT is recognized as an evidence-based practice by the National Registry of Evidence-based Programs and Practices (NREPP, www.nrepp.samhsa.gov) and by the California Evidence-Based Clearinghouse (CEBC) for Child Welfare (www.cebc4cw.org). Specifically, NREPP recognized CPRT as *effective* for child externalizing problems/disruptive disorders and for family functioning (the highest level of evidence for an intervention) and *promising* for child internalizing disorders (next highest level of evidence). CEBC recognized CPRT as *promising* (second highest level of effectiveness) for child disruptive behaviors, attachment intervention, and parent training. CEBC requires follow-up studies to examine long-term effects of treatment in order to give the highest level of effectiveness rating.

Despite the growing recognition of CPRT as an evidence-based practice (EBP), researchers must continue to build an even stronger evidence base using current criteria for research deign and methods that will lead to the recognition of CPRT as an EBP for a broader range of childhood disorders. Noticeably absent are replication studies, with the exception of Opiola and Bratton's (2018) replication of Carnes-Holt and Bratton (2014), and follow-up studies. Follow-up studies are essential to evaluate maintenance of therapeutic gains, and they can provide useful information regarding optimum length of treatment relative to participant characteristics. Replication studies, preferably with independent teams of researchers, provides confidence in study findings for a specific population or presenting issue. Verifying the outcomes of the new CPRT models included in this volume, e.g., toddler and preadolescent, is another area of needed research. Apart from one pilot study investigating the effect of preadolescent-adapted CPRT protocol using a repeated-measures single group design (Swan, Bratton, Ceballos, & Laird, 2019), no studies have examined the effectiveness of CPRT with these populations.

Implications

The empirical support for CPRT holds implications for managed care providers and practitioners, especially in light of the current trend toward brief therapy and short-term interventions. CPRT was designed to increase parent participation and reduce financial and time constraints. It can be provided in a time-limited and group format and therefore aligns with managed care stipulations, while enabling practitioners to provide effective care. Moreover, it is plausible to suggest that training parents in CPRT serves a preventative function by equipping parents with skills that can be infused into their daily interactions with their children, thereby helping them respond to difficulties in the parent-child relationship long after treatment has ended. Based on the research evidence, child therapists should strongly consider the use of CPRT in their practice when clinically appropriate. There are cases in which the presenting concerns or parent or child characteristics would dictate another course of action, initially, such as the use of play therapy with a trained professional over CPRT, or as supplement to. The question is not whether to train parents in CPRT; rather, the question is when and to what extent.

Conclusion

The present evidentiary base of research supports CPRT as an intervention for training parents and other caregivers to utilize Child-Centered Play Therapy skills to address the mental health needs of children. The body of research indicates that parents can be effective change agents under the supervision of a trained and certified CPRT practitioner. Meta-analytic results suggest that treatment outcomes are stronger when parents are fully involved in the delivery of CCPT than for traditional play therapy. CPRT's manualized protocol contributes to its ease of replication by practitioners and researchers. Research findings support its efficacy with a broad range of populations, settings, and presenting concerns and demonstrate CPRT's transportability across settings and its potential for successful application with a variety of clinical populations. The use of CPRT cross-culturally is strongly indicated by the overwhelmingly positive findings from research with several non-dominant groups. The focus on the family and the uniqueness of each individual positions this intervention as especially responsive to cultural variables. The robust findings for CPRT's effectiveness with a variety of problems and populations suggest that if a child and a parent are both suitable candidates, CPRT should be considered as the treatment of choice.

References

Bratton, S., Dafoe, E., Swan, A., Opiola, K., McClintock, D., & Barcenas, G. (2015). *Play therapy outcome database*. Retrieved from www.evidencebasedchildtherapy.com

Bratton, S., & Landreth, G. (1995). Filial therapy with single parents: Effects on parental acceptance, empathy, and stress. *International Journal of Play Therapy, 4*(1), 61–80.

Bratton, S., Landreth, G., Kellum, T., & Blackard, S. (2006). *Child Parent Relationship Therapy (CPRT) treatment manual: An Evidence-Based 10-session filial therapy model for training parents* (2nd ed). New York, NY: Routledge.

Bratton, S., Landreth, G., & Lin, Y. (2010). Child Parent Relationship Therapy (CPRT): A review of controlled outcome research. In J. N. Baggerly, D. C. Ray, & S. C. Bratton (Eds.), *Child-centered play therapy research: The evidence base for effective practice* (pp. 267–294). Hoboken, NJ: Wiley.

Bratton, S., Ray, D., Rhine, T., & Jones, L. (2005). The efficacy of play therapy with children: A meta-analytic review of treatment outcomes. *Professional Psychology: Research and Practice, 36*(4), 376–390.

Brodzinsky, D. M. (2013). *A need to know: Enhancing adoption competence among mental health professionals: Policy perspective*. New York, NY: Donaldson Adoption Institute.

California Evidence-Based Clearinghouse (CEBC). www.cebc4cw.org

Carnes-Holt, K., & Bratton, S. C. (2014). The efficacy of child parent relationship therapy for adopted children with attachment disruptions. *Journal for Counseling and Development, 92*, 328–337.

Center for Play Therapy (CPT). www.cpt.unt.edu

Chorpita, B., Daleiden, E., Ebesutani, C., Young, J., Becker, K., Nakamura, B., & Starace, N. (2011). Evidence-based treatments for children and adolescents: An updated review of indicators of efficacy and effectiveness. *Clinical Psychology Science and Practice, 18*(2), 154–172.

Cohen, J. (1988). *Statistical power analysis for the behavioral sciences* (2nd ed.). New York, NY: Academic Press.

Guerney, L. (1975). *Follow-up study on filial therapy*. Paper presented at the annual convention of the Eastern Psychological Association, New York, NY.

Guerney, L., & Ryan, V. (2013). *Group filial therapy: The complete guide to teaching parents to play therapeutically with their children*. London: Jessica Kingsley Publishers.

Guerney, B. G., Jr., & Stover, L. (1971). *Filial therapy: Final report on MH 18264-01*. Unpublished manuscript, Pennsylvania State University, University Park.

Landreth, G., & Bratton, S. (2006). *Child Parent Relationship Therapy (CPRT): An Evidence-Based 10-session filial therapy model* (2nd ed). New York, NY: Routledge.

LeBlanc, M., & Ritchie, M. (2001). A meta-analysis of play therapy outcomes. *Counseling Psychology Quarterly, 14*(2), 149–163.

Lin, Y. D., & Bratton, S. (2015). A meta-analytic review of child-centered play therapy approaches. *Journal of Counseling and Development, 93*(1), 45–58. (IF = .669; 5 yr. impact = .91)

National Registry of Evidence-based Programs and Practices (NREPP). www.nrepp.samhsa.gov

Nezu, A., & Nezu, C. (2008). *Evidence-based outcome research*. New York, NY: Oxford Press.

Lindo, N. A., Bratton, S. C., & Landreth, G. L. (2015). Child parent relationship therapy: Theory, research, and intervention process. In L. A. Reddy, T. M. Files-Hall, & C. E. Schaefer (Eds.), *Empirically based play interventions for children* (2nd ed) (pp. 241–261). Washington, D.C.: American Psychological Association.

Opiola, K., & Bratton, S. (2018). The efficacy of child parent relationship therapy for adopted children with attachment disruptions. *Journal for Counseling and Development, 96*(4), 155–166.

Oxman, L. (1972). The effectiveness of filial therapy: A controlled study (Doctoral dissertation, Rutgers The State University of New Jersey, 1972). *Dissertation Abstracts International, B, 32*(11), 6656.

Stover, L., & Guerney, B. (1967). The efficacy of training procedures for mothers in filial therapy. *Psychotherapy: Theory, Research, and Practice, 4*(3), 110–115.

Swan, A., Bratton, S., Ceballos, P., & Laird, A. (2019). Effect of Child-Parent relationship therapy (CPRT) with adoptive parents of preadolescents: A pilot study. *International Journal of Play Therapy, 28*(2), 107–122.

Weisz, J. R., & Kazdin, A. E. (2010). The present and future of evidenced-based psychotherapies for children and adolescents. In J. R. Weisz & A. E. Kazdin (Eds.), *Evidenced-based psychotherapies for children and adolescents* (2nd ed) (pp. 557–572). New York, NY: Guilford Press.

INDEX

Note: *Italicized* numbers indicate figures, and **bold** numbers tables on the corresponding pages.